*Study Guide*

# *Pharmacology for Nursing Care*

## Study Guide

# Pharmacology for Nursing Care

*Sixth Edition*

RICHARD A. LEHNE, PhD

*Prepared by*
**Sherry Neely,** MSN, RN, CRNP
Associate Professor
Butler County Community College
Butler, Pennsylvania

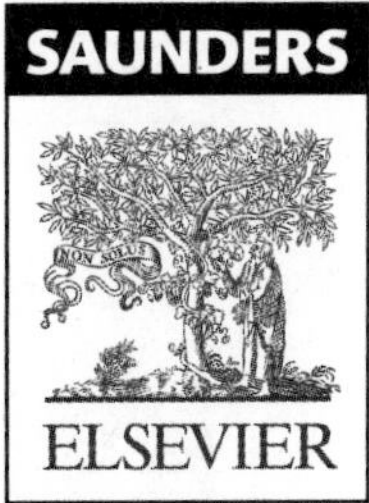

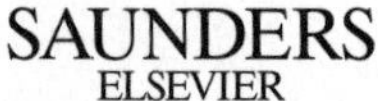

SAUNDERS
ELSEVIER

11830 Westline Industrial Drive
St. Louis, Missouri 63146

STUDY GUIDE FOR PHARMACOLOGY FOR NURSING CARE ISBN-13: 978-1-4160-3025-6
ISBN-10: 1-4160-3025-5



**Notice**

Knowledge and best practice in this field are constantly changing. As new research and experience broaden our knowledge, changes in practice, treatment and drug therapy may become necessary or appropriate. Readers are advised to check the most current information provided (i) on procedures featured or (ii) by the manufacturer of each product to be administered, to verify the recommended dose or formula, the method and duration of administration, and contraindications. It is the responsibility of the practitioner, relying on their own experience and knowledge of the patient, to make diagnoses, to determine dosages and the best treatment for each individual patient, and to take all appropriate safety precautions. To the fullest extent of the law, neither the Publisher nor the [Editors/Authors] assumes any liability for any injury and/or damage to persons or property arising out or related to any use of the material contained in this book.

The Publisher

Previous editions copyrighted 2004, 2000, 1999.

ISBN-13: 978-1-4160-3025-6
ISBN-10: 1-4160-3025-5

*Acquisitions Editor:* Kristin Geen
*Senior Developmental Editor:* Lauren Borstell
*Publishing Services Manager:* Jeff Patterson

Printed in the United States of America

Last digit is the print number: 9 8 7 6 5 4 3 2 1

# Reviewers

**Jo Ann Acierno,** RN, BSN
Instructor
Clarkson College
Omaha, Nebraska

**Jo Anne Wozniak,** MSN, RN, CCRN
Clinical Research Coordinator
Sewickley Valley Medical Group, Cardiology
Leetsdale, Pennsylvania

# Introduction

The critical thinking and study questions in this study guide include review of knowledge, application of knowledge to nursing care, and critical thinking for data analysis and decision-making related to patient care. Some of the questions have a ▸ near them. Answering these questions will require more than repetition of the information in the textbook. The student will have to integrate other nursing knowledge such as developmental considerations, laboratory values, and symptoms of adverse effects. Identifying the correct answer to these questions requires careful examination of the data and reflection on the patient in a holistic manner.

When using this book as a study guide, the questions that do not have a ▸ are excellent tools to augment the initial reading of the textbook before attending class and for review immediately following classroom discussion. The ▸ critical thinking questions reflect the reasoning that students and new graduate nurses need to be able to perform in order to safely administer pharmacotherapy. These questions are an excellent source of review when preparing for the NCLEX® examination.

Critical thinking by the student nurse requires assimilating classroom learning and clinical experience. No two experiences are the same. Sometimes the student integrates information into questions that is not directly stated, based on his/her own nursing experiences. The student may find that he/she disagrees with an answer provided in the study guide. When this occurs, the student should first review the question looking for key words and for its main point. Then, the student should identify information that substantiates his/her thoughts. This is an opportunity for additional critical thinking. Discuss the question with faculty and peers; be prepared to substantiate the rationale. In other words, explain your thinking. It will enrich your learning experience.

# Contents

*Study Guide*

# *Pharmacology for Nursing Care*

# 1 Orientation to Pharmacology

## OBJECTIVES

After reading and studying the corresponding chapter and completing the critical thinking and study questions, the student will be able to:

1. Describe the basic factors that the nurse and patient must consider when deciding whether to administer or withhold a prescribed drug.
2. List factors across the life span that can alter patient adherence to the prescribed drug regime.
3. Identify nursing interventions that address barriers to adherence to the prescribed drug regime.

## CRITICAL THINKING AND STUDY QUESTIONS

1. The following questions must be considered when the nurse administers medications. Describe the actions the nurse must take to answer each question relating to the properties of an ideal drug.
   a. Effectiveness—Is the drug doing what it is supposed to do?
   b. Safety—Is there any reason why this drug should not be administered?
   c. Selectivity—What effects in addition to the intended effect is the drug producing?
   d. Reversible action—When will the effects of the drug start, peak, and stop?
   e. Predictability—What individual factors will affect how this patient will respond to this drug?
   f. Ease of administration—What characteristics of the medication will promote or hinder the patient taking the medication as prescribed? What can the nurse do to make it easier for the patient to take the medication as prescribed?
   g. Freedoms from drug interactions—What possible interactions with the combination of drugs that the patient is taking are likely to occur?

h. Low cost—Can the patient afford this drug? What can the nurse do if the patient states that he or she cannot afford the prescribed medication?

i. Chemical stability—What can the nurse teach to ensure that the patient stores a medication so that it does not loose potency or become toxic?

j. Possession of simple generic name—What should the nurse do to ensure that the patient knows the name and desired action of the drug?

▶ 2. The nurse is providing discharge teaching for a patient who has had outpatient surgery and who has been prescribed oxycodone and acetaminophen (Percocet) 2 tablets every 4 to 6 hours as needed for pain. What should the nurse include in the teaching to prevent liver damage from excessive acetaminophen ingestion?

# 2 Application of Pharmacology in Nursing Practice

## OBJECTIVES

After reading and studying the corresponding chapter and completing the critical thinking and study questions, the student will be able to:

1. Describe how the nurse fulfills the responsibility for the five rights of drug administration.
2. Develop a teaching plan for a newly prescribed drug.
3. Describe the use of the nursing process in drug administration.
4. List the data that should be obtained in a preadministration assessment.
5. Recognize the importance of the liver and kidneys in pharmacokinetics.
6. Differentiate nursing actions for drug contraindications versus drug precautions.
7. Describe interventions to overcome self-care obstacles for drug therapy adherence.

## CRITICAL THINKING AND STUDY QUESTIONS

1. The nurse is preparing to administer prescribed drugs to a patient in a hospital. Describe how the nurse ensures that these rights occur.
   a. Right drug

b. Right route

c. Right dose

d. Right time

e. Right patient

2. Why does the nurse need to know the mechanism of action of an antihypertensive drug before administering the medication?

3. Research the drug furosemide (Lasix). Use the following chart to create a patient teaching handout using wording that the average adult patient could understand.

| **Furosemide (Lasix, Apo-furosemide)** | |
|---|---|
| Therapeutic category and action | |
| Dosage, route, and time schedule | |
| Expected therapeutic response | |
| Nondrug measures to enhance therapeutic response | |
| Duration of treatment | |
| Method of drug storage | |
| Symptoms of common adverse effects | |
| Symptoms of early toxicity | |
| Measures to minimize harm | |
| Major adverse drug-drug and drug-food interactions | |
| When to contact the prescriber | |

4. Describe the needed nursing actions for each step of the nursing process for administering a medication for pain (analgesic) to a patient who is postoperative following gallbladder removal (cholecystectomy) and who does not want to cough and deep breathe because of the pain.
   a. Assessment

   b. Analysis: nursing diagnosis

   c. Planning

d. Implementation

e. Evaluation

5. List the data that should be obtained in a preadministration assessment.

6. The nurse is preparing to administer an antihypertensive drug (medication that lowers the blood pressure). The nurse assesses the patient's blood pressure, and it is 110/70 mm Hg, which is within normal limits. What action should the nurse take to determine if it is safe to administer the drug?
   a. Call the prescriber, report the current blood pressure, and ask if the medication should be administered.
   b. Hold the medication because the patient's blood pressure is too low to administer an antihypertensive drug.
   c. Administer the medication because the antihypertensive medication is prescribed.
   d. Assess the patient's baseline blood pressure and the blood pressure before and after the last dose of this medication to determine if the medication should be administered.

7. Why are liver and kidney function so important to assess before administering any drug?

8. The nurse is administering medications. The medication administration record (MAR) has cefazolin sodium (Ancef) prescribed for two different patients. One patient's chart states that the patient is allergic to cephalosporin. The other states that the patient is allergic to penicillin. Allergy to cephalosporin is a contraindication for cefazolin. Allergy to penicillin is a precaution for cefazolin. The nurse should assess both patients for their allergic symptoms and:
   a. hold both medications and notify the prescriber.
   b. administer the medication to the patient who is allergic to penicillin because cefazolin is not a penicillin.
   c. notify the prescriber of the allergy and administer the cefazolin cautiously to the patient who is allergic to penicillin because there is sometimes a cross allergy between penicillins and first-generation cephalosporins.
   d. administer both medications if the patient did not have a life-threatening reaction with the previous drug reaction.

9. State interventions to overcome these factors that may interfere with a patient's ability to perform self-care with a medication regime.
   a. Unable to remember what they are supposed to do.
   b. Lack money to pay for medications.
   c. Believe drug is not needed.

# 3 Drug Regulation, Development, Names, and Information

## OBJECTIVES

After reading and studying the corresponding chapter and completing the critical thinking and study questions, the student will be able to:

1. Discuss the characteristics of reliable research studies.
2. Describe the role of the nurse in clinical testing of a new drug.
3. Apply information about new drugs to a patient's situation.
4. Describe the three types of names of drugs.
5. Recognize the benefit of knowing the generic name of drugs.
6. Explain the problems with use of trade names to identify drugs.
7. Recognize the characteristics of generic drugs.

## CRITICAL THINKING AND STUDY QUESTIONS

1. The nurse is caring for a patient who has high blood cholesterol (hyperlipidemia). The patient states that she became worried about her high cholesterol when her sister had a "heart attack." She went to a health food store to see if they had any natural product that could help lower her cholesterol. She noticed a sign on the counter asking for volunteers to enter a study. Volunteers are to submit a copy of their blood cholesterol results and again at the end of a year after taking the product as directed for a full year. Explain why the results of this study may not be reliable based on these factors.
   a. Control
   b. Randomization
   c. Blinding
2. Some drugs have been approved by the Food and Drug Administration (FDA) and have been released but later withdrawn from the market. Describe the role of the nurse in Phase IV of clinical testing of a new drug: postmarketing surveillance of drugs.
3. Angiotensin-converting enzyme inhibitor (ACEI) drugs are used for high blood pressure (hypertension). These drugs can cause a dry cough in approximately 40% of patients. Newer, more expensive angiotensin II receptor blocker (ARB) drugs have been developed that produce essentially the same therapeutic effect but do not the cause the same cough. A patient who is receiving an ACEI explains to the nurse that her friend is getting a new drug (ARB) and that

she is sure it is better because it is new. Discuss how the nurse should respond.

4. Describe the three types of names of drugs.
   a. Chemical name

   b. Generic name

   c. Trade name

5. Why is it important for the nurse to learn the generic names of drugs? (Select all that apply.)
   a. The same generic name is never used for more than one medication.
   b. Generic names tell the nurse the chemical ingredients of the drug.
   c. The generic name of a drug will be the same no matter which company produces the drug.
   d. Generic names are easy to recall and pronounce.
   e. Generic names often suggest the action of the drug.
   f. Generic names of drugs in the same therapeutic class often have a similar suffix making them easy to identify.

6. When preparing discharge instructions for a patient the nurse should:
   a. review the prescriptions written for discharge and include the stated trade name and generic name in discharge teaching.
   b. write and explain the generic name so the patient does not become confused.
   c. write and explain the trade name because it is easier for the patient to remember.
   d. ask the patient which name he or she uses for the drug and only use that name in discharge teaching.

7. A patient has been taking a brand-name drug for a chronic condition for several years. Recent changes in his insurance plan require the use of generic drugs whenever they are available. The patient asks the nurse if he should pay out of his pocket to continue receiving the brand-name drug. The nurse's response should be based on the fact that:
   a. trade name drugs contain different active ingredients than generic drugs.
   b. generic drugs are equal in their therapeutic equivalency to their brand-name counterparts.
   c. generic drugs usually are not absorbed at the same rate as brand-name drugs.
   d. continuing to use the brand-name drug will prevent confusion.

# 4 Pharmacokinetics

## OBJECTIVES

After reading and studying the corresponding chapter and completing the critical thinking and study questions, the student will be able to:

1. Define pharmacokinetics.
2. Identify nursing responsibilities when administering drugs.
3. Employ knowledge of factors that affect drug movement when administering drugs.
4. Use critical thinking to develop measures that prevent drug administration errors.
5. Identify nursing considerations for timing and routes of drug administration.
6. Research the metabolism and excretion of a drug and apply the information to nursing care.
7. Apply the principles of narrow therapeutic range, half-life, peak, and trough to nursing responsibilities when administering drugs.
8. Explain the clinical significance between a narrow and wide therapeutic range.

## CRITICAL THINKING AND STUDY QUESTIONS

1. Define the four processes of pharmacokinetics.
   a. Absorption

   b. Distribution

   c. Metabolism (biotransformation)

   d. Excretion

▶ 2. The nurse is preparing to administer Clarinex (desloratadine) to an adult patient who is experiencing severe symptoms of seasonal allergies. The medication administration record (MAR) lists the patient's dosage as 15 mg once a day. The nurse's drug handbook lists the acceptable dosage for adults as 5 mg once a day. Which of the following actions should the nurse initially employ?
   a. Hold the medication and check the original prescriber's order.
   b. Hold the medication and question the prescriber about the dose.
   c. Ask the patient if this is the pill that he usually receives.
   d. Administer the dose because that was the dose prescribed.

3. Drugs can cross cell membranes in three ways. Match the method of movement with characteristics for that method of movement.

| | | |
|---|---|---|
| ___ | a. Passage through channels | 1. May require energy or pores |
| ___ | b. Direct penetration of the membrane | 2. Requires small size |
| ___ | c. Passage with the aid of a transport system | 3. Requires lipid solubility |

4. The four processes of pharmacokinetics have which of the following characteristics in common?
   a. Stimulation of receptors
   b. Blocking of processes
   c. Dose-response relationship
   d. Movement

5. Insulin is a hormone that is available as a drug. It combines with receptors on cardiac and skeletal muscle and fat cells to facilitate the transport mechanism that allows the glucose ($C_6H_{12}O_6$) molecule to enter the cell. Why does glucose require a transport mechanism to enter these cells? (Select all that apply.)
   a. Glucose is water soluble.
   b. Glucose is fat soluble.
   c. Glucose is too large to cross the cell membrane through a channel.
   d. Glucose is an ion.
   e. Glucose is a quaternary ammonium compound.

6. The nurse is caring for a patient who has recently been diagnosed with asthma and is prescribed an inhaled bronchodilator drug that is a quaternary ammonium compound. The patient does not like using the inhaler and asks the nurse why the physician did not just prescribe a pill. The nurse's response would be based on knowledge that the:
   a. oral drug would not produce the desired effect.
   b. oral drug would be absorbed too quickly.
   c. inhaled drug and oral drug produce the same effects.
   d. inhaled drug has very limited absorption into the bloodstream and should cause less adverse effects.

▶ 7. The nurse has a heavy assignment including caring for a hospitalized patient who has been prescribed the following medications: 0800 glyburide (DiaBeta) 10 mg; 0900 quinapril HCl (Accupril) 20 mg. Breakfast is served at 0810. Hospital policy states that medications may be administered 30 minutes before and after the designated time. To save time the nurse plans to administer both of these medications at 0830. Research these medications and describe why this is not a good plan.

8. Explain if the following factors would increase or decrease the absorption of an oral medication.
   a. Administer a chewable aspirin (acetylsalicylic acid) instead of an enteric-coated aspirin.

   b. The patient has an ileostomy.

   c. Take a medication immediately before or after vigorous exercise.

9. Describe why chemotherapy for cancer is administered through a central intravenous line instead of a peripherally inserted intravenous line.

10. Heparin sodium is available in pre-filled syringes in two concentrations. Heparin sodium 100 units/mL is for flushing intravenous lines, and heparin sodium 5000 units/mL is for subcutaneous administration. Identify measures that prevent accidental administration of the wrong concentration of this drug.

11. Describe administration techniques for intravenous drugs that can decrease the chance of adverse reactions.

12. What steps does the nurse need to take before administering any intravenous (IV) medication?

13. A 15-year-old young woman comes to a family planning clinic and is diagnosed with primary syphilis. Based on knowledge that developmentally this patient is not likely to adhere to a lengthy treatment plan, the best route for administering an antibiotic to this patient is:
   a. a once-a-day oral pill.
   b. a depot intramuscular injection.
   c. an intravenous infusion.
   d. a topical cream.

14. The home health nurse notes that a family member has been crushing all of the patient's medications, including enteric-coated preparations, and mixing them in pudding so that they are easier to swallow. The nurse should explain that enteric-coated drugs should not be crushed because:
   a. they must be taken on an empty stomach.
   b. crushing these preparations destroys the medication.
   c. crushing these preparations can cause stomach distress or cause the acid in the stomach to alter the drug.
   d. crushing these preparations can delay medication absorption.

15. The nurse is teaching a patient how to take the medication nitroglycerin for anginal chest pain. Teaching on the route of administration should be based on the fact that nitroglycerin has an extensive first-pass effect, which means: (Select all that apply.)
   a. most of the drug is inactivated by the liver before it reaches circulation when administered orally.
   b. most of the drug is activated by the liver, so it must be administered orally.
   c. once absorbed, the drug stays in systemic circulation for a long time because it is not metabolized by the liver.
   d. administration by dissolving under the tongue (sublingually) allows the drug to be absorbed directly into systemic circulation bypassing first pass in the liver.
   e. the drug can only be administered as a topical patch.

16. The nurse is preparing to administer the medication digoxin (Lanoxin) to a patient who has been receiving the drug for chronic heart failure (HF) and who recently went into renal failure. Research the metabolism and excretion of this drug and explain why the nurse needs to be cautious when administering digoxin to this patient.

17. Digoxin (Lanoxin) is a drug that has a narrow therapeutic range. When administering this drug the nurse needs to: (Select all that apply.)
   a. administer the medication only on an as needed (PRN) basis.
   b. carefully monitor the patient for therapeutic and toxic effects.
   c. be diligent about administering the medication exactly as prescribed.
   d. monitor blood levels of the drugs to assess if they are in the therapeutic range.

18. Research the drugs heparin sodium and warfarin (Coumadin). Based on the action and half-life of these drugs, explain why heparin sodium administered subcutaneously can be administered the day before elective surgery, but the surgeon may delay elective surgery for several days to a week if a patient is receiving warfarin.

19. A patient stopped taking levothyroxine (Synthroid) 3 days ago. This drug has a half-life of 9 to 10 days. He tells the nurse that the drug must not have been necessary because he does not feel any different. The basis of the nurse's explanation on why the patient has not noticed any difference is the:
    a. drug's previous doses are still in the patient's body.
    b. drug probably was not needed if the patient has not experienced any symptoms.
    c. patient's dose was probably too high, so the drug is still working.
    d. patient could not have been taking the drug as prescribed before stopping the drug 3 days ago.

20. A patient is receiving vancomycin 500 mg every 6 hours intravenously for a serious infection. Vancomycin IV has an immediate onset Vancomycin can be neurotoxic, but adequate levels of the drug are needed to treat the infection. The prescriber has ordered peak and trough levels to be drawn. When would the nurse expect the peak and trough levels to be drawn?
    a. Peak level 1.5 hours before infusion started and trough level immediately after infusion of the drug is complete.
    b. Peak level 1.5 hours after infusion and trough level 30 minutes before next dose.
    c. Peak level while the drug is infusing and trough level immediately after infusion of the drug is complete.
    d. Peak level while the drug is infusing and trough level 30 minutes before next dose.

21. Phenytoin (Dilantin) is a drug that has a narrow therapeutic range. Serum levels of these drugs are monitored periodically because the:
    a. drug is very potent.
    b. drug is used for patients who have critical illnesses.
    c. dose of the drug that is needed to produce the desired effect is very high.
    d. difference between the dose that produces the desired effect and the dose that is toxic to the patient is very small.

# 5 Pharmacodynamics

## OBJECTIVES

After reading and studying the corresponding chapter and completing the critical thinking and study questions, the student will be able to:

1. Explain why knowledge of pharmacodynamics is needed for drug administration.
2. Describe the three phases of the dose-response relationship.
3. Recognize the significance of potency and drug-receptor interactions.
4. Identify the relationship of the type of receptor to onset of therapeutic effect.
5. Differentiate between appropriate and inappropriate nursing actions based on expected effects of a drug.
6. Compare the intrinsic activity and affinity of selected drugs.
7. Anticipate possible adverse effects of a drug based on excessive individual response.
8. Apply pharmacodynamic principles to nursing clinical decision making.

## CRITICAL THINKING AND STUDY QUESTIONS

1. Increasing urinary fluid excretion, vasodilation, and decreasing heart rate are different mechanisms of action of drugs used to treat hypertension. Why does the nurse need to know the mechanism of action of an antihypertensive drug?

2. Describe the three phases of the dose-response relationship.
   a. Phase 1

   b. Phase 2

   c. Phase 3

3. The nurse is reading research about a drug. The literature states that the drug is potent. This means the drug:
   a. produces its effects at low doses.
   b. produces strong effects at any dose.
   c. requires high doses to produce its effects.
   d. is very likely to cause adverse effects.

4. Except for gene therapy, which of the following statements are true about drug-receptor interactions? (Select all that apply.)
   a. Drugs can mimic the actions of endogenous molecules.
   b. Receptors for drugs do not respond to hormones and neurotransmitters produced by the body.
   c. Binding of a drug to its receptor is usually irreversible.
   d. Drugs can block the actions of endogenous molecules.
   e. Drugs can give the cell new functions.

5. A patient has been diagnosed with hypothyroidism and has been prescribed levothyroxine (Synthroid), a synthetic thyroid hormone replacement. An explanation of why the drug does not reach a peak therapeutic effect until taken regularly for 3 to 4 weeks is that thyroid hormone stimulates the family of receptors that are:
   a. located on the cell surface (cell membrane–embedded enzymes).
   b. located on the cell surface and regulate the flow of ions in and out of the cell (ligand-gated channels).
   c. found within the cell and function to regulate protein synthesis (transcription factors).
   d. folded receptors that activate a G protein that then activates the effector (G protein–coupled receptor systems).

▶ 6. The nurse is administering morphine sulfate for moderate to severe postoperative pain. Based on the effect of modulating processes that are affected by morphine the nurse should: (Select all that apply.)
   a. assess respirations and hold the medication if adventitious breath sounds are present.
   b. assess respiratory rate and hold the medication if respirations are weak or less than 12/min.
   c. maintain the patient on complete bed rest with all four side rails elevated to prevent injury.
   d. assist the patient when ambulating to prevent injury.
   e. do not administer the medication if the patient's behavior does not suggest that he is having moderate to severe pain.
   f. restrict fluids to prevent nausea.
   g. encourage ambulation if not contraindicated to promote bowel motility.

7. A patient has been receiving intravenous hydromorphone HCl (Dilaudid) 1 mg every 4 hours as needed for severe pain. The patient has been progressing and is experiencing less pain. The prescriber has discontinued the hydromorphone and prescribed intravenous pentazocine (Talwin) 30 mg every 4 hours as needed for moderate pain. This suggests that hydromorphine:
   a. and pentazocine are agonists and have equally high affinity and intrinsic activity.
   b. and pentazocine are agonist-antagonist and have equally moderate affinity and intrinsic activity.

c. is an agonist with a higher affinity and intrinsic activity than the agonist-antagonist pentazocine.
d. is an agonist-antagonist with a lower affinity and intrinsic activity than the agonist pentazocine.

8. Metoprolol (Lopressor, Betaloc) is a drug that is a selective antagonist for beta$_1$ ($\beta_1$) adrenergic receptors. When stimulated, ($\beta_1$) receptors of the heart increase the heart rate. The nurse should assess the patient receiving metoprolol for excessive response, which would be seen as:
   a. hypertension and tachycardia.
   b. hypertension and bradycardia.
   c. hypotension and tachycardia.
   d. hypotension and bradycardia.

9. Research the pharmacokinetics of methadone HCl (Metadol), an opiate, and naloxone HCl (Narcan), a narcotic antagonist. A patient who has overdosed on methadone HCl is brought into the emergency department unresponsive with severely depressed respirations. The patient receives intravenous naloxone HCl with a dramatic improvement in the level of consciousness and respiratory rate and effort within minutes. What must the nurse be prepared to do 45 to 60 minutes after the naloxone HCl is administered?
   a. Assess for return of pain because the effect of the naloxone HCl should be peaking.
   b. Administer another dose of naloxone HCl because respiratory and CNS depression might occur as the naloxone HCl effect is ending.
   c. Prepare to administer the drug intramuscularly if the drug has not taken effect.
   d. Counteract effects of opiate withdrawal.

10. Ibuprofen is a nonsteroidal anti-inflammatory drug (NSAID) that is available over-the-counter. Based on the dose instructions on the label (or a drug handbook), what is the $ED_{50}$ for mild to moderate pain relief?

11. The pediatrician has prescribed amoxicillin suspension 150 mg twice daily for a child who weighs 22 lb (10 kg). The nurse's drug handbook states that the recommended dosage of amoxicillin for a child weighing less than 20 kg is 20 to 40/kg/day divided into three equal doses. The recommended dosage for this child is 200 to 400 mg/day divided into 67-to 133-mg doses 3 times daily. The nurse should:
   a. hold the medication and notify the pediatrician that the dose is more than the recommended dose.
   b. hold the medication and notify the pediatrician that the dose is less than the recommended dose.
   c. administer the medication and continue to assess the child.
   d. administer no more than 133 mg per dose.

12. When the therapeutic index of a drug is narrow, the nurse would expect:
   a. the drug would produce the desired effect at low doses.
   b. blood levels of the drug to be monitored throughout therapy.
   c. the drug would produce many adverse effects at low doses.
   d. the drug should only be used in an emergency.

# 6 Drug Interactions

## OBJECTIVES

After reading and studying the corresponding chapter and completing the critical thinking and study questions, the student will be able to:

1. Identify common substances that can alter the effect, metabolism, and/or excretion of other drugs.
2. Describe the purpose of additive ingredients in drugs.
3. Explain a disulfiram (Antabuse) reaction.
4. Evaluate the process of drug administration and order transcription for common errors that can cause drug interactions.
5. Apply knowledge of pH-dependent ionization and partitioning to therapeutic uses.
6. Use knowledge of the effects of the hepatic microsomal enzyme system and P-glycoprotein on drug levels.
7. Research situations that can cause altered drug absorption, metabolism, and excretion.
8. Identify assessment data that suggests drug accumulation.
9. Solve drug administration problems that relate to interactions.

## CRITICAL THINKING AND STUDY QUESTIONS

1. Identify which of the following substances can cause drug interactions. (Select all that apply.)
   a. Beer
   b. Chocolate
   c. Garlic
   d. Over-the-counter drugs
   e. Potassium
   f. Prescription drugs
   g. Tea
   h. Tobacco

2. A mother asks the nurse why her son was prescribed amoxicillin and potassium clavulanate (Augmentin) for otitis media if amoxicillin has not worked in the past. The nurse's response is based on:

3. The nurse is providing discharge teaching for a patient who will be taking metronidazole (Flagyl) after discharge. The drug information states to caution the patient that a disulfiram (Antabuse) reaction can occur. This means:
   a. adverse reactions can occur if the patient takes metronidazole and the drug disulfiram.
   b. adverse reactions can occur if the patient ingests or absorbs alcohol while taking metronidazole.
   c. metronidazole must be taken with disulfiram to prevent adverse reactions.
   d. disulfiram is frequently prescribed for patients who are receiving metronidazole.

▸ 4. List some examples of how the nurse can inadvertently mix two drugs together during medication administration and possibly produce adverse effects.

5. It is the nurse's responsibility at this institution to decide what time a medication will be administered. Cholestyramine (Questran) has been

prescribed for a patient who takes many drugs for diabetes and hypertension. The patient takes the other drugs at 0900 and 1700. Medications can be given up to 1 hour before or after the assigned time. When should the cholestyramine be administered?

6. A patient has toxic levels of an alkaline drug in his blood. The drug is excreted unchanged in the urine. Which of the following substances would be the best choice to increase the excretion of the alkaline substance?
   a. Sodium bicarbonate
   b. Antacids
   c. Acetylsalacylic acid (aspirin)
   d. Ascorbic acid (Vitamin C)

7. Patients receiving certain drugs that are metabolized by the CYP3A4 enzyme should not drink grapefruit juice because it inhibits the CYP3A4 enzyme and might inhibit the drug transporter P-glycoprotein. The patient asks what might happen if she drinks grapefruit juice and takes the medication. The nurse's response is based on knowledge that the effect could be:
   a. lack of response to the drug because it does not get to the site of action.
   b. possible toxicity because metabolism and excretion of the drug can be impaired, and absorption may be increased.
   c. lack of response because the drug will not be absorbed.
   d. liver damage because the CYP3A4 enzyme destroys the liver.

8. Smoking induces the CYP1A2 liver enzyme. Coumadin (warfarin), an anticoagulant blood thinner, is metabolized by the CYP1A2 enzyme. Because of this interaction, the nurse needs to be alert for what response in the patient receiving warfarin who also smokes tobacco?
   a. More than expected response to the warfarin
   b. Decreased need for the medication warfarin
   c. Increased bruising and bleeding gums
   d. Inadequate response to the warfarin

9. A patient is taking digoxin (Lanoxin), a drug that is excreted by the kidneys in the active state. The nurse notes that the patient's laboratory values include significantly elevated creatinine levels suggesting renal failure. Research digoxin and list symptoms that the nurse should assess for in this patient.

10. The nurse is caring for a 92-year-old female who was admitted yesterday with pneumonia. Past history includes hypertension and heart failure. The patient is exhibiting signs that she is experiencing hallucinations. What information does the nurse need to provide to the prescriber to help determine if the behavior is related to a drug interaction?

11. A patient has been having severe diarrhea for the past 5 days after receiving a new antibiotic. He takes an anticonvulsant orally. What is the possible effect on the blood level of the anticonvulsant?

12. The nurse is getting ready to give two IV antibiotics. Both are scheduled at 0900. The nurse cannot find any information about the compatibility of these two drugs, but knows that it is important to stay on schedule to keep plasma levels stable. One drug (drug X) can be given over 20 minutes, and the other (drug Y) requires 1 hour to infuse. Describe the steps of safely administering these drugs.

13. Describe how the nurse should respond to these possible drug-food interactions.
    a. The patient wants to take tetracycline with milk because it upsets his stomach.
    b. The patient takes digoxin (Lanoxin) in the morning with breakfast.
    c. A patient who is HIV positive has a poor appetite and is prescribed saquinavir (Invirase).
    d. A patient who is taking a calcium channel blocker states that he does not drink grapefruit juice with his medication, only later in the day.
    e. The patient has been prescribed tranylcypromine (Parnate), an MAO inhibitor for depression.
    f. The patient has started taking warfarin (Coumadin) and only eats green vegetables occasionally.

# 7 Adverse Drug Reactions and Medication Errors

## OBJECTIVES

After reading and studying the corresponding chapter and completing the critical thinking and study questions, the student will be able to:

1. Identify patients who are at risk for drug reactions.
2. Assess the necessary nursing response when an adverse drug reaction occurs.
3. Anticipate the effect of sudden withdrawal from a drug for which the patient has developed a physical dependence.
4. Describe common symptoms of nephrotoxicity, neurotoxicity, and ototoxicity.
5. Research drugs for potential adverse effects.
6. Incorporate laboratory test analysis in nursing decision making relating to drug administration.
7. Apply knowledge of drug-induced long QT-syndrome to nursing care.

8. Determine appropriate nursing actions when adverse effects are probable.
9. Recognize the importance of correct dose calculation.
10. Apply the appropriate scope of nursing practice to medication administration situations.
11. Develop strategies that reduce the incidence of medication errors.
12. Summarize nursing responsibilities when a medication error occurs.

## CRITICAL THINKING AND STUDY QUESTIONS

1. Adverse drug reactions occur more often in: (Select all that apply.)
   a. patients taking multiple drugs.
   b. patients taking potent drugs.
   c. situations where a drug error occurs.
   d. patients over 60 years of age.
   e. patients younger than 1 year of age.
   f. malnourished patients.
   g. accidental poisonings.

▶ 2. The nurse has administered quinapril (Accupril). One hour after administration, the patient reports a tingling sensation of the lips. The nurse notes perioral edema. The nursing action with the highest priority is to:
   a. hold the next dose of the medication.
   b. document the finding and continue to assess the patient.
   c. notify the prescriber STAT.
   d. withhold all food and water.

3. The nurse is administering metoprolol tartrate (Lopressor, Toprol), a $beta_1$-adrenergic receptor blocking drug that slows the heart rate and lowers the blood pressure. The nurse must teach the patient not to stop taking the drug suddenly because this could cause:
   a. bradycardia and hypotension
   b. bradycardia and hypertension.
   c. tachycardia and hypotension.
   d. tachycardia and hypertension.

4. Because the drug handbook lists gentamicin sulfate (Garamycin) as being ototoxic, the nurse should teach the patient to report:
   a. dizziness.
   b. tinnitus.
   c. palpitations.
   d. rash.

5. A public health crisis occurred when many patients who ate at a specific restaurant developed hepatitis A from contaminated, imported green onions. A common factor in two of the patients for whom the hepatitis was fatal was treatment of the illness symptoms with:
   a. acetaminophen (Tylenol).
   b. acetylsalicylic acid (Aspirin).
   c. ibuprofen (Motrin).
   d. naproxen (Aleve).

▶ 6. Before administering lovastatin (Mevacor), a potentially hepatotoxic lipid-lowering medication, the nurse reviews the patient's laboratory tests. Test results include alanine aminotransferase (ALT) 334 International Units/L and aspartate aminotransferase (AST) 197 units/L. The nurse should:
   a. administer the medication.
   b. assess the vital signs before administering the medication.
   c. hold the medication and report the results to the prescriber.
   d. notify the prescriber STAT.

7. The nurse is teaching a patient who has been prescribed terbinafine HCl (Lamisil) tablets 250 mg once a day for 12 weeks for toenail onychomycosis. Because the drug can be hepatotoxic, the nurse teaches the patient to report: (Select all that apply.)
   a. constipation.
   b. light-colored stool.
   c. rash.
   d. yellow-colored skin.
   e. pale conjunctiva.
   f. anorexia.
   g. angioedema.
   h. nausea and vomiting.
   i. tarry stool.

▶ 8. The nurse is administering a drug that has been known to cause long-QT syndrome to a female patient. Assessment findings that would warrant consultation with the prescriber include: (Select all that apply.)
   a. lightheadedness or dizziness.
   b. palpitations.
   c. serum magnesium 1.9 mEq/L.
   d. serum potassium 4.7 mEq/L.
   e. medication regime includes three drugs known to prolong QT interval.
   f. nausea and vomiting.
   g. constipation.

h. heart rate 58 beats/min.
i. heart rate 122 beats/min and BP 80/46 mm Hg.

9. A patient who is prescribed a medication for degenerative joint disease experiences edema and shortness of breath (SOB) within 24 hours after a new medication is started. Drug information does not include these symptoms as adverse effects. The medication is discontinued, and the edema and SOB disappear, but the joint symptoms return. The prescriber restarts the medication, and the edema and SOB occur again. The nurse should:
   a. administer the medication because edema and SOB are not known adverse effects.
   b. administer the medication because it has been prescribed by the prescriber.
   c. report the event to www.fda.gov/medwatch.
   d. hold all medications until the cause of the edema and SOB are identified.

10. The nurse is mentoring a student nurse. The student complains that it is unfair that the nursing program requires 100% proficiency in dose calculation on a dose calculation examination during the last semester. The student complains that students may be stressed by test taking and should not be expected to meet that level of proficiency. The basis of the nurses response to the student is to:
   a. support the student's efforts to overturn the policy because it is unrealistic.
   b. share with the student the policy that existed when the nurse was in school.
   c. support the school policy because 100% proficiency on dose calculations is required on the state board National Council Licensure Examination (NCLEX) examination.
   d. explain to the student that students must be able to calculate drug doses under stress because emergency situations are very stressful and that drug dose errors in these situations can be fatal.

11. The nurse is caring for a patient who is experiencing severe pain. Morphine sulfate 10 mg intramuscular (IM) is ordered every 4 hours as needed. The patient asks the nurse to administer the medication via an existing intravenous (IV) cap because he hates the pain of an IM injection. The nurse should:
   a. explain to the patient that the nurse cannot change the route of a medication and that the patient can receive the medication IM as prescribed now or wait until the nurse pages the prescriber for the patient's request.
   b. administer the medication IM.
   c. administer the medication via the intravenous cap.
   d. determine if the dose is safe for IV administration and administer it via the IV cap if it is safe.

12. The nurse is preparing to administer 0900 medications on an assigned patient. The medication administration record states Celebrex 20 mg once a day. The medication supplied is Celexa 20-mg tablets. What should the nurse do? (Select all that apply.)
   a. Research the original drug order.
   b. Inform the prescriber and pharmacy of the discrepancy.
   c. Follow the institution policy to complete an internal incident report describing the discrepancy.
   d. Research the error to determine how future errors can be prevented.
   e. Report the error to www.usp.org.

13. Describe measures that the nurse can take to prevent medication errors including specific actions for the three most common types of fatal medication errors.
   a. Measures that apply to all types of errors

   b. Giving an overdose

   c. Giving the wrong drug

   d. Using the wrong route

# 8 Individual Variation in Drug Responses

## OBJECTIVES

After reading and studying the corresponding chapter and completing the critical thinking and study questions, the student will be able to:

1. Identify the most accurate method for determining appropriate drug doses.
2. Specify nursing assessments that reflect renal functioning.
3. Describe the effect of alterations in acid-base balance on drug distribution.
4. Examine the relationship of serum potassium levels and digoxin toxicity.
5. Compare pharmacodynamic and metabolic (pharmacokinetic) tolerance.
6. Determine the best nursing action when tachyphylaxis occurs.
7. Develop a teaching plan for a drug with a narrow therapeutic index and factors that can vary drug absorption and concentration.
8. Recognize appropriate nursing actions when adverse effects are probably caused by genetic variations.
9. Contrast differences in select drug metabolism between the sexes.
10. Predict the effect of nutritional status on drugs that are highly protein bound.

## CRITICAL THINKING AND STUDY QUESTIONS

1. Dose requirements for drugs with a narrow therapeutic range are most accurately calculated based on:
   a. age.
   b. body surface area.
   c. sex.
   d. weight.

2. Aminoglycoside antibiotics are potentially nephrotoxic antibiotics. What assessments and laboratory tests should the nurse monitor when a patient is receiving aminoglycoside antibiotics?

3. A patient is totally dependent on a respirator to initiate respirations. Recent laboratory values include pH 7.48, $PCO_2$ 32 mm Hg, and $HCO_3$ 20 mEq/L indicating respiratory alkalosis. The effect of this acid-base imbalance on acidic drugs would be:
   a. ionization of the drug in the blood, increasing the blood level of the drug.
   b. trapping of the drug in the cells, decreasing the blood level of the drug.

4. A terminal cancer patient has been receiving narcotic analgesics for severe pain for more than 6 months. The prescriber has increased the dose of the long-acting opiate and added an "as needed" opiate for breakthrough pain. The nurse should:
   a. recognize that the higher dose is needed because the patient would have undergone down-regulation of opiate receptors.
   b. recognize that the additional medication is needed because cancer causes an up-regulation of opiate receptors.
   c. question the higher dose of medication because the patient is at risk for narcotic addiction.
   d. question why the medication is being prescribed on a regular and as needed basis.

5. The difference between pharmacodynamic and metabolic (pharmacokinetic) tolerance is that there is a decreased response to the drug in tolerance and:
   a. both involve high levels of the drug, but pharmacodynamic tolerance involves lack of response, and metabolic tolerance involves normal response.
   b. both involve high levels of the drug, but metabolic tolerance involves lack of response, and pharmacodynamic tolerance involves excessive response.
   c. pharmacodynamic tolerance is lack of response to high levels of the drug, and metabolic tolerance is lack of response because of low levels of the drug.
   d. pharmacodynamic tolerance is excessive response to low levels of the drug, and metabolic tolerance is lack of response to high levels of the drug.

▶ 6. Nitroglycerin transdermal patch is ordered to be applied at 0900 and removed at 2100. The patch from the previous day is still in place when the nurse is preparing to administer the 0900 patch. The best action by the nurse is:
   a. leave the old patch on and apply the new one in a different site.
   b. remove the old patch and apply the new one in a different site.
   c. remove the old patch and do not apply a new patch until tomorrow.
   d. remove the old patch and consult with the prescriber for further directions.

7. Research the drug lithium carbonate (Eskalith) and identify important teaching points about the administration of the drug.

8. The nurse is caring for a 57-year-old black man who has been prescribed sulfamethoxazole and trimethoprim (Septra IV) and whose history includes a G-6-PD deficiency. Because this enzyme deficiency can cause hemolytic anemia in patients receiving sulfonamide, penicillin, and cephalosporin antibiotics, the nurse will monitor which laboratory tests?
   a. BUN and creatinine
   b. Hematocrit and hemoglobin
   c. AST and ALT
   d. PT and INR

9. Based on differences in metabolism of alcohol between the sexes, if both a man and woman consume the same amount of alcohol (on a weight-adjusted basis) and take the drug metronidazole (Flagyl), the disulfiram reaction between alcohol and the drug in the woman should: (Select all that apply.)
   a. last longer than the man.
   b. abate sooner than the man.
   c. be more intense than the man.
   d. be less intense than the man.

10. Warfarin sodium (Coumadin) is a drug that slows the formation of clots. It is highly protein bound. Only the unbound fraction of the drug is active. If the nurse is administering warfarin to a malnourished patient with a serum protein level of 4.9 gm/dL, the nurse would expect the patient's response to the drug to be:
    a. more intense with a greater risk for bleeding.
    b. less intense with a greater risk for bleeding.
    c. more intense with a lesser risk for bleeding.
    d. less intense with a lesser risk for bleeding.

# 9 Drug Therapy During Pregnancy and Breast-Feeding

## OBJECTIVES

After reading and studying the corresponding chapter and completing the critical thinking and study questions, the student will be able to:

1. Apply knowledge of drug safety during pregnancy and lactation to clinical cases.
2. State principles that guide prescribing of drugs during pregnancy.
3. Employ principles of pharmacokinetics to drug transfer to a fetus.
4. Recognize symptoms of opiate addiction in a neonate.
5. Formulate nursing interventions that can decrease the incidence of exposure of pregnant women to teratogenic substances.
6. Identify factors that make it difficult to detect teratogens.
7. Use the FDA pregnancy category of drugs in nursing practice.
8. Determine why a drug may be needed during pregnancy.
9. Recognize the role of the nurse in situations where exposure to a teratogen has occurred.
10. Teach interventions to decrease the risk of adverse effects from maternally administered drugs to the fetus and breast-fed neonate.

## CRITICAL THINKING AND STUDY QUESTIONS

1. The nurse is working in an obstetric office. A pregnant patient states that she has stopped taking all of her medications because she has heard that medications are harmful to the developing baby. The nurse's response should be based on:
   a. pregnant women should not take any drugs.
   b. the health of the fetus depends on the health of the mother.
   c. drugs have been tested and the prescriber will know which drugs are harmful to the fetus.
   d. the health of the fetus is always the first consideration when drugs are prescribed to pregnant women.

2. Principles that are considered when a drug is prescribed for a pregnant woman include:

3. Based on pharmacokinetics, drugs are most likely to pass into fetal circulation if they are:
   a. highly polar.
   b. ionized.
   c. protein bound.
   d. lipid soluble.

4. A mother with a history of heroin addiction has delivered a full-term infant. Which signs and symptoms suggest the infant is experiencing withdrawal symptoms?
   a. Shrill cry and irritability
   b. Respiratory depression and lethargy
   c. Peripheral cyanosis and hypotension
   d. APGAR score of 3 at 1 minute and 4 at 5 minutes

5. A mother with a history of heroin addiction has delivered a full-term infant. What should be included in the nursing care of this neonate?

6. Exposure to teratogens during the embryonic period can produce gross malformation in the fetus. What are nursing actions that can decrease teratogenesis during this period?

7. A mother is grieving because her newborn has an anatomic defect. She asks why scientists have not been able to identify all substances that cause birth defects. What factors make it difficult to identify teratogens?

8. A pregnant woman with a history of hypertension asks the nurse why the physician changed her high blood pressure medication from quinapril (Accupril) to methyldopa (Aldomet). The nurse's response should be based on:
   a. methyldopa is more effective for treating hypertension during pregnancy.
   b. methyldopa is pregnancy category B and quinapril is pregnancy category C in the first trimester and category D in the second and third trimesters.
   c. the dose of quinapril is more potent than the dose of methyldopa.
   d. quinapril crosses the placenta, but methyldopa does not.

9. Recommendations for levothyroxine state that the drug should be continued and increased during pregnancy. Research the drug and propose why this is recommended.

10. An important role of the nurse when a pregnant woman has a known exposure to a known teratogen during week 4 of the pregnancy would be:
    a. ordering an ultrasound.
    b. providing the diagnosis from the ultrasound to the parents.
    c. recommending termination of pregnancy if a severe malformation is detected.
    d. providing information and emotional support.

11. The nurse is providing discharge teaching to a postpartum mother who is breast-feeding her neonate. The mother has a chronic condition that requires drug therapy. Teaching about taking these drugs should include:

# 10 Drug Therapy in Pediatric Patients

## OBJECTIVES

After reading and studying the corresponding chapter and completing the questions and the case studies, the student will be able to:

1. Identify the effects of organ system immaturity on drug doses and responses.
2. Apply knowledge of pharmacokinetics to pediatric cases.
3. Determine needed assessments relating to potential adverse effects.
4. Recognize drugs that are uniquely contraindicated for pediatric patients
5. Use body surface area to calculate safe drug doses.
6. Employ knowledge of developmental characteristics of pediatric development and family centered care to increase adherence to the drug therapy regimen.
7. Accurately measure pediatric doses.
8. Compare differences in infant and adult blood-brain barriers.

## CRITICAL THINKING AND STUDY QUESTIONS

1. Premature infants are at risk for:
   a. inadequate and short-lived response to drugs.
   b. intense and prolonged response to drugs.
   c. inadequate but prolonged response to drugs.
   d. intense but short-lived response to drugs.

2. An infant is diagnosed with scurvy caused by vitamin C deficiency. Based on the principles of pH-dependent ionization and ion trapping and the differences in gastrointestinal physiology in the infant, the nurse would expect that the prescribed dose of vitamin C (ascorbic acid) adjusted for weight would be:
   a. less than an adult dose.
   b. equal to an adult dose.
   c. more than an adult dose.

3. A pregnant patient received morphine sulfate late in labor. The neonate was born 22 minutes later. Because the drug crosses the placenta and the characteristics of the blood-brain barrier of the neonate, it is important to assess the neonate for:
   a. vomiting.
   b. irritability.
   c. tachycardia.
   d. respiratory depression.

4. In general terms, describe the capacity of the liver to metabolize drugs from birth through puberty.

5. The nurse is administering a drug that is excreted primarily unchanged in the urine to a 15-month-old child. The nurse would expect the dose of this drug, adjusted for weight, to be:
   a. less than an adult dose.
   b. equal to an adult dose.
   c. more than an adult dose.

6. Which over-the-counter drugs would be contraindicated in children younger than 19 years

of age because of the danger of Reye's syndrome? (Select all that apply.)
a. Acne cleansers
b. Alka-Seltzer
c. Anacin
d. Ascriptin
e. Astringents
f. Kaopectate
g. Dristan
h. Pepto-Bismol
i. Robitussin
j. Sudafed
k. St Joseph's baby aspirin
l. TUMs
m. Tylenol
n. Vitamin C

7. The nurse is preparing to administer 10 mL of medication to a 5-year-old child. Which of the following nursing interventions is most likely to gain cooperation from the child with taking the drug?
   a. Mix the medication in a 6-ounce glass of juice to mask the taste.
   b. Use a syringe to accurately measure the medication and squirt the medication into the child's mouth.
   c. Place the medication in a large empty glass so that the child can see that there is only a small amount of medication.
   d. Ask the parents if they have any special technique for administering medication that has been effective with this child.

8. The nurse is preparing to administer a drug with a narrow therapeutic range to a toddler. The dose equals 0.75 mL of the medication. The nurse will measure the medication using a:
   a. calibrated plastic medicine cup.
   b. 1-mL syringe.
   c. 3-mL syringe.
   d. measuring spoon.

9. Drugs do not readily cross into an adult's central nervous system (CNS). This is not true in neonates. What difference between the adult and the neonate makes what drug characteristics more of a concern in neonates than in adults?

10. A new mother says it is impossible to get her infant to take an oral suspension of an antibiotic. She tells you that she has been putting the medicine in the baby's formula. What can the nurse do to increase adherence to the drug regime?

## CASE STUDIES AND PATIENT TEACHING

*(Use a separate piece of paper for your responses.)*

### Case Study 1

*The recommended adult dose of a drug is 500 mg twice a day.*

1. Based on body surface area, what is the recommended dose for a child who is 43 inches tall and 48 lbs in weight?

2. The prescriber has prescribed 225 mg of the drug above twice a day for this child. Is this a safe dose for this child?

3. The drug is available in an elixir of 250 mg/5 mL. How much medication will the nurse administer?

# 11 Drug Therapy in Geriatric Patients

## OBJECTIVES

After reading and studying the corresponding chapter and completing the critical thinking and study questions, the student will be able to:

1. Identify factors that increase the risk of adverse effects from drugs in the older adult.
2. Develop nursing interventions that can decrease the incidence of adverse drug reactions and drug-drug interactions in the older adult.
3. Incorporate laboratory test interpretation in the nursing role in drug therapy for the older adult.
4. Assist the older adult with overcoming obstacles to adherence to the prescribed drug regimen.

## CRITICAL THINKING AND STUDY QUESTIONS

1. Which statements about older adults and pharmacotherapy are generally true? (Select all that apply.)
   a. The goal of therapy is to cure the disease.
   b. There is a wider individual variation in drug response.
   c. They are less sensitive to drugs.
   d. They absorb less of the dose of medication than younger individuals.
   e. Absorption of many drugs is slowed.
   f. Changes in body fat and lean body mass can cause lipid-soluble drugs to decrease in effect and water-soluble drugs to have a more intense effect.
   g. Liver enzyme activity may be increased.
   h. Drug accumulation secondary to decreased renal excretion is the most common cause of adverse reactions in older adults.
   i. A reduction in the number of receptors and/or decreased affinity for receptors may decrease the response to drugs that work by receptor interactions.

2. When evaluating kidney function in the older, debilitated adult, it is most important for the nurse to review the results of the:
   a. serum blood urea nitrogen (BUN).
   b. serum creatinine.
   c. creatinine clearance.
   d. renal ultrasound.

3. How can the nurse decrease the incidence of adverse drug reactions and drug-drug interactions based on these factors?
   a. Altered pharmacokinetics

   b. Multiple severe illnesses and multiple-drug therapy

   c. Poor adherence

▶ 4. An older adult with liver disease is receiving several drugs that are normally highly protein bound. The patient's serum albumin is 2.8 mg/dL (normal 3.5 to 5 mg/dL). The nurse needs to assess the patient for symptoms of:
   a. excessive action of the drugs.
   b. inadequate action of the drugs.

▶ 5. A 76-year-old patient, who has mild arthritis and a cataract of the left eye, has been prescribed four medications with varied time intervals. Identify the steps that the nurse would use to promote adherence to a prescribed drug regimen.

# OBJECTIVES

## (CHAPTERS 12-109)

The following are the overall objectives for this workbook. After reading and studying the corresponding chapters and completing the questions and the case studies, the student will be able to:

- □ Recognize common suffixes of generic names of drugs.
- □ Apply knowledge of pathophysiology of diseases and chronic conditions to nursing clinical decision making for teaching and safe administration of prescribed drug therapy.
- □ Use the nursing process to develop a plan of nursing care for patients receiving drug therapy.
- □ Incorporate knowledge of pharmacokinetics and pharmacodynamics when planning, providing, and evaluating nursing care.
- □ Recognize situations that can cause altered drug absorption, metabolism, and excretion.
- □ Identify patients who are at risk for drug reactions.
- □ Evaluate the factors that the nurse, patient, or caregiver must consider when deciding whether to administer or withhold a prescribed drug.
- □ Review the patient history for significant data relating to drug therapy.
- □ Incorporate developmental, genetic, gender, economic, and other issues that affect drug therapy in nursing care.
- □ Evaluate laboratory test results for needed nursing responses.
- □ Differentiate among normal, abnormal, and critical assessment findings and test results.
- □ Respond appropriately when abnormal data is identified.
- □ Interpret the significance of laboratory values as they relate to drug therapy and nursing care.
- □ Differentiate between critical and noncritical situations.
- □ Communicate pertinent data to the prescriber in an appropriate time frame.
- □ Recognize common factors at different developmental stages that affect adherence to prescribed drug regimen.
- □ Work with patients to develop realistic goals for drug therapy.
- □ Prioritize nursing actions relating to drug therapy.
- □ Calculate safe and therapeutic drug doses.
- □ Use critical thinking to develop measures that prevent drug administration errors.
- □ Safely administer prescribed drugs.
- □ Assess for adverse effects of drug therapy.
- □ Differentiate between medically acceptable and significant adverse effects.
- □ Develop interventions to minimize adverse effects.
- □ Apply knowledge of routes of administration to clinical cases.
- □ Develop a teaching plan for a prescribed drug.

# 12 Basic Principles of Neuropharmacology

## OBJECTIVES

See page 26 for the Objectives.

## CRITICAL THINKING AND STUDY QUESTIONS

1. Two drugs that alter synaptic transmission are in the same therapeutic class. Which would the nurse expect to have more adverse effects?
   a. Selective drug
   b. Nonselective drug

2. The nurse can identify possible adverse effects of drugs that alter synaptic transmission by identifying: (Select all that apply.)
   a. normal responses to receptor activation.
   b. whether the drug increases or decreases receptor activation.
   c. the dose of the drug.
   d. the target cell.
   e. whether the drug is selective or nonselective for specific receptors.
   f. the axon that is affected.
   g. the body cells that have receptors for the drug.

3. Selective serotonin reuptake inhibitors are a class of antidepressant drugs. Their mechanism of action is to:
   a. increase the release of serotonin from the vesicles into the synapse.
   b. decrease the synthesis of serotonin in the axon.
   c. decrease the pumping of serotonin back into the axon from which it was released.
   d. stimulate receptors for serotonin.

4. A cholinergic (mimics the action of acetylcholine) drug would cause the heart rate to slow because the drug:
   a. stimulates cardiac receptors for acetylcholine.
   b. causes an increased release of acetylcholine.
   c. causes a decreased release of acetylcholine.
   d. blocks receptors for acetylcholine.

5. What characteristics allow naloxone (Narcan) to take the place of the opiate at opiate receptors and reverse respiratory depression caused by an opiate (narcotic) analgesic? (Select all that apply.)
   a. Binding of naloxone and opiates to opiate receptors is reversible.
   b. Naloxone has a longer half-life than opiates.
   c. Naloxone has a stronger affinity for the receptor.
   d. Naloxone is selective for opiate receptors.
   e. The dose of naloxone is larger than the dose of the opiate.

6. What would be the possible adverse effects on these organs and/or processes of a nonselective drug that is administered to slow the heart rate that acts by blocking stimulation of $beta_1$ and $beta_2$ sympathetic nervous system receptors? (Think of the opposite of fight or flight.)
   a. Eyes

   b. Respiratory rate

   c. Airway

   d. GI motility

   e. Production of glucose by the liver and release into the blood

7. Based on the adverse effects that are possible above in question 6, the nurse would be especially cautious when administering a nonselective blocker of $beta_1$ and $beta_2$ receptors to patients with which chronic disorders?

# 13 Physiology of the Peripheral Nervous System

## OBJECTIVES

See page 26 for the Objectives.

## CRITICAL THINKING AND STUDY QUESTIONS

1. Match the divisions of the nervous system to functions that can be influenced by drugs.

| | |
|---|---|
| 5 a. Autonomic | 1. Involuntary process and skeletal muscle |
| 3 b. Central | 2. Thinking, emotion, and processing data |
| 3 c. Parasympathetic | 3. Skeletal muscle and parasympathetic |
| 4 d. Peripheral | 4. Heart, secretory glands, and smooth muscle |
| 1 e. Somatic | 5. Involuntary processes |

2. From head to toe, list the seven regulatory functions that are relevant to drug therapy that occur with stimulation of the parasympathetic nervous system.

3. The nurse would assess for which common adverse effects if a patient has experienced exposure to insecticides, nerve gas, or toxic mushrooms (cholinesterase inhibitors)?

4. Sympathetic nervous stimulation ("fight or flight") can cause which of the following? (Select all that apply.)
   a. Increase heart rate
   b. Dilate bronchi
   c. Constrict pupils
   d. Inhibit the release of epinephrine from the adrenal gland
   e. Maintain blood flow to the brain
   f. Compensate for blood loss by vasodilation
   g. Constrict surface blood vessels
   h. Dilate surface blood vessels
   i. Stimulate sweating
   j. Shunt blood from muscles to vital organs during exercise
   k. Decrease blood pressure
   l. Increase blood glucose

5. The nurse is caring for a patient whose temperature is 102.4°F. The nurse notes that the patient's skin is flushed and sweaty. Vital signs include pulse 96 beats/min and respirations 25/min. Describe why stimulation of the sympathetic nervous system would respond to fever in this way.
   a. Dilate surface vessels and sweating

   b. Increase heart and respiratory rate

6. A patient asks the nurse why so many drugs have the adverse effect of impairing male sexual functioning. The nurse's response is based on:

7. A patient with a blood pressure (BP) of 188/104 mm Hg takes a potent vasodilating drug to lower the blood pressure. One hour after administration, the BP has dropped to 140/78 mm Hg in response to the drug. What change in pulse would the nurse expect with this rapid drop in blood pressure?

8. Most drugs that affect muscarinic receptors of the parasympathetic nervous system produce adverse effects because:
   a. high doses are needed to get therapeutic effects.
   b. muscarinic receptors are present on all postganglionic neurons.
   c. most drugs that affect muscarinic receptors are nonselective.
   d. muscarinic receptors are stimulated by epinephrine, which is secreted by the adrenal gland.

9. Why would stimulation of nicotinic$_N$ ($N_n$) receptors cause widespread effects?

10. Complete this chart.

| Effects of parasympathetic muscarinic receptor stimulation and blocking | | |
|---|---|---|
| Location | Cholinergic (Muscarinic) Substances that stimulate muscarinic receptors | Anticholinergic (Antimuscarinic) Substances that block muscarinic receptors |
| Eye | | |
| Heart | | |
| Lungs | | |
| Bladder | | |
| GI tract | | |
| Sweat glands | | |
| Sex organs | | |
| Blood vessels | (not caused by nervous system activation) | |

11. Based on the chart that you created, what would be logical therapeutic uses for:
   a. cholinergic (muscarinic) drugs?

   b. anticholinergic (antimuscarinic) drugs?

12. What are reasons why there might not be a drug developed for these conditions?

13. Complete this chart.

| Effects of sympathetic (adrenergic) receptor stimulation and blocking | | | |
|---|---|---|---|
| Receptor | Location | Adrenergic *Substances that stimulate adrenergic receptors* | Adrenergic blocker *Substances that block adrenergic receptors* |
| Alpha$_1$ $\alpha_1$ | Eye | | |
| | Arterioles of skin, organs, and mucous membranes | | |
| | Veins | | |
| | Male sex organs | | |
| | Prostate capsule | | |
| | Bladder | | |
| Alpha$_2$ $\alpha_2$ | Presynaptic nerve terminals | | |
| Beta$_1$ $\beta_1$ | Heart | | |
| | Kidney | | |
| Beta$_2$ $\beta_2$ | Arterioles of heart, lungs, and skeletal muscle | | |
| | Bronchi | | |
| | Uterus | | |
| | Liver | | |
| | Skeletal muscle | | |

14. Based on the chart that you created, what would be logical therapeutic uses for:
   a. alpha$_1$-($\alpha_1$) adrenergic drugs?
   b. alpha$_1$-($\alpha_1$) adrenergic blocking drugs?
   c. beta$_1$-($\beta_1$) adrenergic drugs?
   d. beta$_1$-($\beta_1$) adrenergic blocking drugs?

e. $beta_2$-($\beta_2$) adrenergic drugs?

f. $beta_2$-($\beta_2$) adrenergic blocking drugs?

15. Which adrenergic receptor is the "brakes" of the system that prevents excessive sympathetic effects?

16. What would be the possible adverse effects on these organs and/or processes of a nonselective drug that acts by blocking stimulation of $beta_1$ and $beta_2$ sympathetic nervous system receptors?
    a. Eyes
    b. Respiratory rate
    c. Airway
    d. GI motility
    e. Production of glucose by the liver and release into the blood

▶ 17. Based on the possible adverse effects, the nurse would be especially cautious when administering a nonselective blocker of $beta_1$ and $beta_2$ receptors to patients with which chronic disorders?

18. Despite the fact that no nerves terminate at muscarinic receptors on blood vessels, what is the effect of muscarinic drugs on the blood pressure?

19. What three factors determine adrenergic receptor stimulation by a drug?

20. The only transmitter that activates $beta_2$-($\beta_2$) adrenergic receptors is:
    a. acetylcholine.
    b. dopamine.
    c. epinephrine.
    d. norepinephrine.

21. Nerve gas is deadly because it can be absorbed through the skin and has an irreversible effect on cholinesterase. The victim experiences increased bronchial secretions, tight chest, dimming of vision, drooling, involuntary defecation and urination, muscle tremors, convulsions, coma, and death. Based on these symptoms, does nerve gas induce or inhibit cholinesterase?

▶ 22. Monoamine oxidase (MAO) inhibitors are a class of antidepressants that inhibit the breakdown of norepinephrine by MAO. The nurse is caring for a patient who has been taking an MAO inhibitor and consumed large amounts of foods containing tyramine. What symptoms would the nurse expect and why? (See Fig. 13-8 in the textbook.)

23. What three factors must be considered when studying drugs that work by receptor interaction?

# 14 Muscarinic Agonists and Antagonists

## OBJECTIVES

See page 26 for the Objectives.

## CRITICAL THINKING AND STUDY QUESTIONS

1. Define these terms.
   a. Agonist

   b. Antagonist

2. The nurse is preparing to administer bethanechol (Urecholine). Which of the following findings would warrant the nurse holding the medication and contacting the prescriber?
   a. Pulse 110 beats/min
   b. BP 100/60
   c. Wheezing
   d. Patient is drooling
   e. Postoperative abdominal distention
   f. Recent bowel resection
   g. Recent vaginal delivery of a 7-lb neonate
   h. 62-year-old male with postvoid residual of 350 mL of urine
   i. Positive hemoccult of stool
   j. TSH 0.2 microunits/mL; $T_4$ 18 mcg/dL

3. A 48-year-old woman with a history of rheumatoid arthritis has been diagnosed with Sjögren's syndrome. Cevimeline (Evoxac) 30-mg capsule, three times daily has been prescribed. Why is it important to assess this patient for electrolyte imbalances?

4. A group of students go camping. One student finds some wild mushrooms and eats them with his lunch. Which of the following symptoms would you expect if he is experiencing muscarinic poisoning? (Select all that apply.)
   a. Tachycardia
   b. Hypertension
   c. Profuse salivation and lacrimation
   d. Constipation
   e. Dilated pupils that do not respond to light
   f. Wheezing

5. The emergency department nurse receives a patient brought in by an ambulance with suspected poisoning from exposure to muscarinic insecticide. A priority nursing action is to prepare:
   a. to relieve the pain of muscle spasms.
   b. for possible respiratory arrest.
   c. to place the patient in a side-lying position because the patient is likely to vomit.
   d. to administer intravenous fluids.

6. Why is antimuscarinic drug a better term than anticholinergic drug?

7. Why might excessive doses of atropine cause sympathetic nervous system stimulation symptoms?

▶ 8. The nurse has administered atropine as a preoperative medication. The patient complains of a sudden feeling of warmth. Her skin is warm and dry, and her face is flushed. The nurse should:
   a. notify the surgeon STAT.
   b. asses the patient's vital signs and notify the surgeon.
   c. assess the patient's vital signs and mental status and notify the OR that surgery must be postponed.
   d. assess the patient's vital signs and mental status and, if within normal limits, document the findings and continue the preoperative protocol.

9. What form of atropine would be prescribed for a person who is at risk to be exposed to toxic levels of insecticide or nerve gas?
   a. Extended-release tablet
   b. Enteric-coated tablet
   c. Self-injectable pen
   d. Intravenous solution

10. Oxybutynin (Ditropan) is an anticholinergic drug prescribed that is available in four formulations. A patient has experienced many adverse effects when taking oxybutynin immediate-release tablets (Ditropan IR) for overactive bladder (OAB). She asks the nurse how the transdermal patch could cause less adverse effects if it is essentially the same drug. The nurse's response should be based on:
   a. transdermal absorption bypasses metabolism in the intestinal wall.
   b. the transdermal form is water soluble and poorly absorbed.
   c. the transdermal form is a different drug than oral oxybutynin.
   d. the transdermal form is less effective than the ER oral form.

11. The nurse is teaching a patient about darifenacin (Enablex), a newly prescribed drug for overactive bladder (OAB) that selectively blocks muscarinic$_3$ ($M_3$) receptors. The nurse should teach the patient that likely adverse effects include: (Select all that apply.)
   a. blurred vision.
   b. confusion.
   c. diarrhea.
   d. dry eyes.
   e. photophobia.
   f. sleepiness.
   g. tachycardia.

▶ 12. Emergency room physician's orders for a patient with advanced HIV admitted with a mycobacterium infection include clarithromycin (Biaxin) 500 mg PO twice a day and continue with all home medications. The patient's regimen includes darifenacin (Enablex) ER 15 mg once a day, delavirdine 400 mg, three times daily, nevirapine 200 mg twice a day, and ritonavir 600 mg twice a day. Based on possible drug interaction with darifenacin, the nurse should:
   a. give the medications with food to prevent GI distress.
   b. administer the medications so that there is at least 1 hour between each medication.
   c. review the home medications and the medication order with the prescriber.
   d. hold all of the medications.

13. The nurse should review the results of the ECG and the history for unexplained fainting or long-QT syndrome before administering:
   a. darifenacin (Enablex).
   b. oxybutynin (Ditropan, Oxytrol).
   c. solifenacin (VESIcare).
   d. tolterodine (Detrol).
   e. trospium (Sanctura).

14. What response to tolterodine (Detrol) would the nurse expect if a patient lacks the P450 cytochrome CYP2D6 isoenzyme?
   a. More adverse effects
   b. Lack of therapeutic response
   c. Prolonged drug action
   d. Need to take the drug on an empty stomach

15. Trospium (Sanctura) 20 mg once a day is prescribed for an older adult patient with overactive bladder (OAB). The nurse instructs the patient to take the medication:
    a. one hour before breakfast.
    b. one hour after breakfast.
    c. with the first bite of breakfast.
    d. anytime during the day as long as it is at the same time each day.

16. The nurse is caring for a patient who has taken an overdose of a tricyclic antidepressant drug that has pronounced antimuscarinic properties. The nurse should prepare to: (Select all that apply.)
    a. support breathing.
    b. administer atropine.
    c. administer drugs for hypotension.
    d. administer phenothiazine antipsychotic drugs to treat delirium.
    e. administer physostigmine.

▸ 17. A patient has received a mydriatic medication as part of an eye examination. Before leaving the office, what instructions would be most useful for the patient's comfort and safety?

## CASE STUDIES AND PATIENT TEACHING

*(Use a separate piece of paper for your responses.)*

### Case Study 1

*A frail-appearing, 66-year-old female with a history of type 2 diabetes mellitus, hypertension, depression, and overactive bladder is admitted to a medical unit with the diagnosis of altered mental status. Assessment findings include BP 182/110 mm Hg, P 118, R 14, and T 102.4°F. The patient is becoming confused and is exhibiting symptoms that suggest she is hallucinating. The patient resists efforts to open her eyes for pupil assessment. Skin is flushed and warm; mucous membranes are dry. Bowel sounds are hypoactive, and there are multiple areas of dullness when percussing the abdomen. The bladder is palpable above the pubic symphysis, with bladder scan reading 350 mL. Admission laboratory test results include BUN 32 mg/dL; creatinine 2.3 mg/dL; glucose 178 mg/dL; WBC 12,400/mm$^3$. Creatinine clearance has been ordered, and the collection was started at 0600. The nurse is preparing the patient's 0900 medications including tolterodine (Detrol).*

1. What do laboratory tests suggest?
2. What concern does the nurse have about administering tolterodine?
3. What symptoms suggest antimuscarinic toxicity?
4. What should the nurse do?
5. The physician discontinues the tolterodine. The patient's condition improves. The patient is concerned about bladder control. What teaching can the nurse provide to assist a patient with overactive bladder (OAB) to attain bladder control?

### Case Study 2

*The recommended subcutaneous dose of atropine for a child is 0.01 mg/kg, not to exceed 0.4 mg.*

1. What is the recommended dose for a child who is 32 inches long and weighs 24 lbs?
2. Based on the recommended dose, how much medication will the nurse draw into the syringe if atropine is available as 0.5 mg/mL?

### Case Study 3

Complete this patient teaching handout for Cevimeline (Evoxac).

| Cevimeline (Evoxac) | |
|---|---|
| Reason for taking this drug | |
| Dose and administration directions | |
| Teaching relating to possible adverse effects | |
| Things to report to your prescriber | |
| Drug interactions | |

# 15 Cholinesterase Inhibitors and Their Use in Myasthenia Gravis

## OBJECTIVES

See page 26 for the Objectives.

## CRITICAL THINKING AND STUDY QUESTIONS

1. Cholinesterase inhibitors can:
   a. intensify transmission at neuromuscular junctions.
   b. intensify transmission at muscarinic, ganglionic, and neuromuscular junctions.
   c. prevent transmission at neuromuscular junctions.
   d. prevent transmission at muscarinic, ganglionic, and neuromuscular junctions.

2. The principle reason why physostigmine is preferred over neostigmine for reversing muscarinic toxicity is related to:
   a. pharmacokinetics
   b. pharmacodynamics.

3. ▸ A 66-year-old male has been taking ambenonium (Mytelase) for myasthenia gravis for 4 years. He is admitted to the hospital for a prostate biopsy after his PSA laboratory test was elevated. The ambelonium (Mytelase) is scheduled to be administered. The nurse should:
   a. administer the medication.
   b. hold the medication.
   c. assess for urine retention before administering the medication.
   d. consult with the urologist.

4. The nurse is caring for a patient who is prescribed pyridostigmine (Mestinon) 240 mg, three times daily for myasthenia gravis. The patient states that he is experiencing an extreme increase in muscle weakness and that he needs the nurse to administer 300-mg doses. The nurse should:
   a. administer 240 mg because that is the dose ordered by the prescriber.
   b. administer 300-mg doses because myasthenia gravis patients often need to adjust their dose of medication according to symptoms.
   c. call the prescriber and request an order for the increased dose.
   d. immediately assess the patient for other symptoms including excessive muscarinic stimulation, such as increased secretion, increased bowel sounds, bradycardia, and wheezing, and contact prescriber with patient's request and assessment findings.

5. Matching

_____ a. Atropine
_____ b. Echothiophate
_____ c. Edrophonium
_____ d. Malathion
_____ e. Neostigmine
_____ f. Physostigmine
_____ g. Pralidoxime
_____ h. Tabun

1. Used to diagnose myasthenia gravis
2. Antidote for poisoning by organophosphate insecticides
3. Used to treat drug-induced muscarinic blockade
4. Irreversible cholinesterase inhibitor used to treat glaucoma
5. Irreversible cholinesterase inhibitor nerve gas that can be used in bioterrorism
6. Antidote for cholinergic crisis
7. Short-acting reversible cholinesterase inhibitor that does not cross blood-brain barrier
8. Organophosphate insecticide

## CASE STUDIES AND PATIENT TEACHING

*(Use a separate piece of paper for your responses.)*

### Case Study 1

*A patient who is receiving a reversible cholinesterase inhibitor for myasthenia gravis is brought into the emergency department by his family because of extreme muscle weakness and difficulty breathing.*

1. In this situation, why is it important to determine if the cause of the weakness is myasthenic crisis versus cholinergic crisis?

2. a. What assessments should the nurse perform?
   b. What questions should the nurse ask the patient and family?
   c. Why?

3. The physician is unsure by history if the patient is experiencing myasthenic crisis or cholinergic crisis. He orders administration of edrophonium to differentiate. What should the nurse do along with preparing to administer the edrophonium?

4. The nurse is doing discharge teaching for this patient. What teaching should the nurse do to help the patient monitor the response to medication for his myasthenia gravis?

### Case Study 2

*The nurse has been asked to speak to a 4-H group in a farming community on preventing poisoning by organophosphate insecticides. The nurse has stressed the importance of following all directions provided and seeking clarification if anything is unclear.*

1. What information should the nurse include to prevent:
   a. exposure when using insecticides through the skin or eyes?
   b. exposure when using insecticides through the respiratory tract?
   c. oral exposure?

2. What symptoms warrant seeking immediate medical attention when using pesticides?

3. What is the treatment for pesticide poisoning?

# 16 Drugs That Block Nicotinic Cholinergic Transmission: Neuromuscular Blocking Agents and Ganglionic Blocking Agents

## OBJECTIVES

See page 26 for the Objectives.

## CRITICAL THINKING AND STUDY QUESTIONS

1. A woman who is 8 weeks pregnant must have surgery. The anesthesiologist administers vecuronium (Norcuron), a quaternary ammonium compound, to achieve muscle relaxation. The most likely effect of this medication on the developing fetus is:
   a. no detectable effect.
   b. respiratory depression.
   c. bradycardia.
   d. teratogenesis.

2. Neuromuscular blocking agents: (Select all that apply.)
   a. block $nicotinic_M$ ($N_M$) receptors on the motor end-plate.
   b. block the sensation of pain.
   c. can be administered orally, intramuscularly, and intravenously.
   d. can cause respiratory arrest.
   e. cross the blood-brain barrier.
   f. do not cause loss of consciousness.
   g. may lower BP by vasodilation.
   h. have a primary effect of spastic paralysis.

▶ 3. The nurse is aware that neuromuscular blocking agents do not alter consciousness or pain perception. The nurse instructs a patient who has received tubocurarine to blink her eyes to indicate if she is experiencing pain. Is this an appropriate assessment technique? Why?

4. Preoperative laboratory test results include potassium 3.2 mg/dL. It is important for the nurse to inform the anesthesiologist of this result because it can cause normal doses of tubocurarine to cause:
   a. tachycardia.
   b. inability to reverse the blockade.
   c. respiratory arrest.
   d. the patient to sense pain during the procedure.

5. The nurse should assess for and plan interventions to relieve muscle pain 12 to 24 hours after surgery for patients who have received:
   a. succinylcholine.
   b. atracurium.
   c. pancuronium.
   d. tubocurarine.

▶ 6. An anesthesia resident is supervising the reversal of the neuromuscular blockade for a patient who has received succinylcholine. She asks the nurse to administer 0.5 mg of neostigmine (Prostigmin) intravenously. The nurse should:
   a. administer the medication slowly to prevent respiratory depression.
   b. question the resident because neostigmine intensifies the neuromuscular blockade caused by succinylcholine, a depolarizing neuromuscular blocker.
   c. only administer the medication if mechanical assistance for ventilation is available.
   d. question the resident as to whether atropine should also be administered to prevent respiratory depression.

▶ 7. A patient will be receiving succinylcholine before electroconvulsive therapy. A nursing priority is:
   a. administering the succinylcholine.
   b. administering atropine if toxicity occurs.
   c. performing the electroconvulsive therapy.
   d. preparing for possible respiratory arrest.

8. Succinylcholine is routinely administered to patients during certain endoscopic procedures. The endoscopy nurse reviews each patient history before the procedure. What information should the nurse look for because it would be a concern and should be reported to the physician or anesthesiologist relating to succinylcholine use?

## CASE STUDIES AND PATIENT TEACHING

*(Use a separate piece of paper for your responses.)*

### Case Study 1

*The postanesthesia care unit (PACU) nurse is caring for a patient who received tubocurarine during surgery to remove a cancerous section of the bowel. The patient is admitted to the PACU with mechanical ventilation and an NG tube to low-intermittent suction.*

1. What are priority assessments that the PACU nurse must monitor while the patient is still under the effects of tubocurarine?

2. The NG tube is draining a large amount of bile-colored liquid. How does this affect potassium levels and nursing care?

3. As the patient regains neuromuscular functioning, the nurse instructs the patient to take deep breaths. How does deep breathing counteract the adverse effects of histamine release stimulated by the tubocurarine?

## Case Study 2

*A patient is receiving a neuromuscular blocker for prolonged paralysis during mechanical ventilation.*

1. Describe measures that should be included in nursing care and their rationale.

2. The patient spikes a temperature of 102° F within an hour after the neuromuscular agent infusion is begun. The infusion of the neuromuscular blocking agent is stopped, and the patient receives a dose of acetaminophen (Tylenol). The patient's temperature continues to rise despite being medicated with the antipyretics. Dantrolene (Dantrium) is prescribed, and the patient's temperature begins to drop. Why would dantrolene be effective in lowering this patient's temperature, but not acetaminophen?

# 17 Adrenergic Agonists

## OBJECTIVES

See page 26 for the Objectives.

## CRITICAL THINKING AND STUDY QUESTIONS

1. What is a common term for adrenergic agonists that reflects that their effects mimic sympathetic nervous system stimulation?

2. Direct-acting adrenergic drugs mimic the action of: (Select all that apply.)
   a. acetylcholine.
   b. dopamine.
   c. epinephrine (epi).
   d. norepinephrine (NE).

3. Matching: Mechanism of action (Some will have more than one answer.).

| | | |
|---|---|---|
| _____ | a. Amphetamines | 1. Promotion of NE release |
| _____ | b. Cocaine | 2. Inhibition of NE reuptake |
| _____ | c. Ephedrine | 3. Inhibition of NE inactivation |
| _____ | d. MAO inhibitors | 4. Direct receptor activation |
| _____ | e. Most sympathomimetics | |
| _____ | f. Tricyclic antidepressants | |

4. Catecholamines: (Select all that apply.)
   a. are inactivated before reaching systemic circulation if administered orally.
   b. cross the blood-brain barrier activating the central nervous system (CNS).
   c. include the drugs epinephrine, norepinephrine, isoproterenol, dopamine, and dobutamine.
   d. are effective when administered by any parenteral route.
   e. have a long half-life.
   f. are polar molecules.
   g. are destroyed by MAO and COMT enzymes in the liver and intestinal wall.
   h. usually have a duration of 3 to 6 hours.

5. The nurse is caring for a patient who is receiving a dopamine intravenous drip. The nurse has been assessing her patient every 15 minutes. The nurse notes that since the last assessment the intravenous dopamine solution has turned pink. The nurse should:
   a. stop the intravenous infusion, assess the patient for adverse effects, and notify the prescriber.
   b. stop the infusion, notify the pharmacy for an immediate replacement, and assess the patient.
   c. continue to assess the patient and infuse the solution as prescribed.
   d. continue to assess the patient and infuse the solution as prescribed for up to 24 hours after being hung.

6. Based on Table 17-2, which catecholamine would stimulate the heart while producing the least unintended effects?

7. A woman who is pregnant at 30 weeks of gestation is receiving terbutaline. The drug book states that it is a drug used to bronchodilate. The patient does not have a history of asthma and denies any problems with bronchoconstriction. What would be a logical problem for which she is receiving the terbutaline?

▸ 8. Based on the general principles of pharmacokinetics and relative specificity, patients with what chronic diseases would be at most risk for adverse effects from adrenergic agonists? (Select all that apply.)
   a. Chronic obstructive pulmonary disease
   b. Cirrhosis of the liver
   c. Hypertension
   d. End-stage renal disease
   e. Osteoarthritis

9. A patient experiences sudden AV block. Intravenous epinephrine is ordered STAT. Nursing care for administration of this drug should include:

10. The nurse is working in the emergency department. A local anesthetic combined with epinephrine is often used when performing procedures on extremities that need a small area of anesthesia and are likely to bleed. Assessment findings that would warrant caution before administering a drug containing epinephrine include: (Select all that apply.)
   a. blood pressure 86/50 mm Hg.
   b. blood pressure 175/90 mm Hg.
   c. history of angina pectoris.
   d. history of AV heart block.
   e. poor capillary refill.
   f. palpitations.
   g. pulse 50 beats/min.
   h. pulse 110 beats/min.
   i. weak peripheral pulse.

▸ 11. The nurse is administering terbutaline to a patient in preterm labor who has a history of asthma and gestational diabetes. It is important to assess this patient for which possible adverse effect of terbutaline?
   a. Hot, dry, flushed skin
   b. Hypotension
   c. Sensitivity to light
   d. Urinary output of 50 mL/hr

12. A patient has a history of depression. Treatment by which of the following antidepressants is most likely to decrease the inactivation of dopamine and increase the risk of toxicity?
   a. bupropion (Wellbutrin)
   b. nortriptyline (Pamelor)
   c. sertraline (Zoloft)
   d. tranylcypromine (Parnate)

13. Dobutamine HCl (Dobutrex) is available in a vial of 250 mg/20 mL. The prescribed dose for a patient weighing 110 lbs is 250 mcg/min. To administer this medication the nurse must:
   a. administer it by intravenous push over 5 minutes.

b. infuse the vial by intravenous piggyback over 20 minutes.
c. dilute the vial in at least 50 mL of diluent and infuse at a rate of 30 mL/hr.
d. dilute the vial in 250 mL and infuse at a rate of 150 mL/hr.

14. Phenylephrine (NeoSynephrine) is available over the counter (OTC) as a nasal decongestant. A patient states that he understands why the label says it should not be used if he has high blood pressure, but he does not understand why it should not be used by diabetics. The nurse's response is based on knowledge that phenylephrine can cause: (Select all that apply.)
a. hypoglycemia in the diabetic patient.
b. hyperglycemia in the diabetic patient.
c. a tremor, which the patient may interpret as hypoglycemia.

▶ 15. The nurse is performing discharge teaching for a patient who was hospitalized with newly diagnosed hyperthyroidism. What teaching should the nurse include regarding commonly used over-the-counter medications?

## CASE STUDIES AND PATIENT TEACHING

*(Use a separate piece of paper for your responses.)*

### Case Study 1

*A female in cardiogenic shock is ordered an intravenous infusion of dopamine at a rate of 400 mcg/min. The patient weighs 154 lbs.*

1. What does the nurse need to do before beginning the infusion?

2. The prescriber decreases the prescribed dose to 300 mcg/min. The dopamine infusion is available in a dilution of 100 mg/250 mL. The infusion pump is calculated in mL/hr. What is the flow rate that the nurse will program into the infusion pump?

3. The nurse is administering the intravenous dopamine infusion. The nurse assesses the large antecubital vein and notes the site is swollen, cold, and extremely pale. The basis of the nurse's response is:
a. dopamine can only be infused through a central vein.
b. a clot has formed and can break off and become an embolus.
c. the intravenous infusion must continue at this site until another IV is successfully started.
d. vasoconstriction can cause tissue necrosis at the site of extravasation.

4. What treatment can prevent necrosis if dopamine extravasation occurs? How is it administered? How does it work?

### Case Study 2

*A 4-year-old child comes to the emergency department with angioedema, wheezing, and hypotension after eating a peanut butter cookie. Epinephrine is administered.*

1. Describe how it treats the symptoms of anaphylactic shock.

2. The child is prescribed an epinephrine auto-injector (EpiPen Jr). What should the nurse teach the parents and child about administering the medication?

3. How can the parents ensure that the child of this age has his pen available at all times?

# 18 Adrenergic Antagonists

## OBJECTIVES

See page 26 for the Objectives.

## CRITICAL THINKING AND STUDY QUESTIONS

1. An advantage of alpha antagonists is that they:
   a. are more potent.
   b. work on specific receptors.
   c. have irreversible action.
   d. are capable of treating a wide variety of illnesses.

2. Matching: Outcome with use (Answers may be used more than once.)

| | | |
|---|---|---|
| _____ | a. $Alpha_1$ agonist toxicity | 1. BP 90/60 mm Hg to 120/80 mm Hg |
| _____ | b. BPH | 2. Warm, pink tissue |
| _____ | c. Essential HTN | 3. Pain less than 2 on a scale of 1-10 in toes and fingers |
| _____ | d. Pheochromocytoma | 4. Brisk capillary refill |
| _____ | e. Raynaud's disease | 5. Post-void residual less than 75 mL |

3. The generic name of $alpha_1$ receptor antagonists share the common suffix:
   a. (-azole).
   b. (-lol).
   c. (-osin).
   d. (-sartan).

▸ 4. Before administering alfuzosin (Uroxatral) to a patient, which of these laboratory values is most important to be checked by the nurse?
   a. AST/ALT
   b. BUN/Creatinine
   c. FBS/$HbA_{1C}$
   d. $Na^+/K^+$

5. A patient has just been prescribed prazosin (Minipress). Which of the following statements would indicate a need for further teaching?
   a. "I should avoid driving and other hazardous activities for 12 to 24 hours after I first take this medication or have a dose increase."
   b. "I should take the medication first thing in the morning."
   c. "I should sit on the edge of the bed for a few minutes before standing up when I get up in the morning."
   d. "I should be sitting down 30 to 60 minutes after I take the first dose of this medication."

6. A patient is receiving terazosin (Hytrin) for hypertension. An adverse effect that may warrant the prescriber changing to another drug in the same class is:
   a. hypotension.
   b. nasal congestion.
   c. headache.
   d. reflex tachycardia.

7. A patient asks why his physician told him he should not take sildenafil (Viagra) for erectile dysfunction when he is taking an $alpha_1$-adrenergic antagonist for his high blood pressure. The basis of the nurse's response is the concern that this combination of drugs can cause:
   a. atrial fibrillation.
   b. migraine headache.
   c. prolonged erection.
   d. severe hypotension and vascular collapse.

8. When administering tamsulosin (Flomax), which of the following assessments would indicate that therapy has achieved the desired effect?
   a. Palpable bladder after voiding
   b. Voiding 250 mL every 2 to 3 hours while awake
   c. Nocturia
   d. Decrease in force of urinary stream

9. Tamulosin (Flomax) should be administered:
   a. with food.
   b. thirty minutes after the same meal each day.
   c. one hour before or 2 hours after the same meal each day.
   d. with a full glass of water and remain upright for 30 minutes.

10. Which of these factors, if identified in the history of a patient who has just been prescribed alfuzosin (Uroxatral), would be a concern to the nurse? (Select all that apply.)
   a. Angina pectoris
   b. Advanced HIV infection
   c. Diabetes mellitus type 2
   d. Erectile dysfunction
   e. Frequent urinary tract infections
   f. Hepatitis B
   g. Hypertension
   h. Ventricular dysrhythmia

11. A patient who is receiving phenoxybenzamine (Dibenzyline) to treat pheochromocytoma faints. BP is 75/40 mm Hg, P 135 beats/min. The nurse contacts the physician and plans to administer:
   a. epinephrine.
   b. norepinephrine.
   c. intravenous fluids.
   d. metoprolol.

12. The generic name of beta$_1$ and beta$_2$ receptor antagonists share the common suffix:
   a. (-azole).
   b. (-lol).
   c. (-zosin).
   d. (-sartan).

▶ 13. An assessment finding that would warrant holding a beta blocker and consulting the prescribing physician is?
   a. Apical pulse 50 beats/min
   b. Blood pressure 110/70 mm Hg
   c. 2+ ankle edema
   d. Capillary blood sugar 90 mg/dL

▶ 14. Which of these assessment findings, if identified 1 hour after administering metoprolol (Lopressor), should the nurse report to the prescriber immediately?
   a. Drop in apical pulse from 80 to 65 beats/min
   b. Warm, flushed, dry skin
   c. Crackles throughout lung fields and peripheral edema
   d. Headache

▶ 15. Which of these conditions, if identified in the history of a patient receiving a drug that blocks beta$_1$-adrenergic receptors, would be a concern to the nurse? (Select all that apply.)
   a. Anxiety
   b. AV heart block
   c. Benign prostatic hyperplasia (BPH)
   d. Chronic obstructive pulmonary disease (COPD)
   e. Depression
   f. Diabetes insipidus
   g. Diabetes mellitus
   h. Hypertension
   i. Hypothyroidism
   j. Migraine headaches
   k. Severe allergic reaction to bee stings

▶ 16. Which of these laboratory findings, if identified in a patient who is prescribed metoprolol (Lopressor), should the nurse report to the prescriber immediately?
   a. Creatinine 1.2 mg/dL
   b. Ejection fraction on echocardiogram of 20%
   c. Hemoglobin $A_{IC}$ (glycosylated hemoglobin) 5.5%
   d. Sinus rhythm on ECG

▶ 17. Which of these findings would be most significant if a patient was prescribed propranolol (Inderal)?
   a. Apical pulse 100 beats/min
   b. Expiratory wheezing
   c. Blood pressure 160/90 mm Hg
   d. Urinary

18. Which adrenergic antagonists block alpha$_1$, beta$_1$, and beta$_2$ receptors?
   a. Atenolol and bisoprolol
   b. Acebutolol and pindolol
   c. Carvedilol and labetalol
   d. Propranolol and timolol

19. The nurse should be especially vigilant to monitor for excessive cardiosuppression in a patient who is receiving metoprolol and:
   a. atorvastatin (Lipitor).
   b. hydrochlorothiazide (HydroDIURIL).
   c. terazosin (Hytrin).
   d. verapamil (Calan).

## CASE STUDIES AND PATIENT TEACHING

*(Use a separate piece of paper for your responses.)*

### Case Study 1

*A 58-year-old male has just been prescribed prazosin (Minipress) for hypertension.*

1. Explain the common adverse effects and nursing teaching needed to provide both comfort and safety for this patient.

2. What assessments should be performed before the nurse administers an alpha$_1$-adrenergic antagonist for hypertension, and what assessment findings would warrant not administering the medication and notifying the prescriber?

3. The patient's blood pressure is not controlled by his prescribed alpha$_1$ antagonist. The physician has added a loop diuretic and a beta$_1$ blocker. The patient asks, "Why do I have to take three different medications for my blood pressure? Can't I just have a higher dose of one medication?" How should the nurse explain the rationale for this drug regimen?

4. Why is it important to address ejaculation problems and other adverse effects with this patient?

### Case Study 2

*A 45-year-old male is being treated for hypertension. Several types of antihypertensive medications have been tried without success. He also has been taking glargine insulin (Lantus) 22 units every morning and aspart insulin (NovoLog) on a sliding scale according to blood sugar for diabetes. His physician prescribes metoprolol 50 mg once a day. When the patient tries to fill the prescription using his insurance, the pharmacist notifies him that his insurance only covers the less expensive beta blocker, propranolol, unless the patient experiences adverse effects or has an absolute contraindication for the use of propranolol. The prescriber can appeal to the insurance company and justify the use of the more expensive decision. The physician asks the office nurse to initiate the insurance appeal form.*

1. Describe and explain the adverse effects that this patient might experience relating to his diabetes diagnosis and propranolol.

2. The insurance appeal is approved, and the patient receives metoprolol, a beta$_1$-selective adrenergic antagonist. The patient states "I'm glad I do not have to take propranolol. I have had frequent episodes of hypoglycemia because with my job I cannot always eat when I should." What should the nurse do and why?

3. The nurse discovers that this patient has a history of poor adherence to medication regimens. Why are beta-adrenergic blockers poor choices for this patient?

# 19 Indirect-Acting Antiadrenergic Agents

## OBJECTIVES

See page 26 for the Objectives.

## CRITICAL THINKING AND STUDY QUESTIONS

1. Matching (Select all that apply.)

| | | |
|---|---|---|
| _____ | a. Clonidine | 1. Depletes NE from adrenergic neurons |
| _____ | b. Guanethidine | 2. Activates $alpha_2$ receptors |
| _____ | c. Methyldopa | 3. Blocks NE release and depletes NE storage |
| _____ | d. Reserpine | 4. Adverse effects of orthostatic hypotension and diarrhea |
| | | 5. Adverse effects of hemolytic anemia and liver damage |
| | | 6. Adverse effects of drowsiness and dry mouth |
| | | 7. Less likely to cause orthostatic hypotension |
| | | 8. Rebound hypertension if stopped abruptly |

2. Depletion of neurotransmitters norepinephrine and serotonin by reserpine makes it a priority for the nurse to assess the patient's:
   a. blood count.
   b. bowel sounds.
   c. mental status.
   d. stool for blood.

3. Which of these factors would be most significant if a patient was receiving clonidine?
   a. Also taking a tricyclic antidepressant
   b. Need to operate complex machinery
   c. Positive Coombs' test
   d. Woman of child-bearing age

4. The nurse is caring for a patient who is receiving reserpine for hypertension. The patient is passive, has poor eye contact and appetite, and is difficult to engage in conversation. The nurse is concerned that the patient is experiencing a drug-induced depression. The nurse should share her concern with the:
   a. patient.
   b. patient and the prescriber.
   c. prescriber and the family.
   d. patient, the prescriber, and the family.

5. A patient was started on reserpine 0.5 mg once a day 4 days ago for hypertension unresponsive to other antihypertensive agents. The nurse assesses the patient's blood pressure which is 155/72 mm Hg. The patient is discouraged. The nurse's response should be based on which of the following?
   a. It takes 1 to 2 weeks for norepinephrine depletion to occur.
   b. At first reserpine promotes norepinephrine release, which can elevate the BP temporarily.
   c. Ensure that the medication is being taken on an empty stomach.
   d. Reserpine primarily affects systolic blood pressure.

▸ 6. A patient is receiving guanethidine for uncontrolled hypertension. Which of the following laboratory test results should be reported to the prescriber immediately?
   a. ALT 35 U/L BUN 20 mg/dL
   b. Creatinine clearance 100 mL/min
   c. Urine catecholamines 870 mcg/24 hr

▸ 7. A patient is receiving methyldopa. Which of the following laboratory tests should be monitored throughout therapy? (Select all that apply.)
   a. Albumin
   b. ALT
   c. Bilirubin
   d. Coombs' test

e. Glucose
f. Hematocrit
g. Hemoglobin
h. LDH
i. Potassium
j. Sodium
k. Troponin T

8. The nurse is teaching a 56-year-old truck driver about taking clonidine. It is very important to explain that he should take the:
   a. two doses 12 hours apart.
   b. larger dose at bedtime.
   c. medication with food.
   d. medication on an empty stomach.

9. Match the drug with the contraindications and/or precautions. (Answers may be used more than once.)

| | Drug | Contraindication/Precaution |
|---|---|---|
| _____ | a. Clonidine | 1. Active peptic ulcer disease |
| _____ | b. Guanethidine | 2. Tricyclic antidepressants |
| _____ | c. Methyldopa | 3. Pregnancy |
| _____ | d. Reserpine | 4. Pheochromocytoma |
| | | 5. History of depression |
| | | 6. Hepatitis |

▶ 10. A patient is receiving methyldopa 250 mg twice a day. Vital signs are 170/90 mm Hg, P 92, and R 20. The nurse is reviewing new laboratory test results, which include ALT 35 International Units/L, creatinine 0.8 mg/dL, BUN 20 mg/dL, Coombs' test positive, sodium 145 mEq/L, and potassium 4.8 mEq/L. The nurse should:
   a. administer the medication and continue to assess the patient.
   b. administer the medication and notify the prescriber of the vital signs and laboratory results.
   c. hold the medication and notify the prescriber of the vital signs and laboratory results.
   d. hold the medication and page the prescriber STAT.

## CASE STUDIES AND PATIENT TEACHING

*(Use a separate piece of paper for your responses.)*

### Case Study 1

*A 68-year-old active retired woman who plays tennis has been prescribed guanethidine 10 mg once a day for hypertension not controlled by other agents. The prescriber asks the office nurse to do teaching regarding this medication.*

1. What teaching should the nurse provide?

2. The patient returns to the office 1 week after initiation of therapy. Her pulse has increased to 88 beats/min, up from a baseline of 80 beats/min and BP 170/78 mm Hg, up from a baseline of 165/70 mm Hg. What could be causing this elevation?

3. Why are anticholinergic antidiarrheal agents appropriate for diarrhea caused by this medication, and when would the patient expect to experience diarrhea as an adverse effect?

# 20 Introduction to Central Nervous System Pharmacology

## OBJECTIVES

See page 26 for the Objectives.

## CRITICAL THINKING AND STUDY QUESTIONS

1. Which of the following are characteristics of drugs that can affect the brain? (Select all that apply.)
   a. Lipid soluble
   b. Highly ionized
   c. Move via transport systems
   d. Protein bound
   e. Water soluble

2. A 3-month-old infant is infected with meningitis. Why would the nurse expect the infant to be more responsive to the prescribed antibiotic than a college student?

3. A patient who has been taking a medication at the same dose for a period of time for a seizure disorder experiences an increase in seizure activity. The physician increases the dose of the medication. This may be an example of:
   a. addiction.
   b. physical dependence.
   c. tolerance.

## CASE STUDIES AND PATIENT TEACHING

*(Use a separate piece of paper for your responses.)*

### Case Study 1

*A patient has recently been diagnosed with major depression. Medication has just been prescribed that alters CNS neurotransmission. The patient verbalizes concerns to the nurse because the medication "is not working." She is also experiencing some daytime sedation.*

1. How should the nurse respond?

2. The patient asks why drug companies have not been able to develop new psychotherapeutic drugs that do not have adverse effects. What would be the basis of the nurse's response?

3. There are many psychotherapeutic drugs that are effective in treating patient symptoms. What factors decrease patient adherence with these medications?

# 21 Drugs for Parkinson's Disease

## OBJECTIVES

See page 26 for the Objectives.

## CRITICAL THINKING AND STUDY QUESTIONS

1. Select all of the following that apply to Parkinson's disease (PD).
   a. Cause of symptoms is degeneration of neurons that supply dopamine to the striatum
   b. Causes a slowing of movement
   c. Current drug treatment prevents further neuronal degeneration and controls symptoms
   d. Findings on autopsy include neurotoxic fibrin strands (Lewy bodies)
   e. Involves blocking of excitatory effects of acetylcholine
   f. Involves excessive dopaminergic stimulation of neurons that release GABA
   g. May be caused by impaired metabolism of a potentially toxic protein synthesized by dopaminergic neurons
   h. Symptoms are called extrapyramidal adverse effects when they are drug induced
   i. Symptoms include tremor when attempting movement
   j. Symptoms may include depression, dementia, and memory loss
   k. Symptoms occur as a result of stimulation of dopamine receptors on striatal GABAergic neurons that cause them to fire at a more rapid rate
   l. Symptoms of tremor and rigidity are most disabling
   m. Usually is not recognized until approximately ¾ of the neurons that supply dopamine to the striatum are lost

2. Matching

_____ a. Amantadine (Symmetrel)
_____ b. Apomorphine (Apokyn)
_____ c. Bromocriptine (Parlodel)
_____ d. Entacapone (Comtan)
_____ e. Levodopa (L-Dopa)
_____ f. Levodopa/ Carbidopa
_____ g. Pergolide (Permax)
_____ h. Pramipexole (Mirapex)
_____ i. Ropinirole (Requip)
_____ j. Selegiline (Eldepryl)
_____ k. Tolcapone (Tasmar)

1. Are not dependent on enzyme conversion to become active
2. Inhibit COMT degradation of dopamine
3. Inhibit dopamine breakdown by MAO-B
4. Promote dopamine release
5. Promote dopamine synthesis
6. Stimulate dopamine receptors (Sinemet/ Paracopa)

▶ 3. A realistic outcome for a patient receiving drug therapy for PD is:
   a. Absence of tremor.
   b. To attain a normal gait.
   c. To improve ability to perform activities of daily living.
   d. To reverse neurodegeneration.

4. Expected beneficial effects of levodopa on Parkinson's disease usually are:
   a. dramatic relief of symptoms that stay suppressed with continued use.
   b. gradual relief of symptoms, peaking in approximately 5 years.
   c. relief of symptoms that increase over 1 to 2 years then decline as tolerance develops.
   d. relief of symptoms that steadily increase over months but decline to pretreatment state within 5 years.

5. The nurse has explained the medication levodopa to a patient who was recently diagnosed with PD. The patient has researched the disease and asks why dopamine is not prescribed. The basis of the nurse's response is:
   a. dopamine cannot cross the blood-brain barrier.
   b. dopamine has significant adverse effects.
   c. dopamine requires decarboxylase to be absorbed and levels of this enzyme are depleted as a person ages.
   d. drug manufacturers have not been able to develop dopamine as a drug.

6. A PD patient who is receiving levodopa displays violent, twisting, jerking movements of the extremities. The nurse holds the medications, notifies the prescriber, and documents this adverse effect as:
   a. ballismus.
   b. choreoathetosis.
   c. fasciculation.
   d. tremor.

7. Which of these findings would be most significant if the nurse is preparing to administer levodopa?
   a. Blood pressure 140/85 mm Hg
   b. Dark-colored urine
   c. Pulse 110 beats/min
   d. Tics

8. A PD patient complains that he has episodes that last from 10 minutes to 2 or 3 hours where PD symptoms are intense. These occur at any time and are different from the feeling that he gets that the drug is loosing effectiveness before the next dose is due. Dietary teaching that may help this "on-off" phenomenon includes avoidance near the time of medication administration of:
   a. foods with a high glycemic index.
   b. high-fat meals.
   c. high-protein foods.
   d. refined carbohydrates.

9. Psychotic symptoms caused by treatment with levodopa are often treated with:
   a. chlorpromazine (Thorazine).
   b. clozapine (Clozaril).
   c. haloperidol (Haldol).
   d. risperidone (Risperdal).

10. The nurse should instruct patients who are prescribed levodopa to avoid dietary supplementation of:
   a. ascorbic acid (vitamin C).
   b. biotin.
   c. niacin.
   d. pyroxidine (vitamin $B_6$).

▶ 11. The nurse is bathing a patient who is receiving levodopa for Parkinson's disease and notes an asymmetrical, irregular darkly pigmented mole on the patient's back. The nurse should:
   a. continue to assess the patient.
   b. notify the prescriber immediately.
   c. tell the patient that he should consult a dermatologist.
   d. stop administering the levodopa until the prescriber can be contacted.

12. Sinemet and Paracopa are levodopa-carbidopa combinations used when a patient has decreased responsiveness to levodopa. Addition of carbidopa to the regimen: (Select all that apply.)
   a. adds to the therapeutic effect because carbidopa more readily crosses the blood-brain barrier than levodopa.
   b. allows for an increase in levodopa dosage without significant adverse effects.
   c. decreases adverse effects, such as nausea and vomiting.
   d. decreases the risk of adverse effects of abnormal movements and psychiatric symptoms.
   e. inhibits decarboxylation of levodopa in the CNS.
   f. inhibits the conversion of levodopa to dopamine in the intestines and in tissue outside the CNS.
   g. stimulates decarboxylation of levodopa by pyroxidine (vitamin $B_6$).

▶ 13. A hospitalized patient is prescribed Paracopa (25 mg levodopa/100 mg carbidopa). The hospital pharmacy substitutes the equivalent Sinemet product. A priority nursing assessment that would warrant further investigation before administering the Sinemet is:
   a. anorexia.
   b. drooling.
   c. hypertension.
   d. tremor.

14. A patient is being switched from levodopa to a levodopa-carbidopa preparation. The nurse instructs the patient to:
   a. allow at least 8 hours to pass after the last dose of levodopa before starting the new medication.
   b. start taking the new medications when symptoms of the old drug wearing off begin.
   c. take the new medication on an empty stomach.
   d. take the new medication within 3 hours after the last dose of the levodopa to prevent return of PD symptoms.

15. It is important for the nurse to teach the patient who is prescribed pramipexole (Mirapex) to avoid use of which OTC medication for heartburn?
   a. axid (nizatidine)
   b. pepcid (famotidine)
   c. tagamet (cimetidine)
   d. zantac (ranitidine)

▶ 16. A patient is prescribed pramipexole (Mirapex) 1.5 mg. The hospital pharmacy stocks pramipexole 0.25 mg. How many tablets should the nurse administer?
   a. ½ tablet
   b. 2 tablets
   c. 4 tablets
   d. 6 tablets

▶ 17. Which of these laboratory test findings would be most significant when a patient is receiving ropinirole (Requip)?
   a. ALT 85 International Units/L
   b. BUN 22 mg/dL
   c. Creatinine 1.4 mg/dL
   d. Creatinine clearance 400 mg/24 hr

18. The medication administration record (MAR) for a patient with PD lists apomorphine (Apokyn) 1 mg subcutaneous with trimethobenzamide (Tigan) 300 mg, up to three doses per day as needed. The nurse should administer these medications if the patient experiences:
   a. a sleep attack.
   b. an "off" episode.
   c. nausea.
   d. psychotic symptoms.

19. A common early complication of most drugs prescribed for PD that the nurse should consider when developing a plan of care for a PD patient is:
   a. confusion.
   b. hypertension.
   c. nausea.
   d. somnolence.

▶ 20. Which of these lung findings would be most significant if a patient was receiving pergolide (Permax)?
   a. Abnormal movements
   b. Confusion
   c. Dizziness when changing positions
   d. Shortness of breath

▶ 21. A patient who is receiving tolcapone (Tasmar) complains of nausea and abdominal pain. His urine is dark amber. Which of the following laboratory test results would be most significant when the nurse reports these symptoms to the prescriber?
   a. ALT 75 International Units/L; AST 59 International Units/L
   b. BUN 22 mg/dL; Creatinine 1.1 mg/dL
   c. Hb 12 g/dL; Hct 39%
   d. $Na^+$ 142 mEq/L; $K^+$ 4.8 mEq/L

▶ 22. The nurse notes an orange color to the urine of a PD patient who is scheduled to receive a dose of entacapone (Comtan). The nurse should:
   a. assess for symptoms of liver failure.
   b. consult with the prescriber.
   c. continue nursing care including administration of the medication.
   d. hold the medication and contact the prescriber immediately.

23. Selegiline (Eldepryl) should not be administered if a patient is receiving: (Select all that apply.)
   a. butorphanol (Stadol).
   b. fluoxetine (Prozac).
   c. hydromorphone (Dilaudid).
   d. meperidine (Demerol).
   e. paroxetine (Paxil).
   f. sertraline (Zoloft).

## CASE STUDIES AND PATIENT TEACHING

*(Use a separate piece of paper for your responses.)*

### Case Study 1

*A 54-year-old male welder who is married and has two adult children and one in college has recently been diagnosed with Parkinson's disease.*

1. What assessments does the nurse need to make to aid in determining the needed therapy for this patient?

2. The patient is prescribed levodopa 0.5 gm twice daily and amantadine 100 mg twice daily. What teaching regarding administration of levodopa can the nurse provide that prevents or minimizes nausea and vomiting while maximizing drug absorption?

3. The nurse is teaching the patient and his wife about adverse effects of levodopa and amantadine. What teaching should be provided regarding possible postural hypotension, psychotic symptoms, and dermatologic changes?

4. Eighteen months after diagnosis the patient is admitted to a medical unit for a 10-day "drug holiday" because of significant adverse effects. It is anticipated that the patient will have a severe return of symptoms including rigidity and postural instability. What are probable nursing issues, and what interventions will the nurse employ to address these problems?

5. The patient's major complaint is increased dyskinesias. The family provides the nurse with a history of progressive memory loss, increased tremors, mottled discoloration of the skin, and the inability to walk straight. He took his last dose of levodopa at 1200. The physician orders Sinemet (25 mg carbidopa with 100 mg levodopa) twice daily. What are the advantages of administering carbidopa to this patient?

6. Describe the precautions needed when switching a patient from levodopa to carbidopa with levodopa/carbidopa (Sinemet).

# 22 Alzheimer's Disease

## OBJECTIVES

See page 26 for the Objectives.

## CRITICAL THINKING AND STUDY QUESTIONS

1. The daughter of a patient asks about the pathophysiology and pharmacologic treatment of Alzheimer's disease (AD). Which of the following information could be included in the nurse's explanation? (Select all that apply.)
   a. An early symptom of AD is loss of appetite.
   b. Current drug therapy for AD is not highly effective for relieving symptoms.
   c. High levels of the neurotransmitter acetylcholine are found in patients with AD.
   d. Neuritic plaques composed of a core beta-amyloid are found in the hippocampus and cerebral cortex of patients with AD.
   e. In AD, the orderly arrangement of microtubules is disrupted forming neurofibrillar tangles.
   f. Neurotoxic effects of beta-amyloid can be blocked by blocking the action of endoplasmic reticulum-associated binding protein (ERAB), which is found in high levels in patients with AD.
   g. Research suggests that individuals with copies of the gene that codes for apolipoprotein E2 (apoE2) are at increased risk for AD.
   h. The American Academy of Neurology recommends trying a cholinesterase inhibitor in all patients with mild to moderate AD.

i. The neuronal damage occurring with AD is reversible if diagnosed early in the disease.
j. A blood test can confirm the diagnosis of AD.
k. Effects of drugs are long lasting.

▶ 2. High levels of homocysteine are associated with an increased risk of AD and other disorders. The nurse can teach patients to lower their homocysteine levels by eating a diet high in vitamins $B_6$ and folate found in:
a. citrus fruits and meat.
b. fruits and vegetables.
c. dairy products and eggs.
d. green leafy vegetables and legumes.

3. Research suggests that some patients with AD regularly display more intense symptoms:
a. in the morning.
b. before meals.
c. in the evening.
d. during the night.

▶ 4. The nurse is caring for a patient who is receiving rivastigmine (Excelon) for AD. Because of common adverse effects, a nursing priority would be:
a. orthostatic BP precautions.
b. ensuring adequate fluids and nutrition.
c. assessing for bleeding.
d. reviewing other prescribed drugs for drug interactions.

5. Research suggests cholinesterase inhibitors:
a. enhance transmission by central cholinergic neurons.
b. decrease the formation of neuritic plaque.
c. maintain the orderly arrangement of microtubules.
d. prevent the degeneration of cortical neurons.

6. Adverse effects of cholinesterase inhibitors come from parasympathetic stimulation. Common adverse effects include:
a. blurred vision.
b. diarrhea.
c. fatigue.
d. tachycardia.

▶ 7. The nurse should be particularly cautious when administering a cholinesterase inhibitor drug to any patient with a history of: (Select all that apply.)
a. asthma.
b. COPD.
c. CHF.
d. hypertension.
e. peptic ulcer disease.
f. peripheral vascular disease.

8. Which of the following treatments for dyspepsia could potentially decrease the renal excretion of memantine (Namenda) and cause toxicity?
a. Calcium carbonate (TUMS)
b. Lansoprazole (Prevacid)
c. Ranitidine (Zantac)
d. Sodium bicarbonate (baking soda)

9. A son of an AD patient asks about taking nonsteroidal anti-inflammatory drugs (NSAIDs) to decrease the risk of developing AD. Research has suggested that they need to be:
a. taken at the prescription-strength dose.
b. taken for at least 2 years starting 4 years before symptom onset.
c. nonaspirin.
d. taken at the first onset of symptoms.

▶ 10. The nurse is assigned an 87-year-old woman who was admitted from an extended care facility with pneumonia. The nursing report reveals that the patient is extremely confused and combative. Why is it important for the nurse to not assume that the patient has AD?

## CASE STUDIES AND PATIENT TEACHING

*(Use a separate piece of paper for your responses.)*

### Case Study 1

*A 77-year-old male who has a history of AD, DM, hypertension, and seasonal allergies has been admitted with a hip fracture that occurred when wandering around the house at night. He is scheduled for an open reduction and internal fixation of the fracture the next morning. On admission the nurse discovers that the patient's wife had been administering Ginkgo biloba for the past 8 months in hope that it would improve his memory.*

1. Why is it important for the nurse to report this to the orthopedic surgeon?

2. The patient's wife is concerned that his confusion, memory loss, and wandering has not improved much and that he seems to have gotten worse since the weather got warm. The wife provided a list of all of the patient's prescribed medications, which include hydrochlorothiazide (HydroDIURIL), metformin (Glucophage), and tacrine, (Cognex). Based on the patient history, what class of over-the-counter (OTC) medication does the nurse need to specifically ask the wife about that could contribute to the patient's sudden decline in functioning?

3. What assessments (including reviewing laboratory tests) should the nurse perform before administering the tacrine, (Cognex) and what findings would warrant consulting the prescriber?

4. The patient's ALT is 178 International Units/L, and his bilirubin is 3.2 mg/mL. The prescriber instructs the wife and patient to discontinue the tacrine (Cognex), not take any OTC antihistamines, and to start donepezil (Aricept). The wife asks the nurse why the physician changed the medication to a medication in the same class if the tacrine is not working well and is hurting her husband's liver.

5. The wife asks why the prescriber is giving her husband less medication (5 mg once a day versus 40 mg, four times a day). The nurse's response should include:

6. What should the nurse teach the wife to assess for before administering donepezil (Aricept) to her husband?

7. The patient's wife heard from friends of something sold in the health food store to cure AD. The friend said that the store provided results of research that states that the supplement is effective in improving memory in AD patients. She is on a limited budget and asks the opinion of the nurse. How should the nurse respond?

# 23 Drugs for Multiple Sclerosis

## OBJECTIVES

See page 26 for the Objectives.

## CRITICAL THINKING AND STUDY QUESTIONS

1. A 26-year-old woman seeks medical care for blurred vision and severe muscle weakness. Which of the following from her history are possible risk factors for multiple sclerosis (MS)? (Select all that apply.)
   a. She smokes.
   b. She is overweight.
   c. She lives in North Carolina.
   d. She has had mononucleosis twice while in college.
   e. Her father has had a cerebral vascular accident (CVA, stroke).
   f. Her paternal grandparents were German immigrants.

2. Matching: Diagnostic tests

| | | |
|---|---|---|
| _____ | a. CSF analysis | 1. Detects areas of demyelination |
| _____ | b. MRI | 2. Measures how quickly the brain responds to visual stimuli |
| _____ | c. VEP | 3. Assesses immune activity in CNS |

3. Current drug therapy for MS can: (Select all that apply.)
   a. cure the disease.
   b. modify the disease process.

c. relieve symptoms.
d. treat relapses.
e. work for all patients.

4. Treatment with immunomodulators for relapsing-remitting MS should: (Select all that apply.)
a. also include the immunosuppressant mitoxantrone.
b. begin as soon as possible after MS is diagnosed.
c. only be used if attacks last more than 1 week.
d. only be used during periods of relapse.
e. continue indefinitely.

▶ 5. The nurse is administering high-dose intravenous methylprednisolone to a patient who is experiencing an acute relapse of MS. The nurse would need to be especially careful of monitoring the patient who has the chronic condition of:
a. asthma.
b. COPD.
c. DM.
d. hypertension.

▶ 6. A patient with MS is started on the immunomodulator interferon beta-1a (Avonex) IM 30 mcg once a week. It is important to teach the patient the importance of complying with scheduled laboratory tests that would include: (Select all that apply.)
a. ALT.
b. amylase.
c. CBC.
d. hemoglobin $A_{1C}$.
e. INR.
f. TSH.

▶ 7. A patient is experiencing flu-like symptoms when therapy with beta interferon is started. Because the drug can injure the liver, the prescriber may recommend that which of the following OTC products not be used to relieve symptoms?
a. Acetylsalicylic acid (aspirin)
b. Acetaminophen (Tylenol)
c. Ibuprofen (Motrin)
d. Naproxen (Aleve)

▶ 8. A patient is prescribed an initial subcutaneous dose of 8.8 mcg of interferon 1a (Refib) for the first 2 weeks of therapy. The drug is supplied as 22 mcg/0.5 mL. How much drug should the patient administer with each dose?

9. A patient receiving interferon 1a (Refib) experiences nausea, vomiting, tea-colored urine, clay-colored stool, and RUQ tenderness. ALT results are 200 International Units/L. The nurse would consult with the prescriber if the medication order was changed from Refib to:
a. betaseron.
b. copaxone.
c. mitoxantrone.

10. Which of the forms of MS is resistant to current drug therapy?
a. Relapsing-remitting MS
b. Secondary progressive MS
c. Primary progressive MS
d. Progressive-relapsing MS

▶ 11. The nurse is administering mitoxantrone (Novantrone) to a patient who was unresponsive to other immunomodulating drugs for MS. The nurse should hold the medication and contact the prescriber if the patient exhibits:
a. diaphoresis and low blood sugar.
b. dizziness and orthostatic hypotension.
c. headache and elevated blood pressure.
d. weight gain of 3 lbs in 24 hours and shortness of breath.

12. When a patient is receiving mitoxantrone (Novantrone), liver function tests (LFT) should be assessed once:
a. a month.
b. every 3 months.
c. every 6 months.
d. a year.

▶ 13. A patient is scheduled to receive mitoxantrone (Novantrone). Which of the following would be definite reasons to withhold the medication and contact the prescriber?
  a. ALT 100 International Units/L
  b. Amenorrhea
  c. Blue-green colored urine
  d. LVEF 65%
  e. HCG 35 International Units/L
  f. Neutrophils 1000 cells/mm$^3$
  g. Yellow-tinged skin

▶ 14. A patient who is receiving mitoxantrone (Novantrone) should not receive which of the following immunizations?
  a. Hepatitis A vaccine
  b. Hepatitis B vaccine
  c. Influenza vaccine
  d. Measles, mumps, and rubella (MMR)
  e. Pneumococcal polysaccharide vaccine (Pneumovax)
  f. Tetanus plus diphtheria toxoids for adults (Td)
  g. Varicella virus vaccine

15. Match the symptoms of MS to the drugs used to manage them. (May use more than one answer.)

| |  | |  |
|---|---|---|---|
| ______ | a. Amantadine (Symmetrel) | 1. | Ataxia and tremor |
| ______ | b. Baclofen (Lioresal) | 2. | Constipation |
| ______ | c. Bethanechol (Urecholine) | 3. | Depression |
| ______ | d. Botulinum toxin | 4. | Difficulty starting or stopping urination and incomplete bladder emptying |
| ______ | e. Docusate sodium | 5. | Dizziness and vertigo |
| ______ | f. Donepezil (Aricept) | 6. | Fatigue |
| ______ | g. Enemeez | 7. | Fecal incontinence |
| ______ | h. Fluoxetine (Prozac) | 8. | Impaired bladder emptying |
| ______ | i. Gabapentin (Neurontin) | 9. | Memory impairment |
| ______ | j. Hyoscyamine | 10. | Neuropathic pain |
| ______ | k. K-Y jelly | 11. | Sexual dysfunction |
| ______ | l. Meclazine (Antivert) | 12. | Sleep disturbances |
| ______ | m. Modafinil (Provigil) | 13. | Spasticity |
| ______ | n. Nortriptyline (Pamelor) | 14. | Urinary frequency, urgency, and incontinence |
| ______ | o. Primidone (Mysoline) | | |
| ______ | p. Psyllium (Metamucil) | | |
| ______ | q. Terazosin (Hytrin) | | |
| ______ | r. Tolterodine (Detrol) | | |
| ______ | s. Vardenafil (Levitra) | | |

## CASE STUDIES AND PATIENT TEACHING

*(Use a separate piece of paper for your responses.)*

### Case Study 1

*A 32-year-old college professor has been diagnosed with relapsing-remitting MS after the birth of her first child.*

1. What assessments are important for the nurse to include when caring for this patient?
2. Her symptoms have significantly resolved. What are the primary factors of the pathophysiologic process of MS that explain how the symptoms can abate but the disease is still present?
3. What are some possible nursing diagnoses for this patient throughout the disease process?
4. When the nurse is administering medications, the patient refuses the drug stating "What's the use? My mom had MS and the drugs didn't help. She died in 1990. She was only 57 years old." What should be the basis of the nurse's response?
5. The patient with MS is started on the immunomodulator interferon beta 1a (Avonex) IM 30 mcg once a week. What should the nurse include in teaching regarding this drug?
6. The patient and her physician have tried treatment with the immunomodulators without success. They have agreed to try the immunosuppressant mitoxantrone (Novantrone). What teaching should the nurse provide this patient?
7. What steps does the nurse need to take before administering the mitoxantrone (Novantrone) by intravenous infusion?
8. The patient is experiencing fecal incontinence. What pharmacologic and nonpharmacologic measures can be employed to prevent this problem?

# 24 Drugs for Epilepsy

## OBJECTIVES

See page 26 for the Objectives.

## CRITICAL THINKING AND STUDY QUESTIONS

1. The experimental procedure called kindling suggests that:
   a. children may outgrow seizure disorders.
   b. early treatment may prevent more serious seizure disorders.
   c. seizures caused by trauma will occur within 24 hours of the trauma.
   d. seizure disorders rarely can be controlled by drugs.

2. Complex partial seizures differ from simple partial seizures in that they involve:
   a. depression.
   b. hallucinations.
   c. loss of consciousness.
   d. motor twitching.

3. The nurse can assist the prescriber with obtaining the effective dose of ethosuximide (Zarontin) for absence seizures by teaching the patient and/or family to:
   a. comply with scheduled lab tests for drug levels.
   b. increase doses if seizure activity increases.
   c. note adverse effects.
   d. observe and record seizure activity.

4. A patient who has been taking valproic acid (Depakene) and carbamazepine (Tegretol) is to begin attempting drug withdrawal. To prevent adverse effects, the nurse reinforces teaching that the:
   a. dose of both drugs should both be gradually decreased.
   b. dose of one drug should be gradually decreased while maintaining the usual dose of the second drug.
   c. carbamazepine should be stopped and the valproic acid continued for at least a week.
   d. valproic acid should be stopped and the carbamazepine continued for at least a week.

▸ 5. When caring for a patient who is receiving phenytoin (Dilantin), which of the following assessments require immediate nursing intervention?
   a. Drowsiness
   b. Gingival hyperplasia
   c. Hirsutism
   d. Nystagmus

6. When administering phenytoin (Dilantin), at what serum level should the nurse consider therapy to be potentially toxic?
   a. greater than 10 mcg/L
   b. greater than 20 mcg/mL
   c. greater than 30 mcg/mL
   d. greater than 40 mcg/mL

7. A 47-year-old patient has been taking phenytoin (Dilantin) for years without significant adverse effects or seizures. Serum levels usually are 12 to 16 mcg/mL. The patient is admitted with sudden onset of multiple seizures. Serum phenytoin levels now are 7 mcg/mL. What question is most important for the nurse to ask?
   a. "Have you changed from brand name to generic phenytoin?"
   b. "Have you noticed a rash anywhere on your body?"
   c. "Have you had any change in or addition of any other medications?"
   d. "Have you been diagnosed with any liver disease?"

8. A parent has received instructions regarding administration of 5 mL twice a day of phenytoin (Dilantin suspension) to their child. Which of these statements made by the parent suggests a need for further teaching?
   a. "I must be sure to shake the medication thoroughly before measuring the dose."
   b. "I should give him a teaspoonful of the drug at each dose."
   c. "I should give him the medication with breakfast and with a snack before bedtime."
   d. "It is important that I space the drug doses as I have been instructed."

▸ 9. When a patient who is receiving carbamazepine (Tegretol) complains of vertigo, which action should the nurse take first?
   a. Ensure patient safety.
   b. Page the prescriber STAT.
   c. Review most recent lab results of CBC, BUN, and electrolytes.
   d. Withhold the medication.

10. The nurse instructs patients who have just received a prescription for carbamazepine (Tegretol) to avoid consuming grapefruit juice for which of the following periods?
   a. Four hours after taking the medication
   b. No more than twice a week when taking the medication
   c. Not at all when taking the medication
   d. Two hours before taking the medication

11. When teaching about adverse effects of valproic acid, the nurse should emphasize the importance of reporting which of the following adverse effects that suggest the possibility of a life-threatening reaction?
   a. Abdominal pain and anorexia
   b. Heartburn and belching
   c. Rash and tremor
   d. Weight gain and hair loss

▸ 12. A woman who is of child-bearing age must take valproic acid to control seizures. Which of the following statements if made by the patient suggest a need for further teaching?
   a. "If I get pregnant, the baby should be okay as long as I stop taking the drug within 2 months of becoming pregnant."
   b. "I need to inform all of my healthcare providers that I am taking valproic acid."
   c. "I need to take folic acid supplements in case I accidentally get pregnant."
   d. "I need to use two reliable forms of birth control."

▸ 13. When administering valproic acid to an elderly patient, the nurse notes the patient chewing the tablet. The nurse should:
   a. ask the pharmacy to send the Depakote sprinkles form of the drug.
   b. contact the prescriber.
   c. crush subsequent doses and put them in applesauce or pudding.
   d. crush subsequent doses and mix them in 5 mL of warm water.

▸ 14. A patient with a history of hypertension and complex partial seizures has been prescribed oxcarbazepine (Trileptal) 100 mg twice a day and spironolactone (Aldactone). It is important for the nurse to assess which of the following symptoms of hyponatremia?
   a. Dry mucous membranes and flushed skin
   b. Hyperactive bowel sounds and tall tented T waves on ECG
   c. Muscle spasms and paresthesias
   d. Weakness and nausea

▸ 15. If a patient who is receiving lamotrigine (Lamictal) develops a rash, the nurse should:
   a. assess vital signs.
   b. continue nursing care.
   c. review laboratory test results.
   d. withhold the medication and contact the prescriber.

▸ 16. Which of the following data, if not known by the prescriber, would be most important for the nurse to communicate to the prescriber when a patient is receiving gabapentin (Neurontin)?
   a. Dizziness
   b. Fasting blood sugar 110 mg/dL
   c. Oliguria
   d. Patient is also receiving phenytoin (Dilantin)

17. Levetiracetam (Keppra):
   a. can cause loss of muscle strength.
   b. can decrease the effectiveness of warfarin (Coumadin).
   c. mechanism of action is blockade of sodium channels.
   d. should be administered with food to decrease GI adverse effects.

▶ 18. It is important for the nurse to monitor laboratory test results for which of the following findings if a patient is prescribed topiramate (Topamax)?
a. Elevated creatinine
b. Elevated liver function tests
c. Low RBC and WBC count
d. Low $HCO_3$

▶ 19. A patient is receiving topiramate (Topamax) in addition to carbamazepine (Tegretol) for tonic-clonic seizures. The nurse should teach the patient to observe for critical adverse effects of toprimate including:
a. ataxia.
b. difficulty concentrating.
c. ocular pain.
d. weight loss.

▶ 20. The nurse notes that tiagabine (Gabitril) is ordered but no other AEDs are prescribed for this patient. The nurse should:
a. administer the medication.
b. administer the medication and ask the patient why they are taking the medication.
c. withhold the medication.
d. withhold the medication and consult the prescriber STAT.

21. The nurse teaches that which of the following AEDs can increase the liver metabolism of contraceptives and increase the risk of unintended pregnancy? (Select all that apply.)
a. carbamazepine (Tegretol)
b. gabapentin (Neurontin)
c. lamotrigine (Lamictal)
d. levetiracetam (Keppra)
e. oxcarbazepine (Trileptal)
f. phenobarbital (Luminal)
g. primidone (Mysoline)
h. phenytoin (Dilantin)
i. topiramate (Topamax)
j. valproic acid (Depakene)
k. zonisamide (Zonegran)

22. It is important for the nurse to assess for suicidal ideation if a patient is prescribed:
a. lamotrigine (Lamictal).
b. levetiracetam (Keppra).
c. topiramate (Topamax).
d. zonisamide (Zonegran).

▶ 23. The nurse would consult the prescriber if the nurse notes that a patient who was prescribed zonisamide (Zonegran) had a known anaphylactic reaction to:
a. acarbose (Precose).
b. insulin aspart (Novolog).
c. glipizide (Glucotrol).
d. metformin (Glucophage).

## CASE STUDIES AND PATIENT TEACHING

*(Use a separate piece of paper for your responses.)*

### Case Study 1

*A 26-year-old female, who is 8 months pregnant, is admitted to the neuro intensive care unit with the diagnosis of head injury. An automobile accident has left the patient unconscious. On admission she has an IV of $D_5$ $\frac{1}{2}$ NS at 50 mL/hr. Within the first 24 hours on the unit, the patient has several tonic-clonic seizures. Standing orders on the unit allow the nurse to administer diazepam (Valium) 5 mg intravenous push. The physician is notified of the seizure and orders an intravenous loading dose of phenytoin (Dilantin) 800 mg followed by 100 mg every 6 hours, a phenytoin level the next day, and intravenous cimetidine 300 mg twice a day.*

1. What nursing precautions are needed when administering phenytoin and cimetidine intravenously?

2. The phenytoin is available for intravenous infusion in a concentration of 50 mg/mL. How long should the nurse take when administering the 800-mg loading dose?

3. What symptoms should the nurse be alert for because of the possible interaction of phenytoin and cimetidine?

4. The next day, the phenytoin level is 14 mcg/mL. Why is it critical for the nurse to closely monitor plasma drug levels of phenytoin?

5. One week later, the patient goes into labor. Based on initiation of phenytoin near the end of the pregnancy, what fetal effects are most likely to occur?

6. What precautions might be taken to protect the fetus during drug therapy, during delivery, and after delivery?

7. Two weeks later, the patient is stabilized and has been transferred to the neuro progressive unit. On admission the nurse notes a fine maculopapular rash on the patient's trunk. What should the nurse do and why?

8. The physician orders the phenytoin (Dilantin) to be discontinued. Carbamazepine (Tegretol) is substituted as the patient's antiseizure drug. The patient is concerned about taking seizure medication because she wants to have more children. She has been advised about possible adverse effects to the fetus. In addition to referring concerns to the physician, what information could the nurse provide about seizures, antiepileptic drugs (AEDs), and pregnancy?

## Case Study 2

*The nurse is working in a neurologic clinic of a major pediatric hospital. One responsibility is obtaining a complete history at the initial visit.*

1. What data would be important for the nurse to collect from the parents of a 3-year-old boy who was referred because of new-onset seizures?

2. The patient weighs 35 lbs and is prescribed phenytoin 20 mg every 12 hours. The suggested initial dose is 2.5 mg/kg/day in divided doses. Is this a safe and effective dose for this child?

3. Phenytoin is available as a suspension of 125 mg/mL. How much drug should be administered at each dose and what measuring device should the nurse teach the parents to use?

4. What care can the nurse teach the parents to provide to minimize the adverse effect of gingival hyperplasia?

5. Despite increasing doses, the child continues to have tonic-clonic seizures. The pediatric neurologist discontinues the phenytoin and orders valproic acid. Based on mechanism of action, why might valproic acid alone be effective when phenytoin was not effective?

## Case Study 3

*A 19-year-old college student has been diagnosed with partial seizures and has been prescribed carbamazepine (Tegretol) 100 mg twice a day. The patient reports his new diagnosis and drug therapy to the nurse at the college health center.*

1. What information would be important for the college health clinic to collect to assist the student with managing his health and illness?

2. What can the nurse teach that enables the patient to assist the prescriber with evaluating the effectiveness of prescribed drug?

3. What should the nurse teach about adverse effects of carbamazepine (Tegretol) including when he should seek medical attention?

4. What should the nurse teach about AEDs and alcohol?

5. At a later visit, the student tells the college health center nurse that he is discouraged because he has been on medication for over a month and continues to have seizures. How should the nurse respond?

6. The student plans to visit home between the fall and spring semester, which is 3000 miles from the college. What teaching should the nurse provide relating to precautions that should be taken with travel?

7. Developmentally, what are common barriers to adherence to drug therapy for this patient, and what are possible nursing interventions to address these barriers?

8. What communication techniques would be most likely to influence this individual?

# 25 Drugs for Muscle Spasm and Spasticity

## OBJECTIVES

See page 26 for the Objectives.

## CRITICAL THINKING AND STUDY QUESTIONS

1. A patient who has chronic back pain asks the nurse why the physician only prescribed ibuprofen instead of a muscle relaxant for his muscle spasms. The basis of the nurse's response is:

2. The only drug that relieves both muscle spasms and is used for the spasticity of MS or cerebral palsy is:
   a. baclofen (Lioresal).
   b. dantrolene (Dantrium).
   c. diazepam (Valium).
   d. tizanidine (Zanaflex).

▸ 3. It is important for the nurse to assess for nausea, vomiting, tea-colored urine, clay-colored stool, RUQ tenderness, yellowish discoloration to eyes or skin, and elevated ALT in patients receiving which of the following drugs? (Select all that apply.)
   a. baclofen (Lioresal)
   b. carisoprodol (Soma)
   c. chlorzoxazone (Paraflex)
   d. cyclobenzaprine (Flexeril)
   e. dantrolene (Dantrium)
   f. diazepam (Valium)
   g. metaxalone (Skelaxin)
   h. methocarbamol (Robaxin)
   i. orphenadrine (Norflex)
   j. tizanidine (Zanaflex)

▸ 4. Nursing interventions and teaching for a patient receiving a central muscle relaxant should focus on:
   a. emotional support.
   b. nutrition.
   c. safety.
   d. skin integrity.

5. Which of the following statements, if made by a patient who has been taking methocarbamol (Robaxin) for 6 months after an accident, would be a concern for the nurse?
   a. "I plan to stop taking this medication on Monday because I have to go back to work."
   b. "My urine has been a funny dark green color."
   c. "I had hepatitis several years ago."
   d. "I have to be careful when I stand up because sometimes I get dizzy."

## CASE STUDIES AND PATIENT TEACHING

*(Use a separate piece of paper for your responses.)*

### Case Study 1

*A 19-year-old male is admitted to the neuro intensive care unit after a motorcycle accident. He is paraplegic with severe lower extremity muscle spasms. He is receiving intrathecal baclofen. A pump is being used to infuse the drug because abrupt discontinuation can cause rhabdomyolysis and multiple organ system failure.*

1. What is rhabdomyolysis, what organ is particularly sensitive to its effects, and what assessment findings would suggest that this is occurring?

2. The patient is transferred to a rehabilitation unit. The physician has prescribed baclofen 20 mg 4 times a day. What assessments should be included in the nurse's plan of care for this patient relating to drug therapy?

3. Developmentally, this patient is at risk for nonadherence to therapy. Why should the patient be discouraged from abrupt discontinuation of baclofen?

4. Dantrolene (Dantrium) would be more convenient for this patient because it only needs to be taken once a day. Why is it not a good choice for this patient?

## Case Study 2

*A patient is receiving cyclobenzaprine (Flexeril) to relieve muscle spasms after experiencing extensive musculoskeletal injuries in a multiple vehicle accident.*

1. What are common anticholinergic adverse effects associated with this drug and nursing interventions relating to these effects?

2. What teaching can the nurse provide to increase muscle strength and prevent further injuries?

## Case Study 3

*A patient returns to the recovery room after general anesthesia. The vital signs have increased from normal to a temperature of 103.6° F, pulse 116, respirations 22, and BP 145/99 mm Hg. The patient is developing muscular rigidity.*

1. Why are antipyretics not appropriate to treat this fever?

2. Dantrolene 150 mg IV push is prescribed. The recommended dose to treat malignant hyperthermia is initially 2 mg/kg to a maximum of 10 mg/kg. The patient weighs 185 lbs, and the initial prescribed dose is 150 mg. Is this a safe and therapeutic dose?

# 26 Local Anesthetics

## OBJECTIVES

See page 26 for the Objectives.

## CRITICAL THINKING AND STUDY QUESTIONS

1. The nurse is assisting the emergency department physician with suturing of a wound on the dorsal aspect of the foot. Which of these findings in the patient's history would be most significant if a patient was receiving lidocaine as the local anesthetic?
   a. Mobitz type I heart block
   b. Peripheral vascular disease
   c. Allergy to tetracaine
   d. Headache with spinal anesthetic

▶ 2. A mother received epidural anesthetic 10 minutes before delivering a 7-lbs 10-ounce girl at 39 weeks of gestation. The neonate is brought to the nursery from the delivery room. Which of the following findings would be a concern to the nursery nurse?
   a. Apical pulse 140 beats/min
   b. Positive Babinski's
   c. Respirations 22 breaths per minute
   d. Temperature 36.8° C

▶ 3. A patient is admitted to a surgical floor at 10 AM (1000) after a total abdominal hysterectomy performed with spinal anesthetic. During the assessment at 4 PM (1600) the nurse notes that the patient has not voided. An appropriate action by the nurse would be to:
   a. administer bethanechol 5 mg subcutaneously ordered as needed for urinary retention.
   b. assist the patient to the bathroom to attempt to void.
   c. sit the patient upright on a bedpan to attempt to void.
   d. perform a bladder scan and notify the physician if the result is greater than 200 mL.

4. Topical local anesthetic should be applied:
   a. using the lowest effective dose.
   b. gently to areas of skin that are abraded.
   c. as a thick film over the entire affected area.
   d. extending approximately ½ inch beyond the affected area.

5. In general anesthetics that are small in the size of particles, highly lipid soluble, and do not readily ionize have a:
   a. fast onset and long duration.
   b. slow onset and long duration.
   c. fast onset and short duration.
   d. slow onset and short duration.

6. Using a vasoconstrictor, such as epinephrine, with a local anesthetic: (Select all that apply.)
   a. Allows for the use of less anesthetic.
   b. Causes local vasoconstriction.
   c. Can cause adverse effects from systemic absorption of the vasoconstrictor.
   d. Causes local vasodilation.
   e. Delays onset of anesthesia.
   f. Delays systemic absorption.
   g. Improves blood flow to the affected area.
   h. Increases the risk of toxicity.
   j. Reduces blood flow to the affected area.
   k. Reduces the risk of toxicity.
   l. Requires the use of a larger dose of anesthetic.

▸ 7. When a patient is receiving a local anesthetic with epinephrine, the nurse should carefully assess for which effects from the epinephrine?
   a. Bradycardia and hypotension
   b. Convulsions and respiratory depression
   c. Headache and urinary retention
   d. Tachycardia and hypertension

8. A patient who has a known allergy to chloroprocaine (Nesacaine) should not receive: (Select all that apply.)
   a. articaine (Septocaine).
   b. prilocaine (Citanest).
   c. lidocaine (Xylocaine).
   d. mepivacaine (Carbocaine).
   e. tetracaine (Pontocaine).

9. Cocaine differs from other ester-type local anesthetics in that it:
   a. can be particularly dangerous if given to a patient with heart failure (HF).
   b. causes intense vasoconstriction.
   c. is known to cause physical dependence.
   d. produces CNS excitement, then depression.

▸ 10. A patient received intravenous regional anesthetic containing lidocaine without epinephrine when he had ankle surgery. At what point during the procedure would the patient be at greatest risk for bradycardia, hypotension, and respiratory depression from the lidocaine?
   a. Immediately after injection of the lidocaine
   b. When the surgeon makes the incision
   c. When the patient is in the postanesthesia unit
   d. When the patient is in his hospital room on the medical-surgical unit

## CASE STUDIES AND PATIENT TEACHING

*(Use a separate piece of paper for your responses.)*

### Case Study 1

*An 8-year-old child, accompanied by both parents, comes to the emergency room with a scalp laceration sustained when he fell off of his bicycle. The physician plans to administer lidocaine with epinephrine to close the wound with 6 to 8 interrupted sutures. The child is tearful but cooperative.*

1. What would be the nursing responsibilities for this procedure?

### Case Study 2

*A patient received lidocaine for the removal of an ingrown toenail. Seeping blood made it difficult for the physician to visualize the area where he was working. Epinephrine is a vasoconstrictor that is often combined with lidocaine to delay systemic absorption of the lidocaine. As a vasoconstrictor, it would have decreased the blood seepage.*

1. Why was it not used in this situation?

2. The patient has had this procedure before and is concerned about pain. She verbalizes a desire to use ice immediately to prevent pain. What precautions should the nurse provide regarding the use of cold?

3. The patient asks if she can use OTC topical lidocaine anesthetic on her toe when sensation returns to relieve discomfort. What teaching should the nurse provide?

# 27 General Anesthetics

## OBJECTIVES

See page 26 for the Objectives.

## CRITICAL THINKING AND STUDY QUESTIONS

1. Anesthesia (aka anaesthesia) involves:
   a. sensibility to pain.
   b. consciousness and sensibility to pain.
   c. consciousness and sensibility to pain and temperature.
   d. consciousness and sensibility to pain, temperature, and taste.

2. Describe the ideal anesthetic.

3. What are the agents included in a balanced anesthetic?

4. Match the class of drugs to the properties of ideal anesthesia that they produce.

| | |
|---|---|
| ___ a. Neuromuscular blocking agents | 1. Analgesia |
| ___ b. Nitrous oxide | 2. Produce state of unconsciousness |
| ___ c. Opioids | 3. Muscle relaxation |
| ___ d. Short-acting barbiturates | |

5. The primary goal of using multiple agents to achieve anesthesia is to:
   a. decrease the pain after the procedure.
   b. make the patient unable to feel pain during the procedure.
   c. permit full anesthesia with less adverse effects.
   d. prevent the patient from remembering the experience.

6. Current data indicates that most inhalation anesthetics:
   a. activate GABA receptors.
   b. activate nicotinic receptors.
   c. activate receptors for glutamate.
   d. increase receptor sensitivity to GABA.

7. Nitrous oxide has an extremely high minimum alveolar concentration (MAC). Because of this:
   a. the drug can be administered at low doses and achieve adequate anesthesia.
   b. surgical anesthesia cannot be obtained with nitrous oxide.
   c. the drug can achieve adequate, safe anesthesia if a high enough dose is administered slowly.
   d. the drug will make the patient unresponsive to painful stimuli.

▸ 8. The nurse is caring for a patient in the postanesthesia care unit. The assessment that the nurse should give the highest priority is:
   a. breathing.
   b. level of consciousness.
   c. pain.
   d. urinary output.

▸ 9. A patient has received succinylcholine during surgery. A priority nursing outcome during nursing care in the postanesthesia care unit is:
   a. blood pressure will be 110/60 to 120/70 mm Hg.
   b. dressing will be dry and intact.

c. patient will void at least 250 mL of clear yellow urine.
d. temperature will be 36.5° C to 37° C.

▶ 10. The nurse is completing the preoperative checklist for a same day surgery patient who has been called to the operating room (OR). The patient makes a comment to the nurse that he hopes they really knock him out because he really needs a lot of a drug to get a good effect. On further discussion the patient reveals that he has been using oxycodone (OxyContin) illegally for 2 years and that his last dose was 6 hours ago. The nurse should:
a. call the OR and cancel the surgery.
b. note the medication on the patient's chart and send the patient to the OR.
c. notify anesthesia and the surgeon of the finding.
d. nothing, the medication should be out of the patient's system.

▶ 11. A male patient who has received midazolam (Versed), a preoperative benzodiazepine, informs the nurse that he needs to "pass his water." The nurse should initially:
a. assist the patient to the bathroom, staying with the patient at all times.
b. provide the patient a urinal and ask him to try to use it while still in bed.
c. provide the patient with a urinal and assist him with standing.
d. insert a Foley catheter.

▶ 12. The most critical assessment before the nurse administers morphine to a postoperative patient is:
a. blood pressure 170/92 mm Hg.
b. pain 9 on a scale of 1 to 10.
c. respirations 8.
d. temperature 37.2° C.

13. A patient has received halothane during surgery. The PACU nurse would be concerned if the patient was unable to be aroused how soon after the halothane inhalation ended?
a. 10 to 15 minutes
b. 15 to 30 minutes
c. 30 to 60 minutes
d. 60 to 90 minutes

▶ 14. A 14-month-old received halothane during surgery. Which of the following immediate postoperative assessment findings would be a concern?
a. Blood pressure 86/54 mm Hg
b. Pulse 68 beats/min
c. Respirations 30 per minute
d. Temperature 39.8° C

▶ 15. The postanesthesia care unit nurse has received a patient who had emergency surgery including general anesthetic with isoflurane (Forane) from the operating room. The family has just arrived, and the nurse has learned that the patient has been taking the calcium channel blocker amlodipine (Norvasc). Because of the similarity in effects of isoflurane and amlodipine on the cardiovascular system, the nurse should assess carefully for early signs of:
a. bradycardia.
b. hypertension.
c. hypotension.
d. tachycardia.

16. Matching: Drug and adverse effects

| Drug | Adverse effect |
|---|---|
| ___ a. Desflurane | 1. High risk of bacterial infection |
| ___ b. Enflurane | 2. Hypotension can occur from vasodilation |
| ___ c. Halothane | 3. Can induce seizures |
| ___ d. Isofloflurane | 4. Delirium and psychotic symptoms can occur post-operatively or days or weeks after surgery |
| ___ e. Ketamine | 5. Can produce heat and fire in administration apparatus |
| ___ f. Propofol | 6. May prolong QT interval T |
| ___ g. Sevoflurane | 7. Tachycardia and hyper-tension can occurs if blood levels drop suddenly |

17. Nitrous oxide is widely used in surgery because:
a. it has significant analgesic effects without significant cardiac or respiratory depression.
b. it can produce a state of unconsciousness at very low doses.
c. full anesthesia can be achieved with nitrous oxide alone.
d. postoperative nausea and vomiting are uncommon.

18. A cataract surgery patient receives midazolam and fentanyl. The nurse would expect these medications to produce: (Select all that apply.)
    a. absence of anxiety.
    b. analgesia.
    c. balanced anesthesia.
    d. flaccid paralysis.
    e. sedation.
    f. unconsciousness.

## CASE STUDIES AND PATIENT TEACHING

*(Use a separate piece of paper for your responses.)*

### Case Study 1

*A 65-year-old white male with a history of lung cancer has been admitted the evening before surgery and is scheduled for a thoracotomy at 8 AM under balanced general anesthetic. He is 5 feet 6 inches and weighs 210 lbs. The patient has a productive cough and admits to tobacco use for the last 40 years, smoking one pack of cigarettes per day. He has hypertension and takes hydrochlorothiazide, which has been effective in keeping his blood pressure under control.*

1. What would be priority concerns of the nurse in the postanesthesia care unit (PACU) for this patient relating to general anesthetic?

### Case Study 2

*The nurse is admitting a patient with a history of diabetes mellitus type 2 and hypertension to the same-day surgery unit who is scheduled for an inguinal herniorrhaphy.*

1. What data is important for the nurse to collect?

2. The patient is in the postanesthesia care unit and has just awakened, but is very drowsy. Describe nursing interventions relating to the effects of inhalation anesthetic that are needed when a patient first awakens.

3. The postoperative patient reports that he awoke during surgery and was in pain, but was unable to tell the surgeon. What should the nurse do?

# 28 Opioid (Narcotic) Analgesics, Opioid Antagonists, and Nonopioid Centrally Acting Analgesics

## OBJECTIVES

See page 26 for the Objectives.

## CRITICAL THINKING AND STUDY QUESTIONS

1. A patient is admitted to the emergency room with chest pain. The ECG indicates inferior wall myocardial infarction. A STAT dose of morphine sulfate is prescribed. What is the most important effect of the morphine in this situation?
   a. Decreases cardiac workload and oxygen consumption
   b. Sedates patient so the patient is not aware of danger of situation
   c. Slows respirations so the patient feels calm
   d. Suppresses awareness of body functioning

▶ 2. The nurse is ambulating a postoperative patient in the hall who is receiving an opioid

analgesic for pain when the patient complains of severe nausea. What should the nurse do first if all options are possible?
a. Administer the prescribed antiemetic.
b. Assist the patient to sit down.
c. Get an emesis basin.
d. Walk the patient back to his room.

▶ 3. A patient who has received morphine becomes slightly disoriented. If this effect is due to the morphine, which intervention by the nurse might aid in reversing this adverse effect?
a. Assist patient to ambulate.
b. Instruct to change positions slowly.
c. Instruct to take slow, deep breaths.
d. Keep the room well lit.

4. A 54-year-old cancer patient asks why his dose of oral morphine is so much higher than the intravenous dose he was receiving postoperatively. The basis of the nurses response is:
a. hepatic first pass metabolizes some of the drug before it reaches the central nervous system.
b. morphine is not lipid soluble and does not readily cross the blood-brain barrier.
c. the kidneys excrete oral morphine faster than intravenous morphine.
d. tolerance develops more rapidly if the patient has first received parenteral morphine.

5. The nurse would expect the dose of morphine for a postoperative patient to be higher than usual for the patient's size and age if prescribed for a patient who routinely uses:
a. alprazolam (Xanax).
b. ethanol (Alcohol).
c. oxycodone (OxyContin).
d. temazepam (Restoril).

▶ 6. A neonate is born to a known heroin addict. The infant is exhibiting symptoms of opioid withdrawal. Which of these nursing issues is of the highest priority as the nurse cares for the neonate in the nursery?
a. Altered nutrition
b. Disturbed sleep
c. Fluid deficit
d. Parenting

7. A cancer patient who is receiving oxycodone (OxyContin) for pain relief develops a rash after being prescribed an antibiotic. The prescriber discontinues the antibiotic and prescribes diphenhydramine (Benadryl). The nurse would include in the plan of care assessment and interventions for which possible effects of this drug combination?
a. Delerium
b. Fever
c. Hypotension
d. Urinary retention

▶ 8. A patient who has overdosed on oxycodone (OxyContin), an opiate, is brought into the emergency department unresponsive with severely depressed respirations. The patient receives intravenous naloxone HCl (Narcan), a narcotic antagonist, with an improvement in level of consciousness and respiratory rate and effort within minutes. A priority nursing concern for this patient is:
a. prevention of abstinence syndrome.
b. short half-life of oxycodone.
c. short half-life of naloxone.
d. substance abuse.

▶ 9. A fentanyl (Duragesic) patch has been prescribed for a patient after multiple musculoskeletal injuries in a car accident. The most important reason why the nurse should teach the patient not to apply heat in the area of the patch is because doing so could cause:
a. inactivation of the drug.
b. loosening of the patch from the skin.
c. prolongation of the drug effect.
d. respiratory depression.

10. Transmucosal fentanyl (Actiq) is not appropriate for acute pain relief in children because the:
a. digestive enzymes in a child's mouth inactivate the drug.
b. dose is too high.
c. onset of effect takes too long.
d. taste is bitter.

11. The nurse should assess for respiratory depression for 24 hours after a patient has discontinued use of:
a. intrathecal morphine.
b. intramuscular meperidine (Demerol).
c. oral methadone (Dolophine).
d. transmucosal fentanyl (Actiq).

▸ 12. An aphasic patient, who has been receiving meperidine 75 mg every 3 to 4 hours for pain for the past 36 hours, has suddenly become restless and irritable. The last dose of meperidine was 4 hours ago. It is important for the nurse to withhold the meperidine, do a complete assessment on the patient, and contact the prescriber with the findings because:
   a. respiratory depression is imminent.
   b. the patient is becoming physiologically dependent on the meperidine.
   c. tolerance to the meperidine has developed.
   d. toxicity from a metabolite may be occurring.

13. A nurse is responsible for obtaining the history for patients undergoing colonoscopy and other procedures in an outpatient gastroenterology department. The most frequently used procedural medications are midazolam (Versed) and meperidine (Demerol). Which of the following antidepressant medications, if taken by a patient, is most critical for the nurse to communicate to the anesthesiologist who will be administering the conscious sedation?
   a. bupropion (Wellbutrin)
   b. nefazodone(Serzone)
   c. phenelzine (Nardil)
   d. venlafaxine (Effexor)

14. A cancer patient has been taking increasing doses of oxycodone (OxyContin) for pain relief. Which of the following adverse effects is most likely to persist with long-term use of this drug?
   a. Constipation
   b. Euphoria
   c. Respiratory depression
   d. Sedation

15. A cancer patient has received instructions regarding administration of oxycodone (OxyContin). Which of these statements made by the client would indicate that the patient needs further teaching?
   a. "I need to inform my doctor if I experience episodes of pain between doses."
   b. "I should tell all of my healthcare providers that I am taking this drug regularly."
   c. "I should not take this drug if I am allergic to Percocet, but not Tylenol."
   d. "If I have difficulty swallowing the pill, I should crush it and take it with a small amount of applesauce."

▸ 16. Which of these findings would be most important for the nurse to report to the prescriber if a patient was receiving propoxyphene?
   a. Anorexia
   b. Drowsiness
   c. Dysphoria
   d. Headache

▸ 17. The nurse is caring for a patient who has just received the first intravenous dose of pentazocine (Talwin). Which of the following, if present within minutes of injecting the drug, would be a reason for the nurse to contact the prescriber immediately?
   a. Constricted pupils
   b. Diaphoresis
   c. Drowsiness
   d. Respirations 18 per minute

18. Because it is an opioid agonist-antagonist, the nurse is less likely to have to administer an opioid antagonist, such as naloxone (Narcan), for respiratory depression when administering which of the following opioid analgesics?
   a. buprenorphine (Buprenex)
   b. fentanyl (Sublimaze)
   c. meperidine (Demerol)
   d. remifentanil (Ultiva)

▸ 19. A patient is admitted to the emergency department after a traumatic injury and is in severe pain from compound fractures. It is most critical that the nurse carefully assess the patient before administering an opioid for evidence of:
   a. asthma.
   b. diabetes.
   c. head injury.
   d. hypertension.

20. The nurse would consult the prescriber if the nurse identified that a patient had which history and was prescribed tramadol (Ultram) for pain relief?
   a. Heart failure (HF)
   b. Chronic obstructive pulmonary disease (COPD)
   c. Dementia
   d. Seizure disorder

21. A cancer patient is prescribed clonidine (Duraclon) for burning pain. Before administering the drug, the nurse should carefully review the patient's history, laboratory

results, and orders and assess for: (Select all that apply.)
a. abuse of opioids.
b. anticoagulant therapy.
c. bradypnea.
d. elevated ALT and/or AST.
e. Elevated serum creatinine.
f. Fever.
g. Hypotension.
h. Tachycardia.

▶ 22. A nursing priority relating to the most common adverse effects for patients receiving intrathecal ziconotide (Prialt) is:
a. breathing.
b. circulation.
c. elimination.
d. safety.

23. The nurse is working in an outpatient cancer center. When a patient is experiencing uncontrolled pain, it is important for the nurse to communicate the quality of pain (sharp, dull, etc.) to the prescriber because it influences analgesic:
a. dose.
b. metabolism.
c. route.
d. timing.

## CASE STUDIES AND PATIENT TEACHING

*(Use a separate piece of paper for your responses.)*

### Case Study 1

*A 67-year-old obese female who has a history of osteoarthritis, type 2 DM, cholecystitis, and hypertension undergoes right knee replacement surgery. Postoperative orders include intravenous morphine 4 mg every 3 hours for pain relief, and continuous passive motion (CPM) apparatus is to be applied at 20° range of motion, 2 cycles per minute, for 10 hours per day, not exceeding 2 hours at a time.*

1. Why is the pain medication ordered every 3 hours instead of every 3 hours as needed?

2. Physical therapy (PT) is prescribed twice a day. Why is it important for the nurse to communicate the timing of the last dose of morphine to the physical therapist when sending the patient for PT?

3. What assessments must the nurse make before administering the morphine and what would be assessment findings that warrant withholding the medication and consulting the prescriber?

4. The pharmacy supplies a morphine solution for injection in a tubex containing 10 mg/mL. The drug handbook recommends that morphine be injected in a dilution of 5 mL administered over 5 minutes. How much morphine will the nurse withdraw from the tubex before diluting with sterile water?

5. What must the nurse do with the additional morphine left in the tubex after the proper dose has been withdrawn?

6. At 2 PM (1400) the patient appears relaxed and is visiting with family. The patient is sitting in a chair, and CPM machine is off. The patient requests morphine for operative site pain (4 of 10). The last dose of morphine was administered at 10 AM (1000). What should the nurse do?

7. Why is it important for the nurse to assist the patient with returning to bed before administering the morphine?

8. What interventions can the nurse provide to a patient who is prescribed an opioid on an as needed basis to achieve the best control of pain?

9. What assessments and nursing interventions might the nurse employ to prevent, identify, and address the following adverse effects of morphine?
a. Constipation
b. Urinary retention
c. Orthostatic hypotension
d. Miosis
e. Nausea and vomiting

10. The patient reports right upper quadrant pain that is worse 30 minutes after receiving a dose of morphine. What in the patient's history could be causing this effect, and what should the nurse do?

### Case Study 2

*The nurse is providing preoperative teaching to a 35-year-old female who has been admitted for an abdominal hysterectomy. Patient-controlled analgesia (PCA) is anticipated as the mechanism of postoperative pain relief.*

1. What preoperative teaching should the nurse provide this patient to enhance pain relief and prevent adverse effects, including respiratory depression?

2. Postoperatively the patient is ordered morphine IV via patient-controlled analgesia (PCA) pump for her postoperative pain. The pump is set to deliver 1 mg of morphine per injection and up to a maximum of 5 mg per hour. What are the advantages and disadvantages of PCA?

3. The patient is resting quietly. The nurse check assesses her respiratory rate as 8 per minute. What other assessments should be performed, and what actions should the nurse take?

4. What measures, other than drug therapy, can the nurse employ to reduce this patient's pain?

## Case Study 3

*A patient continues to require morphine long after the usual time frame for opioids after the type of surgery that was performed. She tells you that she has no tolerance for pain, but the physician has decided that she must stop the morphine. The nurse is concerned that the patient may have been dependent on drugs before coming to the hospital, and withdrawing the morphine may lead to abstinence syndrome.*

1. How should the nurse address these concerns?

2. What are the symptoms of abstinence syndrome that the nurse should include in patient assessment?

3. Is it possible that the patient could be having uncontrolled pain, not be a substance abuser, and not have any other medical problems?

4. How does physical dependence on opioid analgesics differ from abuse and addiction?

5. Describe a situation where physical dependence on opioid analgesics is acceptable.

# 29 Pain Management in Patients with Cancer

## OBJECTIVES

See page 26 for the Objectives.

## CRITICAL THINKING AND STUDY QUESTIONS

1. Match types of pain to cause, origin, or characteristics. (Some may be used more than once.)

| | |
|---|---|
| ___ a. Neuropathic | 1. Adjunctive drugs most effective |
| ___ b. Nociceptive | 2. Bone, joint, muscle |
| ___ c. Somatic | 3. Burning, numb, cold |
| ___ d. Visceral | 4. Diffuse, aching |
| | 5. Opioids most effective |
| | 6. Organ |
| | 7. Peripheral nerve injury |
| | 8. Sharp, localized |
| | 9. Tissue injury |

▶ 2. The most reliable indicator of the need for pain relief is:
   a. changes in vital signs that can occur with pain.
   b. extensiveness of the cancer involvement.
   c. patient's expressions and reluctance to move.
   d. patient's report of a need for pain relief.

▶ 3. When developing a plan of care for pain management for the cancer patient, it is most important for the nurse to identify outcomes based on achieving: (Select all that apply.)
   a. a rating of pain less than 3 on a scale of 0 to 10.
   b. comfort that allows the patient to complete all ADL.
   c. pain relief that is acceptable to the patient.
   d. total pain relief.

4. A cancer patient whose history includes type 2 diabetes mellitus informs the nurse that she is experiencing constant pain in her feet. Based on the type of foot pain commonly experienced by diabetics, the nurse would consult the physician regarding possible prescribing of a/an:
   a. analgesic, such as acetaminophen (Tylenol).
   b. neurologic-acting adjunct drug, such as gabapentin (Neurontin).
   c. nonsteroidal anti-inflammatory drug (NSAID), such as naproxen (Aleve).
   d. opioid agonist analgesic, such as morphine.

▶ 5. Which of these laboratory test results would be of most concern to the nurse when a cancer patient treated with chemotherapy is taking a pain reliever that contains aspirin?
   a. ALT 40 International Units/L
   b. BUN 22 mg/dL
   c. Platelet count 80,000/m$^3$
   d. WBC 4500/m$^3$

6. The nurse is performing a pain assessment on a newly admitted patient with metastatic cancer. The patient describes the pain as sharp and rates it at 5 of 10. Admission orders include acetaminophen 650 mg every 4 hours as needed. The nurse should:
   a. administer the acetaminophen.
   b. consult with the prescriber.
   c. obtain more data regarding the pain and administer the acetaminophen.
   d. obtain more data regarding the pain and consult the prescriber.

7. A postoperative cancer patient was receiving intravenous morphine sulfate 10 mg every 4 hours for pain. The prescriber has discontinued the intravenous morphine and ordered morphine sulfate 20-mg tablet every 4 hours. The nurse recognizes that this is a/an:
   a. dose that cannot be compared with the intravenous dose.
   b. equianalgesic dose.
   c. less potent dose than the intravenous dose.
   d. more potent dose than the intravenous dose.

▶ 8. The nurse knows that respiratory depression is most likely to occur with which of the following pain regimens?
   a. A loading dose of 10 mg of morphine before starting PCA
   b. Increasing long-term intravenous dose of morphine from 5 mg to 7 mg
   c. PCA morphine at 1 mg of morphine per injection and up to a maximum of 5 mg per hour
   d. 60 mg of intravenous morphine every hour to a patient who has been receiving steadily increasing doses of morphine

9. Generally the best pain control regimen for a hospitalized patient who has been known to abuse opioids and who has severe pain is:
   a. agonist-antagonist opioids.
   b. codeine administered orally.
   c. intermittent intravenous dosing of meperidine (Demerol).
   d. intravenous opioid agonist administered by patient-controlled analgesia (PCA).

## CASE STUDIES AND PATIENT TEACHING

*(Use a separate piece of paper for your responses.)*

### Case Study 1

*The nurse is caring for a 68-year-old retired steelworker who is postoperative a right lung lobectomy for lung cancer. The patient is ordered morphine IV via patient-controlled analgesia (PCA) pump for postoperative pain. The pump is set to deliver 1 mg of morphine per injection and up to a maximum of 5 mg per hour. Vital signs are BP 150/92 mm/Hg, pulse 94, respirations 24. Chest tube is intact and draining. Other assessment findings are within expected limits except the patient is restless and grimaces with movement. He is reluctant to use the incentive spirometer. He has not complained of pain.*

1. What actions should the nurse take?

2. What psychosocial issues might influence this patient to be reluctant to use prescribed opioid analgesia?

3. What nursing approaches might increase the chance that the patient will use all available resources to obtain pain relief and increase adherence to prescribed therapy?

4. What teaching can the nurse provide regarding benefits of controlled pain for this patient?

## Case Study 2

*A cancer patient is being discharged on oxycodone and acetaminophen (Percocet).*

1. What teaching should the nurse provide regarding the opioid and nonopioid components of this drug?

*The patient's pain is not relieved by 2 Percocet (oxycodone 10 mg and acetaminophen 325 mg) tablets taken every 4 hours. The prescriber has discontinued the Percocet and ordered oxycodone CR (OxyContin) 40 mg twice a day, oxycodone IR 5 mg every 6 hours as needed, and acetaminophen 650 mg every 6 hours. The patient is overwhelmed by the multiple medications and asks why he cannot just take 3 Percocet tablets every 4 hours.*

2. How should the nurse respond?

3. What interventions can the nurse offer to help the patient understand his analgesic regimen?

4. What teaching should the nurse provide regarding the adverse effect of constipation?

5. What teaching can the nurse provide to enable the patient to assist the physician with decisions regarding analgesic prescription?

## Case Study 3

*A patient who is receiving radiation therapy for metastatic breast cancer complains of pain.*

1. Describe the nurse's role in implementing the clinical approach to pain management recommended by the AHCPR.
   a. Ask and assess
   b. Believe
   c. Choose
   d. Deliver
   e. Empower and enable

2. Describe what the nurse should include when assessing and documenting the patient's pain.

## Case Study 4

*Developmental considerations*

1. Identify the pain scale that would be most effective in evaluating pain for these cancer patients. Explain how it is used and why you think it would be the best method of evaluating this patient's pain.
   a. A 3-month-old infant
   b. A 3-year-old who is shy
   c. A 15-year-old with osteosarcoma
   d. An adult who is nonverbal because of a laryngectomy
   e. An elderly patient with dementia

2. Describe physiologic differences in the infant, child, and elderly that must be considered when pain medication is prescribed.

# 30 Drugs for Headache

## OBJECTIVES

See page 26 for the Objectives.

## CRITICAL THINKING AND STUDY QUESTIONS

1. Migraine headaches: (Select all that apply.)
   a. always start with an abnormal sensation (aura).
   b. cannot be treated effectively after the pain starts.
   c. involve inflammation of intracranial blood vessels.
   d. involve vasoconstriction of intracranial blood vessels.
   e. therapy includes drugs and nonpharmacologic measures to prevent attacks.
   f. therapy should start at the earliest sign of attack.

2. The primary reason why abortive medication for migraine headaches should not be used more than 1 or 2 days a week is:
   a. abuse potential.
   b. development of chest pain.
   c. development of tolerance, and medication is not effective.
   d. medication overuse headache.

▶ 3. Which of these patient assessment findings would be most significant if the nurse was preparing to administer ergotamine to a patient who is experiencing the start of a migraine headache?
   a. ALT 30 International Units/L
   b. Blood pressure 90/58 mm/Hg
   c. Capillary refill 8 seconds
   d. Flashes of light in visual fields

4. A rationale for administering both ergotamine and metoclopramide (Reglan) to a patient to abort a migraine headache includes that the metoclopramide:
   a. minimizes sensitivity to light.
   b. prevents adverse effects of weakness and myalgia from ergotamine.
   c. provides additional vasoconstriction to relieve cranial vessel vasodilation.
   d. reverses gastric stasis, which improves absorption of the ergotamine.

5. Which of the following over-the-counter medications has not demonstrated effectiveness in relieving mild to moderate migraine headache pain?
   a. Aspirin
   b. Acetaminophen
   c. Acetaminophen, aspirin, and caffeine
   d. Ibuprofen

▶ 6. The nurse would consult the prescriber before administering ergotamine or triptan drugs for migraine headache to a patient with: (Select all that apply.)
   a. cardiovascular disease.
   b. diabetes mellitus.
   c. hypertension.
   d. infection.
   e. peptic ulcer disease.
   f. possible pregnancy.

7. A postoperative patient reports experiencing a migraine aura and asks for medication to abort the attack. The patient's migraines usually involve nausea and occasionally vomiting. Ergotamine 2 mg is ordered. Which of the following prescribed drugs should the nurse administer with the ergotamine to prevent nausea and vomiting?
   a. butorphanol nasal spray (Stadol)
   b. meclopromamide (Reglan)
   c. riboflavin (Vitamin $B_2$)
   d. toprimate (Topamax)

8. Which of the following are true about triptan therapy for migraine headaches?
   a. Administering an oral dose of the drug after subcutaneous administration will prevent recurrence of the headache.
   b. One dose provides long-lasting relief for 80% of patients.
   c. It relieves headache, nausea, and sensitivity to sound and light.
   d. Peripheral vasoconstriction is the primary concern with adverse effects.

▶ 9. The nurse has administered sumatriptan (Imitrex) subcutaneously to a 35-year-old nonsmoker who was admitted for depression and is experiencing a migraine headache. One hour after administration the patient complains of heavy arms and chest pressure. The nurse should:
   a. assess vital signs and PQRST the chest pain.
   b. continue care; this is a normal adverse effect.
   c. notify the prescriber STAT.

10. A college student has been prescribed propranolol to prevent migraine headaches and frovatriptan (Frova) 2.5 mg by mouth to treat recurrent migraine headaches. Which statement, if made by the patient, would indicate a need for further teaching?
   a. "I need to lie down in a dark room after taking the Frova because it takes several hours before it relieves the headache."
   b. "I may experience the same number of headaches for the first weeks that I take propranolol because it takes weeks to take effect."
   c. "I should take a double second dose of Frova an hour after the first dose if the first dose is ineffective."
   d. "Propranolol will decrease the number and intensity of my migraine attacks."

11. Matching: Prophylactic treatments for cluster headaches

| | |
|---|---|
| __ a. Lithium | 1. Onset of prevention within days |
| __ b. Prednisone | 2. Less effective, but safer |
| __ c. Verapamil | 3. Narrow therapeutic range |
| | 4. Should not be used for longer than 1 to 2 months |
| | 5. Therapeutic level 0.6 to 1.2 mEq/L |

## CASE STUDIES AND PATIENT TEACHING

*(Use a separate piece of paper for your responses.)*

### Case Study 1

*A registered nurse is working in an ED. A 49-year-old white female nurse has the chief complaint of severe, frequent headaches that begin midmorning and grow progressively worse throughout the day. She admits to occasional nausea and vomiting. Advil has been minimally successful in treating the headaches. Her history includes the following: 2 months ago she is noticed one black, tarry stool; she is on low-dose oral contraceptives for perimenopausal symptoms; and she is frequently asked to work double shifts. Her headaches are pulsatile and usually unilateral. All of the patient's laboratory findings are within normal limits. The attending physician reads the history and proceeds to order sumatriptan (Imitrex) 6 mg subcutaneously now and writes a prescription for Imitrex STATdose Pen 6 mg as directed.*

1. Describe what would need to be included in teaching this patient about using the self-injecting pen.

2. The patient's prescription insurance does not cover sumatriptan. The physician then provides a prescription for ergotamine tartrate, 1 mg PO (10 tablets), take as directed and instructs the patient to seek follow-up with her PCP. What teaching needs to be provided by the ED nurse regarding the prescribed ergotamine?

3. At the appointment with her PCP, the patient asks about Excedrin Migraine. What in the patient's history needs to be explored before the patient begins regular use of a product containing aspirin?

4. The PCP discusses the use of prophylactic drugs to prevent the migraine headaches. What drugs might be considered?

## Case Study 2

*A 20-year-old college student comes to the college health center with a complaint of frequent intense headaches. The nurse is responsible for collecting data before the patient is seen by the nurse practitioner.*

1. What subjective and objective data should the nurse obtain?

2. Teaching of nonpharmacologic measures to prevent migraine headaches should include:

3. The nurse practitioner has prescribed dihydroergotamine. What is the most significant reason why ergotamine or triptan drugs were not prescribed for this patient?

4. What teaching regarding preventing toxicity from dihydroergotamine should be provided to this patient?

# 31 Antipsychotic Agents and Their Use in Schizophrenia

## OBJECTIVES

See page 26 for the Objectives.

## CRITICAL THINKING AND STUDY QUESTIONS

1. Matching: Symptoms

| | |
|---|---|
| ___ a. Cognitive | 1. Diminished emotional response |
| ___ b. Negative | 2. False beliefs |
| ___ c. Positive | 3. Thinking is not logical |
| | 4. Disheveled appearance |
| | 5. Cannot remember |
| | 6. Suspiciousness |
| | 7. Cannot pay attention |
| | 8. Does not interact with others |
| | 9. False perceptions |

2. Atypical antipsychotic drugs are preferred over conventional antipsychotics primarily because they:
   a. cost less.
   b. do not affect thinking.
   c. do not cause significant adverse effects.
   d. treat positive and negative symptoms.

3. A highly potent antipsychotic differs from low potency drugs in that it:
   a. is more likely to cure the disorder.
   b. produces desired effects at low doses.
   c. provides more symptom relief.
   d. treats positive and negative symptoms.

▸ 4. A patient who is receiving chemotherapy for breast cancer is prescribed chlorpromazine (Thorazine). There is no mention of other medical or psychiatric disorders in the patient's history. It is important for the nurse to assess for:
   a. delusions.
   b. hallucinations.
   c. nausea.
   d. tics.

5. Which of the following extrapyramidal adverse effects of antipsychotic drugs would the nurse expect to only occur after an extended period of drug therapy?
   a. Repetitive, slow, twisting movements of the tongue and face
   b. Severe spasms of the mouth, face, neck, or back
   c. Slow movement, tremor, and rigidity
   d. Uncontrollable need to be in motion

▸ 6. The priority nursing focus for a patient experiencing acute dystonia is:
   a. airway clearance.
   b. anxiety.
   c. pain.
   d. safety.

▶ 7. Which of these findings, if identified in a patient who has been receiving a neuroleptic antipsychotic, should the nurse report to the prescriber immediately?
   a. Agitation
   b. Difficulty speaking
   c. Involuntary movements of the tongue
   d. Sudden, whole-body muscle contractions

▶ 8. The nurse is assessing orthostatic blood pressure and pulse of a patient who is prescribed a neuroleptic antipsychotic drug. Which of the following assessment findings would be reason to withhold the drug and consult the prescriber?
   a. BP lying 110/66 mm Hg and pulse 76 beats/min; 1 minute later BP standing 108/70 mm Hg and pulse 80 beats/min
   b. BP lying 116/70 mm Hg and pulse 72 beats/min; 1 minute later BP standing 116/68 mm Hg and pulse 122 beats/min
   c. BP lying 120/84 mm Hg and pulse 70 beats/min; 1 minute later BP standing 110/76 mm Hg; pulse 72 beats/min
   d. BP lying 146/90 mm Hg and pulse 73 beats/min; 1 minute later BP standing 138/88 mm Hg; pulse 78 beats/min

▶ 9. Which of the following symptoms of an adverse effect, if identified in a patient who is receiving haloperidol (Haldol), should the nurse report to the prescriber immediately?
   a. Milk secretion from a male
   b. Red skin
   c. Sore throat
   d. Unexplained fainting, not associated with sudden position changes

10. It is important for the nurse to teach patients who are prescribed any neuroleptic antipsychotic drug to avoid taking which of the following over-the-counter medications?
   a. acetaminophen (Tylenol)
   b. acetylsalicylic acid (aspirin)
   c. diphenhydramine (Benadryl)
   d. pseudoephedrine (Sudafed)

▶ 11. A patient is prescribed haloperidol decanoate (Haldol) 50 mg every 4 weeks. When selecting a site for administration, the nurse knows the site that is no longer recommended for intramuscular (IM) injection is the:
   a. deltoid.
   b. dorsogluteal.
   c. vastus lateralis.
   d. ventrogluteal.

12. Which of the following statements, if made by the husband of a patient receiving haloperidol decanoate (depot preparation of Haldol) would indicate a need for further teaching?
   a. "The doctor has prescribed this injection because she needs a higher dose than is available in the pill."
   b. "Taking Haldol this way decreases the chance that she will develop abnormal mouth movements."
   c. "Taking Haldol this way increases the chance that her symptoms will be controlled."
   d. "This will help achieve a steady level of drug in her body."

▶ 13. Which of these findings would have the most significance for the nurse who is caring for a patient who is receiving clozapine (Clozaril)?
   a. Blood pressure drop of 10 mm Hg systolic when changing from lying to standing position
   b. Residual of 300 mL of urine after voiding
   c. Temperature 104° F (40°C)
   d. Weight gain of 2 lbs in 1 month

▶ 14. A patient who has been receiving glargine (Lantus) insulin for type 2 diabetes mellitus and levodopa (L-Dopa) for Parkinson's disease develops suspiciousness and illogical thinking. The psychiatric resident prescribes clozapine (Clozaril) 150 mg twice a day. The nurse should:
   a. consult the prescriber.
   b. consult the prescriber if the patient's WBC count is less than 10,000/m$^3$.
   c. hold the clozapine if the patient's fasting blood sugar is less than 70 mg/dL.
   d. review the patient's kidney and liver function laboratory results.

▶ 15. Which of these laboratory tests would be most important for the nurse to monitor when a patient is receiving clozapine (Clozaril)?
   a. Eosinophils
   b. Hematocrit and hemoglobin
   c. Platelets
   d. WBC

▶ 16. Risperidone (Risperdal) is prescribed for an elderly patient who has become agitated, disheveled, and inappropriate. Which of the following assessments is most critical to include in the nurse's plan of care relating to this drug therapy?
   a. Bowel sounds
   b. Chest pain
   c. Pedal edema
   d. Peripheral pulses

▶ 17. It is important for the nurse to assess for excessive hunger, thirst, and urination if a patient is prescribed:
   a. chlorpromazine (Thorazine)
   b. haloperidol (Haldol)
   c. molindone (Moban)
   d. olanzapine (Zyprexa)

▶ 18. A bipolar patient has revealed to the nurse that her appearance is very important to her. This patient would most likely be adherent to which of the following atypical drugs?
   a. aripiprazole (Abilify)
   b. clozapine (Clozaril)
   c. olanzapine (Zyprexa)
   d. quetiapine (Seroquel)

19. A patient who has been stabilized on oral risperidone (Risperdal) receives an intramuscular injection of Risperdal Consta before discharge. How long does the patient need to continue oral therapy?
   a. 3 hours
   b. 3 days
   c. 3 weeks
   d. 3 months

20. A patient's daughter has read that clozapine (Clozaril) is the most effective atypical antipsychotic. What should the nurse include in the explanation of why this drug is not used until other agents have failed?
   a. Can cause hypoglycemia
   b. Effect on white blood cell production
   c. High incidence of tardive dyskinesia
   d. Orthostatic hypotension is common

21. What laboratory tests are important for the nurse to monitor when caring for a patient who is prescribed risperidone (Risperdal)? (Select all that apply.)
   a. ALT and/or AST
   b. Cholesterol
   c. Creatinine
   d. Hemoglobin $A_{1C}$
   e. INR
   f. Platelets
   g. Triglycerides
   h. WBC count

22. Why is it important for the nurse to know the half-life of antipsychotic drugs?

## CASE STUDIES AND PATIENT TEACHING

*(Use a separate piece of paper for your responses.)*

### Case Study 1

*An 82-year-old woman who resides in a nursing facility is admitted to the hospital with pneumonia. She has a history of agitation and is ordered haloperidol 0.5 mg every 8 hours as needed when nonpharmacologic measures cannot control agitation. Two hours after administering the drug orally, the nurse notes the patient is moaning. Her eyes are rolled upward, and her back is arched.*

1. What action should the nurse take first?

2. What assessment data are important for the nurse to collect and communicate to the physician?

*Intravenous benzotropine (Cogentin) 1 mg is prescribed STAT. The drug is available as 1 mg/mL and can be administered undiluted over at least 1 minute. The nurse decides to be cautious and administer the drug over 2 minutes.*

3. How much drug should the nurse administer every 10 seconds?

4. What observations during infusion would be a reason to stop infusing the drug?

### Case Study 2

*The nurse is preparing for a group family session focusing on antipsychotic drugs.*

1. What information should be presented regarding prevention, identification, and when to seek medical treatment for these common adverse effects?
   a. Blurred vision
   b. Constipation
   c. Dry mouth
   d. Orthostatic hypotension
   e. Photophobia
   f. Sedation
   g. Sexual dysfunction
   h. Tachycardia\
   i. Urinary hesitancy

## Case Study 3

*A 52-year-old woman is admitted to the hospital for symptoms of schizophrenia. She has been hospitalized previously and was discharged on haloperidol (Haldol) 5 mg 3 times a day. Her husband reports that her symptoms had been controlled until she stopped taking her medication 3 days ago because of blurred vision, dry mouth, and chronic constipation. During the admission procedure she appeared to be responding to voices. The psychiatrist prescribes risperidone (Risperdal) orally disintegrating tablets 1 mg twice a day (day 1) with further orders to follow after laboratory test results are obtained.*

1. What laboratory test results are important for the nurse to communicate to the psychiatrist when consulting for further medication orders?

2. The next day the psychiatrist orders 2 mg twice a day (day 2), and 3 mg twice a day (subsequent days). On the fourth day, the patient's husband discusses with the nurse his concern that his wife does not appear to be improving. How should the nurse respond?

3. After 10 days, the patient reports that the voices have decreased. The nurse is providing drug teaching to the patient and her husband. The patient is concerned about adverse effects and asks how risperidone (Risperdal) is different from haloperidol (Haldol). Because the patient's concentration can be limited, the nurse develops a teaching handout including common adverse effects for the patient and her husband. Complete this teaching handout:

| **risperidone (Risperdal)** | | |
|---|---|---|
| Administration directions: | | |
| **Possible adverse effects** | **How to decrease chance that effect will occur** | **What to do if the effect occurs** |
| | | |
| | | |
| | | |
| | | |
| | | |

4. The patient's husband is concerned about his wife adhering to drug therapy. What information should the nurse offer to increase the likelihood that the patient will take the drug as prescribed?

# 32 Antidepressants

## OBJECTIVES

See page 26 for the Objectives.

## CRITICAL THINKING AND STUDY QUESTIONS

1. When assessing a patient who is receiving an antidepressant, which of the following questions would be most important for the nurse to ask?
   a. "Are you concerned about weight gain when you take medications?"
   b. "Are you having any thoughts about doing anything that could harm yourself?"
   c. "Do you experience dizziness when you stand up?"
   d. "Have you had any difficulty voiding?"

2. Patient compliance with antidepressant drug therapy is most likely to be increased if the nurse explains:
   a. drug interactions.
   b. expected timing of therapeutic response.
   c. the reason for limiting the number of units of the drug dispensed with each prescription.
   d. the seriousness of adverse effects.

▶ 3. When a patient who is receiving an antidepressant verbalizes suicidal ideation, which action should the nurse take first?
   a. Administer the antidepressant.
   b. Ask the patient why he or she feels this way.
   c. Notify the physician.
   d. Provide a safe environment.

4. Tricyclic antidepressants are often the drug of first choice for depression because they are:
   a. effective and inexpensive.
   b. have less adverse effects than other antidepressants.
   c. more effective than other antidepressants.
   d. not toxic if taken in excessive doses.

▶ 5. A patient who did not experience relief of depression after taking a tricyclic antidepressant was instructed to stop taking his prescription for amitriptyline hydrochloride (Elavil) 2 weeks ago. He has now been prescribed an MAO inhibitor. Because of possible interactions if the patient did not stop taking the amitriptyline when instructed, the nurse should assess for which of the following possible reactions?
   a. Complete AV block
   b. Flushed skin
   c. Hypertension
   d. Mydriasis

6. Tricyclic antidepressant (TCA) and selective serotonin reuptake inhibitor (SSRI) properties include: (Select all that apply.)
   a. effect on neurotransmitters occurs rapidly.
   b. effect on neurotransmitters occurs slowly.
   c. serious adverse effects can occur if combined with MAO inhibitor antidepressants.
   d. therapeutic effects occur rapidly.
   e. therapeutic effects occur slowly.

▶ 7. The nursery nurse notes that a neonate, whose mother has been taking fluoxetine (Prozac) for major depression throughout pregnancy, is tremulous and very irritable. Which of the following assessment findings, noted when the neonate is crying, would be of most concern to the nurse?
   a. Difficulty calming
   b. Flexed extremities
   c. Respiratory distress
   d. Tachycardia

8. The nurse notes bruxism in the history of a patient who is prescribed an SSRI. The nurse assesses the patient for:
   a. abnormal mouth movements.
   b. jaw pain.
   c. restlessness.
   d. tremors.

9. The nurse would be most concerned about the potential for hyponatremia if a patient exhibited nausea and anorexia and was prescribed fluoxetine (Prozac) and:
   a. candesartan.
   b. enalapril.
   c. hydrochlorothiazide.
   d. spironolactone.

▶ 10. Which of these laboratory test results, if identified in a patient who is receiving fluoxetine and warfarin, should the nurse report to the prescriber immediately?
   a. AST 30 International Units/L
   b. Creatinine 0.8 mg/dL
   c. INR 4.5
   d. Platelets 250,000/m$^3$

11. The nurse should question which of the following orders?
   a. Fluoxetine (Prozac) 20 mg by mouth once a day HS
   b. Fluoxetine 10 mg twice a day by mouth 8:00 AM and 12:00 PM
   c. Fluoxetine (Serafem) 20 mg by mouth days 14 to 28 of menstrual cycle
   d. Discontinue fluoxetine today (Monday) and start enteric-coated fluoxetine (Prozac Weekly) 90 mg by mouth once a week next Monday

12. Paroxetine (Paxil CR) differs significantly from paroxetine hydrochloride (Paxil) in:
   a. better absorption when administered with food.
   b. dose.
   c. length of action.
   d. less nausea and diarrhea.

13. The nurse would be especially vigilant to assess the patient for unexplained bleeding when a patient is prescribed fluoxetine and:
   a. an antihistamine.
   b. lithium.
   c. low-dose aspirin therapy.
   d. a thiazide diuretic.

14. Which of these factors, if identified in the history of a patient receiving duloxetine (Cymbalta), would be a concern to the nurse?
   a. Diabetic neuropathy
   b. Glaucoma
   c. Hypernatremia
   d. Musculoskeletal pain

15. Which of the following foods could be included in the diet of a patient who is prescribed the MAO inhibitor isocarboxazid (Marplan)?
   a. Cheddar cheese
   b. Chocolate
   c. Fava beans
   d. Roast beef

▶ 16. A patient complains to the nurse that he has been experiencing erectile dysfunction since he was prescribed paroxetine (Paxil). The best response by the nurse would be to:
   a. encourage the patient to share this concern with the prescriber.
   b. instruct the patient to not take the antidepressant on weekends.
   c. suggest the patient ask the prescriber to change his prescription to bupropion (Wellbutrin).
   d. withhold the drug until the issue is resolved.

▶ 17. Which of the following laboratory results would be of greatest concern to the nurse when a patient is receiving nefazodone?
   a. AST 356 International Units/L
   b. BUN 22 mg/dL
   c. Na 146 mEq/L
   d. WBC 11,000/mm$^3$

▶ 18. The nurse has received reports on patients who have recently been prescribed the following antidepressant medication and are experiencing the noted adverse effects. Which patient is of highest priority for the nurse?
   a. Amitriptyline—sleepiness and constipation
   b. Fluoxetine—nausea and diarrhea
   c. Tranylcypromine (Parnate)—headache and vomiting
   d. Venlafaxine—anorexia and sweating

19. It is most important for the nurse to teach a patient who has been prescribed trazodone (Desyrel) to:
   a. drink at least 2500 mL of fluid each day.
   b. increase fluid and fiber in diet to prevent constipation.
   c. report any symptoms of a urinary tract infection.
   d. seek medical care if an erection does not subside after ejaculation with sexual intercourse.

20. A patient has been taking St. John's Wort for minor depression. The nurse should teach the patient that (to):
    a. protect the skin from sun exposure.
    b. research has proven the product is as effective as antidepressant drugs for mild depression.
    c. the substance has not been proven to be effective.
    d. the substance is completely safe because it is natural and not a drug.

21. Matching antidepressants and associated adverse effects.

| | |
|---|---|
| _____ a. Bupropion | 1. Anticholinergic effects |
| _____ b. MAO inhibitors | 2. Cardiotoxicity |
| _____ c. Mirtazapine | 3. CNS stimulation |
| _____ d. SSRI | 4. Headache |
| _____ e. TCA | 5. Hypertensive crisis from eating foods containing tyramine |
| | 6. Hyponatremia |
| | 7. Insomnia |
| | 8. Nausea |
| | 9. Orthostatic hypotension |
| | 10. Sedation |
| | 11. Seizures |
| | 12. Sexual dysfunction |

## CASE STUDIES AND PATIENT TEACHING

*(Use a separate piece of paper for your responses.)*

### Case Study 1

*A 28-year-old mother of two, who is a high school science teacher, comes to the community mental health center at her family's urging because of lack of interest in usual activities, difficulty concentrating, excessive sleepiness, and feeling "down" every day for the past 3 months. Desipramine (Norpramin) 50 mg at bedtime is prescribed.*

1. Developmentally, what are the advantages of this particular TCA for this patient?

2. The patient is hopeful that the medication will help. She asks "If the drugs work, why do I have to meet with the doctor every week?" What is the basis of the response to this question?

3. What symptoms should the patient, family members, and/or caregivers be told to report?

4. The patient asks why the drug is supposed to be taken at bedtime. How should the nurse respond?

5. What teaching should the nurse provide regarding these common adverse effects of tricyclic antidepressants?
    a. Sedation
    b. Orthostatic hypotension
    c. Anticholinergic effects

6. The patient is concerned about cost because the prescriber has only prescribed 1 week's supply at a time. What would be the rationale for such a small prescription amount?

7. The patient is admitted for an inguinal herniorrhaphy. When providing history information, the patient states that she has been taking desipramine (Norpramin) 200 mg at bedtime for 3 months. She tells the nurse that some nights she forgets to take the medication, but does not feel bad the next day. She states that she thinks she must not need the medication any more. How should the nurse respond?

### Case Study 2

*A patient has been experiencing major depression for over 1 year without relief despite compliance with cognitive-behavioral therapy and pharmacotherapy with a TCA. Later the patient was switched to an SSRI antidepressant. The patient has been admitted to the inpatient psychiatric unit and received electroconvulsant therapy 3 times a week for the past 2 weeks.*

1. What should be included in the nurse's assessment and documentation?

2. The psychiatrist has explained that the discharge treatment plan includes prescribing phenelzine (Nardil), an MAO inhibitor antidepressant. The patient discontinued taking fluoxetine (Prozac) before admission and is anxious to start taking the new antidepressant. How should the nurse respond to the patient's concern?

3. What teaching would be important for the nurse to provide to the patient's significant others on discharge?

4. What teaching should the nurse provide about the prescribed phenelzine (Nardil)?

# 33 Drugs for Bipolar Disorder

## OBJECTIVES

See page 26 for the Objectives.

## CRITICAL THINKING AND STUDY QUESTIONS

1. Which of the following statements about bipolar disorder (BPD) are true? (Select all that apply.)
   a. All patients alternate between mania and depression, but length of episodes vary.
   b. Cause is an unstable personality.
   c. It is a chronic condition.
   d. Involves atrophy of brain regions involved with emotion.
   e. Manic episodes are always distressing to the patient.
   f. Requires treatment for life.

2. A patient is admitted with an acute mixed episode of BPD. The patient is started on a valproic acid and bupropion. A priority nursing concern is:
   a. electrolyte imbalances.
   b. hydration.
   c. safety.
   d. toxicity.

3. A nurse is reviewing laboratory tests of a patient receiving lithium carbonate for an acute episode of BPD. Which of the following results should the nurse report to the prescriber immediately?
   a. ALT 30 International Units/L
   b. Creatinine 2.7 mg/dL
   c. Sodium 132 mEq/L
   d. Potassium 4 mEq/L

4. The nurse is caring for a patient on a medical-surgical unit who is receiving lithium for BPD, which is currently not symptomatic. Which of the following treatments could increase lithium levels and cause toxicity? (Select all that apply.)
   a. Colonic cleansing preparation for colonoscopy
   b. Foley catheter insertion
   c. Frequent dressing change on a diabetic wound
   d. Hemodialysis
   e. Nasogastric suctioning
   f. Repeated hypoglycemic episodes with diaphoresis

5. The most common cause of lithium toxicity is:
   a. overdose of medication.
   b. renal failure.
   c. sodium depletion.

6. When administering valproic acid (Depakote), which of the following observations would be a reason to hold the medication and contact the prescriber? (Select all that apply.)
   a. Constant midepigastric pain radiating to the back
   b. LMP 38 days ago
   c. Nausea, vomiting, and very dark colored urine
   d. Pale conjunctiva
   e. Petechiae
   f. Temperature 102.4° F
   g. Warm, hot skin and fruity breath

7. The CBC on a patient who is scheduled to receive the first dose of carbamazepine includes hemoglobin 14.5 gm/dL, platelets 170,000/mm$^3$, reticulocyte count 2%, and WBC 6600/mm$^3$. The nurse should:
   a. administer the medication as ordered.
   b. hold the medication and assess the patient.
   c. hold the medication and consult the prescriber.
   d. hold the medication and page the prescriber STAT.

8. When administering lithium carbonate, which of the following assessments would indicate that therapy has achieved the desired effect?
   a. Flight of ideas
   b. Pressured speech
   c. Sit and watch TV for 8 hours per day
   d. Sleep 8 hours per night

9. A patient has decided to try fish oil to treat her BPD. It is important for this patient to decrease intake of:
   a. dairy products.
   b. processed grains.
   c. red meat.
   d. vegetable oils.

## CASE STUDIES AND PATIENT TEACHING

*(Use a separate piece of paper for your responses.)*

### Case Study 1

*A 35-year-old female who has a history of BPD, hypertension, osteoarthritis, and environmental allergies has stopped taking her prescribed valproic acid (Depakote). She is brought to the hospital because she has become increasingly hyperexcitable over the past 5 days. She has talked on the phone almost continuously because she says she is trying to start a business. She has called friends and relatives all over the country at all hours of the night to tell them her news. She went on a spending spree to buy new clothes and equipment for her business venture and accumulated almost $10,000 worth of bills before she was caught for writing bad checks. Her husband was called when she tried to purchase a car, and the bank reported that she had insufficient funds to cover the check. She was brought to the hospital in an acute manic state. On admission she moves about restlessly, waving her arms in a threatening manner while loudly berating her husband and the hospital staff. She demands to be released from "this jail" and curses the nurse who interviewed her.*

1. Why might this patient have stopped taking her medication?

2. The physician prescribes lithium carbonate 300 mg 4 times a day. Why must lithium be taken in divided daily doses?

3. The patient complains that she cannot play cards or write a letter. What should the nurse do?

4. The nurse has explained the importance of monitoring plasma lithium levels every 2 to 3 days until therapeutic levels have been reached and maintained and every 1 to 3 months once maintenance level dose has been established to the patient and family. What should the nurse teach about other times that the patient should consult her physician about the need for additional monitoring?

5. What measures can the nurse teach the patient to prevent fluctuations in lithium levels?

6. What is the therapeutic range of plasma lithium for maintenance therapy, and at what point are lithium levels critical?

7. Adherence to drug therapy is often an obstacle to managing BPD. How can the nurse increase the likelihood of this patient taking her medication and participate in therapy as prescribed?

8. What teaching does the nurse need to provide to the patient and family relating to prescribed and OTC drugs that relate to the patient's medical history?

# 34 Sedative-Hypnotic Drugs

## OBJECTIVES

See page 26 for the Objectives.

## CRITICAL THINKING AND STUDY QUESTIONS

1. Match the effect of benzodiazepines with the affected area of the brain.

| | | |
|---|---|---|
| _____ | a. Anterograde amnesia | 1. Cerebral cortex and hippocampus |
| _____ | b. Confusion | 2. Cortical areas |
| _____ | c. Muscle relaxation | 3. Limbic system |
| _____ | d. Promote sleep | 4. Supraspinal motor areas |
| _____ | e. Reduce anxiety | |

2. Lipid solubility of benzodiazepines: (Select all that apply.)
   a. causes induction of hepatic metabolizing enzymes.
   b. decreases the risk that the drug will cause congenital defects.
   c. extends plasma half-life.
   d. increases absorption.
   e. improves distribution to CNS.

▶ 3. Although benzodiazepines are weak respiratory depressants, the nurse must be cautious with what situations that increase the risk that respiratory depression will cause significant problems?
   a. Breast-fed infant
   b. COPD
   c. Neonate if given near time of birth
   d. Obstructive sleep apnea
   e. Partial airway obstruction

▶ 4. A patient asks for a sleeping pill at 2200. She states that she can fall asleep but awakens during the night and has difficulty getting back to sleep. The MAR lists triazolam (Halcion) 0.125 mg hs PRN. The nurse should:
   a. administer the triazolam.
   b. administer the triazolam and communicate the need to assess for effectiveness.
   c. contact the prescriber and discuss the need for a slower onset hypnotic.
   d. hold the triazolam because it is not effective in this situation.

5. A patient asks why she cannot use a sleeping pill to help her anxiety if they are both the same kind of medication. The basis of the nurse's explanation is that the principle determinant of the use of specific benzodiazepines is the drug's:
   a. pharmacodynamics.
   b. pharmacokinetics.
   c. potential for abuse.
   d. tolerance profile.

6. A patient is admitted after taking an overdose of a benzodiazepine and alcohol. The nurse would expect to administer which of the following antidotes?
   a. acetylcysteine (Mucomyst)
   b. flumazenil (Romazicon)
   c. naloxone (Narcan)
   d. vitamin $K_1$ (Mephyton)

▶ 7. A priority nursing concern for a patient who is receiving a benzodiazepine is:
   a. gastric distress.
   b. potential for abuse.
   c. respiratory depression.
   d. safety.

8. A patient who is taking zolpidem (Ambien) is at risk for exhibiting which symptoms of common adverse effects?
   a. Dizziness
   b. Hypertension
   c. Sweating
   d. Tremors

9. Characteristics of benzodiazepine-like drug zolpidem (Ambien) include: (Select all that apply.)
   a. can intensify the effects of other CNS depressants.
   b. metabolized into an inactive compound.
   c. moderate muscle relaxation.
   d. prevents seizures.
   e. prolongs periods of uninterrupted sleep.
   f. promotes falling asleep.
   g. rapid onset.
   h. reduces REM sleep.
   i. reduced doses used in people with liver impairment.
   j. significant rebound insomnia if suddenly discontinued.

10. A patient awakens at 0300 and asks the nurse for medication because she cannot fall back to sleep. Which of the following as needed medications, if prescribed for this patient, would be appropriate to administer at this time?
    a. eszopiclone (Lunesta)
    b. temazepam (Restoril)
    c. zaleplon (Sonata)
    d. zolpidem (Ambien)

11. Tolerance to barbiturates does not produces cross-tolerance to:
    a. alcohol.
    b. benzodiazepines.
    c. general anesthetics.
    d. opiates.

12. A child who received a severe head injury is in a barbiturate-induced coma. The child's parents ask the nurse why he is being kept unconscious. They want the drug to be stopped so they can see if he will respond. The best explanation is that this therapy:
    a. decreases the brain's need for oxygen and glucose.
    b. lowers the patient's blood pressure and pulse.
    c. produces amnesia so the child will not remember the accident.
    d. relaxes skeletal muscle so the patient is not uncomfortable.

13. Barbiturates are contraindicated for a patient with porphyria. Symptoms of porphyria include:
    a. confusion, disorientation, and weakness.
    b. hypotension, bradycardia, and bradypnea.
    c. nausea, abdominal colic, behavioral and neuromuscular disturbances.
    d. restlessness, insomnia, and hyperthermia.

▶ 14. The nurse should assess for which symptoms in a patient with a suspected barbiturate overdose?
    a. Apnea and hyperthermia
    b. Bradypnea and constricted pupils
    c. Hypertension and hypothermia
    d. Hypotension and dilated pupils

▶ 15. A nursing priority for a patient during immediate care after overdose on a barbiturate is:
    a. circulation.
    b. hydration.
    c. oxygenation.
    d. safety.

16. Patients with depression sometimes experience insomnia. The nurse recognizes that in addition to being a symptom of the disorder, insomnia is an adverse effect of some antidepressants. Which antidepressant is effective in treating depression-associated insomnia?
    a. bupropion (Wellbutrin)
    b. fluoxetine (Prozac)
    c. fluvoxamine (Luvox)
    d. trazodone (Desyrel)

17. An elderly patient occasionally uses diphenhydramine (Sominex) for insomnia. A nursing teaching to prevent common adverse effects is:
    a. increase fiber in diet.
    b. limit fluids.
    c. low-fat diet.
    d. take medication with food.

18. A patient asks the nurse about use of melatonin for insomnia. Teaching should include: (Select all that apply.)
    a. existing research suggests 2 mg of a controlled-release formula taken 2 hours before bedtime is most effective.
    b. it is a dietary supplement and is not closely regulated.
    c. it relieved insomnia in a study of blind insomniacs.
    d. studies have shown that melatonin is effective in preventing jet lag.
    e. there is no guarantee that product purchased contains the exact amount of melatonin as listed on the label.

## CASE STUDIES AND PATIENT TEACHING

*(Use a separate piece of paper for your responses.)*

### Case Study 1

*An 18-year-old college student comes to the outpatient department of a local mental health center. She expresses worries about upcoming exams, states that she cannot sleep, cannot concentrate on her studies, has felt her heart pound, is dizzy, and has trouble catching her breath. These symptoms are unusual for her and began several weeks ago.*

1. What additional data should the nurse collect about the patient's symptoms?

2. The patient is placed on alprazolam (Xanax) 0.25 mg 3 times a day with instructions to return to the mental health center in 2 weeks. Practically all responses to benzodiazepines, such as Xanax, result from actions in the CNS. Briefly describe the mechanism of action of benzodiazepines and barbiturates and explain why benzodiazepines are preferred over barbiturates and other general CNS depressants for anxiety and insomnia.
   a. Benzodiazepines
   b. Barbiturates

3. Why is it imperative that patients on benzodiazepines be cautioned against combining them with alcohol?

4. What information should be included in your health teaching plan for this patient?

### Case Study 2

*A 73-year-old man who lives alone is brought into the emergency department with multiple contusions and abrasions. He contacted the police and reported an intruder after awakening in the morning and finding his home in disarray, his clothing torn, and bruises aver his body. The police report that there is no evidence of forced entry and all portals of entry were locked. The patient has no memory of what occurred during the night. When taking the history, the nurse discovers that the patient took triazolam (Halcion) 0.25 mg at 0100.*

1. What possible adverse effects of this drug could have caused this situation?

### Case Study 3

*The nurse is preparing to administer an intravenous benzodiazepine for status epilepticus.*

1. Describe precautions that the nurse needs to take in this situation.

### Case Study 4

*A patient with a known history of alcohol abuse is brought into the emergency department unconscious. His wife states that he has been taking chlordiazepoxide (Librium) for alcohol withdrawal. His wife found him unresponsive, smelling of alcohol, with an empty pill bottle beside him. Assessment includes respirations 4 per minute. A decision to administer an antidote to the benzodiazepine is made before blood levels of the drug are available.*

1. Why are blood levels of a benzodiazepine not extremely significant?

2. Flumazenil (Romazicon) 0.2 mg followed by a second dose of 0.3 mg 30 seconds later is prescribed by intravenous push. The drug is available in 0.1 mg/mL. How much drug should the nurse administer every 5 seconds?

3. After the second dose, the patient becomes responsive, and VS stabilize within normal limits. Why is it important for the nurse to continue to closely assess this patient?

## Case Study 5

*A patient who has been receiving benzodiazepine therapy for a long time has been notified that her insurance will no longer cover the medication.*

1. What are possible effects of sudden discontinuation of the drug?

2. What can the nurse do to help this patient?

# 35 Management of Anxiety Disorders

## OBJECTIVES

See page 26 for the Objectives.

## CRITICAL THINKING AND STUDY QUESTIONS

1. Which of the following statements about anxiety disorders and their treatment are true? (Select all that apply.)
   a. Acute anxiety, generalized anxiety, obsessive-compulsive, panic, phobia, and post-traumatic stress disorders are all primary anxiety disorders.
   b. Benzodiazepines are approved for use for three major anxiety disorders—generalized anxiety disorder, obsessive-compulsive disorder, and phobias.
   c. Cognitive behavioral therapy combined with drug therapy is effective for panic disorder.
   d. Depression often co-exists with anxiety disorders.
   e. Generalized anxiety disorder (GAD) is an acute condition.
   f. Onset of relief from anxiety with lorazepam (Ativan) and buspirone (BuSpar) is rapid.
   g. Principle adverse effects of buspirone (BuSpar) include sedation and psychomotor slowing.
   h. Selective serotonin reuptake inhibitors (SSRIs) are effective against anxiety even when depression is not present.
   i. Supportive, cognitive behavioral, and/or relaxation therapy is usually all that is needed in mild to moderate anxiety disorders.
   j. Symptoms of situational anxiety may be intense, but they are temporary.

▶ 2. A nurse is admitting a patient who is scheduled for outpatient cataract surgery. The patient had been instructed to take her levothyroxine (Synthroid) with a sip of water in the morning before coming to the hospital. The patient reveals that she was extremely anxious so she also took a lorazepam (Ativan), but only with the same sip of water "about 1 hour ago." Which of the following nursing actions would be of the greatest priority?
   a. Assessing for abuse of benzodiazepines
   b. Determining if the patient had signed all of the needed consents before coming to the hospital
   c. Ensuring that the patient understands the preoperative teaching
   d. Notifying anesthesia of the medications taken this morning

3. The nurse is preparing to administer buspirone (BuSpar) to a patient who has been taking the drug for 2 months for situational anxiety following a divorce. Important nursing considerations include:
   a. assessing for suicidal ideation because of increased incidence of sucide in patients taking this drug.
   b. safety precautions because of sedation.
   c. teaching to avoid drinking grapefruit juice.
   d. teaching to not discontinue this drug suddenly.

4. Match the drug with the possible effects.

| |  | |  |
|---|---|---|---|
| _____ | a. Atypical antidepressant (venlafaxine) | 1. | Abrupt discontinuance can produce withdrawal |
| _____ | b. Benzodiazepines (alprazolam and lorazepam) | 2. | No abuse potential |
| _____ | c. Buspirone (BuSpar) | 3. | CNS depressant |
| _____ | d. MAO inhibitors | 4. | Can be used as needed (PRN) |
| _____ | e. SSRI (paroxetine and escitalopram) | 5. | Do not use with MAO inhibitor |
| _____ | f. TCA | 6. | Dysrhythmias can occur with overdose |
| | | 7. | Foods can cause hypertensive crisis |
| | | 8. | Hypertension |
| | | 9. | Can increase anxiety early in therapy |
| | | 10. | Nausea common adverse effect |
| | | 11. | Rapid onset |
| | | 12. | Sedates and slows movement |
| | | 13. | Slow onset |
| | | 14. | Spacey feeling |

5. The nurse is caring for a patient who has been diagnosed with panic disorder. Teaching should include:
   a. avoid strenuous exercise because it increases anxiety.
   b. drug therapy helps patient be more comfortable with situations and places they have been avoiding.
   c. importance of adequate, regular sleep habits.
   d. symptoms usually last 1 to 2 hours.

6. The nurse notes that a patient becomes very upset when the nurse rearranges any object in the room. The nurse would expect to find which diagnosis in the patient's history?
   a. Obsessive-compulsive disorder
   b. Panic disorder
   c. Social anxiety disorder
   d. Situational anxiety

▶ 7. When administering sertraline (Zoloft) for OCD, which of the following outcomes would indicate that therapy has achieved the desired effect?
   a. Go to market without experiencing palpitations, chest pain, dizziness, and fear of losing control.
   b. Ride in elevators without experiencing an anxiety attack.
   c. Sleep 7 to 8 hours per night.
   d. Touch people without fear of contamination.

8. Matching

| |  | |  |
|---|---|---|---|
| ▶ _____ | a. Agoraphobia | 1. | Anxiety when thinks cannot leave a room or situation |
| _____ | b. GAD | 2. | Chronic uncontrollable worrying |
| _____ | c. OCD | 3. | Intense irrational fear of embarrassment |
| _____ | d. Panic disorder | 4. | Persistent uncontrollable thinking and repetitive actions |
| _____ | e. PTSD | 5. | Re-experiencing, avoidance and/or emotional, numbing, and hyperarousal |
| _____ | f. Social anxiety disorder | 6. | Sudden anxiety attacks that may include fear of dying or going crazy |

## CASE STUDIES AND PATIENT TEACHING

*(Use a separate piece of paper for your responses.)*

### Case Study 1

*A 58-year-old woman with a history of 70 pack-years of tobacco use is admitted with exacerbated chronic obstructive pulmonary disease. The patient is very demanding. During care the patient states that she constantly worries about things that might go wrong.*

*She has not been sleeping and has difficulty completing daily tasks because of weakness and fatigue.*

1. What should the nurse do?

2. The nurse tries nonpharmacologic interventions to relieve the patient's anxiety without success. The physician orders alprazolam (Xanax) 0.5 mg 3 times a day. What should the nurse include in her teaching about this benzodiazepine drug?

3. A daughter comes to visit and expresses concern about her mother receiving a benzodiazepine drug. She states that her mother has a history of alcohol abuse, but has not had a drink for several years. How should the nurse respond to this information?

4. A consult is ordered, and the patient is diagnosed with generalized anxiety disorder and history of alcohol abuse. Alprazolam (Xanax) is discontinued, and buspirone (BuSpar) 7.5 mg twice a day is ordered. Why is this drug a good choice for this patient?

5. The patient complains that the drug is not working. She asks if she can take an extra dose. How should the nurse respond?

# 36 Central Nervous System Stimulants and Attention-Deficit/Hyperactivity Disorder

## OBJECTIVES

See page 26 for the Objectives.

## CRITICAL THINKING AND STUDY QUESTIONS

1. Indications for the use of CNS stimulants include: (Select all that apply.)
   a. ADHD.
   b. antidote for CNS depressant poisoning.
   c. depression.
   d. narcolepsy.
   e. obesity.

2. An 8-year-old child being treated with methylphenidate (Ritalin) for ADHD is taken back to an examination room by the nurse in the pediatrician's office. What subjective and objective data should the nurse collect?

▸ 3. The elementary school nurse cares for children who receive CNS stimulant drugs for ADHD. The child comes into the office complaining of not feeling well. Which of the following assessment findings would be a concern?
   a. BP 120/84 mm Hg
   b. Heart rate 100 beats/min
   c. Respirations 22 per minute
   d. Weight gain of 2 lbs since last year

4. A patient asks the nurse why her physician will not prescribe amphetamines to help her lose weight. Her mother took them and lost weight. The nurse's response should be based on amphetamines:
   a. are ineffective for weight loss.
   b. can cause hypotension and bradycardia.
   c. can unmask latent bipolar disorder.
   d. causes physical and psychologic dependence.

▸ 5. A patient with a history of narcolepsy, treated with Dexedrine spansules, is first day postoperative after a right knee replacement. He has become agitated and is refusing all treatments including pain medications. He accuses the staff of trying to hurt him. Which of the following most strongly supports that these paranoid ideas are a result of high-dose therapy with an amphetamine?
   a. Symptoms resolve within 24 hours of oral administration of chlorpromazine (Thorazine).
   b. Symptoms resolve when haloperidol (Haldol) is administered intramuscularly.
   c. Symptoms resolve within 48 hours of discontinuation of the Dexedrine.
   d. Symptoms resolve within 1 week of discontinuation of the Dexedrine.

6. A child who has been prescribed Metadate CD for ADHD is having difficulty swallowing the medication. The nurse suggests:
   a. crushing the medication and mixing it in a small amount of applesauce.
   b. notifying the prescriber; the medication must be taken whole.
   c. opening the capsule and sprinkling the beads in a small amount of soft food and telling the child to be careful not to chew the beads.
   d. opening the capsule and mixing the contents with 1 ounce of fluid.

7. A child who has been diagnosed with ADHD responded poorly to methylphenidate (Ritalin) 10 mg twice a day. If the prescriber stops the methylphenidate and prescribes dexmethylphenidate (Focalin), what dose of dexmethylphenidate would be equivalent to the Ritalin?
   a. Equal to the total methylphenidate dose but once a day
   b. One-half the methylphenidate dose
   c. The same as the methylphenidate dose
   d. Twice the methylphenidate dose

8. A nurse's aide is experiencing a headache aura. Caffeine often helps prevent a full-blown migraine. She asks the nurse which of the following beverages has the most caffeine?
   a. Pepsi Cola 12 ounces
   b. Snapple iced tea 12 ounces
   c. Sprite 12 ounces
   d. Sunkist orange soda 12 ounces

9. Research suggests that moderately heavy caffeine consumption (500mg/day) during human pregnancy is associated with:
   a. birth defects.
   b. chromosomal damage.
   c. first trimester spontaneous abortion.
   d. sudden infant death syndrome (SIDS).

▸ 10. A loading dose of caffeine citrate (Cafcit) 60 mg has been prescribed for a neonate who weighs 6 lbs 10 ounces and is experiencing prolonged periods of apnea and bradycardia. The drug comes in a concentration of 20 mg/mL. How much caffeine citrate should the nurse administer?
   a. 0.66 mL
   b. 3 mL
   c. 20 mL
   d. None without consulting the pharmacy and/or prescriber. The dose is higher than the recommended dose.

11. Which of these assessment findings, if identified in a patient who is receiving pemoline (Cylert) should the nurse report to the prescriber immediately?
   a. Anorexia and insomnia
   b. Dark urine and nausea
   c. Headache and abdominal pain
   d. Lethargy and listlessness

12. Modafinil (Provigil) has been prescribed for a 22-year-old woman who works rotating shifts. When teaching about this drug, the nurse should include: (Select all that apply.)
   a. do not take with food because absorption of the drug will be decreased.
   b. orthostatic blood pressure precautions.
   c. take as soon as awakening because the drug can cause insomnia.
   d. use a second form of birth control if using oral contraceptives.

13. Atomoxetine (Strattera) is a newer drug for ADHD. Which of the following statements about this drug are true?
   a. It is approved for use in ADHD in adults.
   b. It has a moderate potential for abuse.
   c. It has a risk of liver injury.
   d. It takes 2 to 3 weeks before therapeutic effects develop.
   e. Patients doing well on stimulant drugs should be switched to Strattera because it is safer and more effective.

f. Patients with an atypical form of the CYP2D6 metabolizing enzyme of cytochrome P450 need higher doses of the drug to be effective.
g. Sexual dysfunction and urinary retention are possible adverse effects in adults.

## CASE STUDIES AND PATEINT TEACHING

*(Use a separate piece of paper for your responses.)*

### Case Study 1

*The school nurse cares for a 7th-grade child who recently was diagnosed with ADHD, combined type. The mother had rejected the diagnosis previously because she does not like the idea of using medication. The child is prescribed methylphenidate (Ritalin) 10 mg 3 times a day. The mother speaks with the nurse when she delivers the medication and forms to the school. She verbalizes concern that she will be "drugging" her son and asks why behavioral therapy would not be sufficient.*

1. Based on current research, how will the nurse explain the rationale for drug therapy?

2. The nurse has been administering the second dose at 11:00 AM. The nurse is planning for the individual education plan (IEP) meeting with teachers, a counselor, and parents. She notes that the child has not been gaining weight. The child admits that he is not very hungry. In the meeting, the nurse learned that the mother gives the child methylphenidate at 6:30 AM before she leaves for work. The child eats his breakfast at school. The last dose is administered at 5:00 PM with dinner. What changes can be made to help improve the appetite of this child?

3. Most teachers at the IEP meeting share that the child's behavior has improved since starting medication. However, his organization and study skills are still very weak. Based on the expected therapeutic response to methylphenidate, what information can the nurse provide?

4. The fourth-period (10:15 to 11:00 AM) teacher states that the child is very sleepy in his class. What could have been happening to cause this sleepiness?

5. Several weeks later the child's mother comes in to see the nurse stating that the pediatrician has recommended that her son be switched to Metadate CD 20 mg once a day. She is concerned because "this is a newer drug, and they don't know enough about it." How should the nurse respond?

6. The child does well at school on Metadate CD but has difficulty once home getting his homework done and socially at after-school activities. The physician puts the child on Concerta. How does the nurse explain the difference between Concerta and Metadate CD?

7. What teaching should be provided about administration of Concerta?

### Case Study 2

*A 25-year-old female is seeking medical help for amphetamine dependence. She was prescribed amphetamines for weight loss several years ago and lost 100 lbs. She is now 5 feet 6 inches and weighs 130 lbs. She continued taking amphetamines after she reached her goal weight and now wants to stop taking the drug, but says she cannot do it alone. When she stops taking the amphetamines, she experiences withdrawal symptoms and becomes frightened so she continues to use the drug.*

1. What is the current medical opinion about taking amphetamines for weight loss?

2. What signs and symptoms would you expect the patient to exhibit when she is using amphetamines?

3. It is important to decrease the amphetamine slowly since the patient has previously experienced withdrawal symptoms. What withdrawal symptoms should the nurse be alert for when a patient is withdrawing from amphetamine use, and what nursing interventions can help the patient cope with these symptoms?

# 37 Drug Abuse I: Basic Considerations

## OBJECTIVES

See page 26 for the Objectives.

## CRITICAL THINKING AND STUDY QUESTIONS

1. Why is it important for nurses to be knowledgeable of the developmental level of patients and the beliefs of different cultures and individuals relating to drugs?

2. Addiction: Addictive behavior: (Select all that apply.)
   a. involves physical, psychologic, or social harm.
   b. involves reinforcement of pleasure or reduction in intensity of an unpleasant experience.
   c. involves activation of the brain's endorphin reward circuit.
   d. is a chronic relapsing illness.
   e. is a treatable disease.
   f. is present if the patient is physically dependent on a psychoactive substance.
   g. requires a pre-existing psychopathology.

3. Matching

| | | |
|---|---|---|
| _____ | a. Cross-dependence | 1. A particular dose elicits a less intense response |
| _____ | b. Cross-tolerance | 2. Abstinence syndrome will develop if drug is stopped |
| _____ | c. Physical dependence | 3. Intense subjective need for a drug |
| _____ | d. Psychologic dependence | 4. Symptoms often opposite of the normal effects of the drug |
| _____ | e. Tolerance | 5. When higher doses of a drug are needed because the person has abused another drug—usually in the same class |
| _____ | f. Withdrawal syndrome | 6. When one drug can prevent withdrawal from another drug |

4. Psychologic factors that have been associated with tendencies toward drug abuse would make it important for the nurse to provide drug abuse prevention for children who have been diagnosed with: (Select all that apply.)
   a. ADHD.
   b. anxiety.
   c. depression.
   d. developmental delay.

5. An example of addiction is an individual who experiences abstinence if he stops taking:
   a. amphetamines used to reduce symptoms of ADHD.
   b. OxyContin used for cancer pain.
   c. phenobarbital used to prevent seizures.
   d. tobacco used to reduce stress.

6. Drugs that the nurse can administer that have the highest potential for abuse and dependence are classified by the Controlled Substances Act as:
   a. schedule I.
   b. schedule II.
   c. schedule III.
   d. schedule IV.
   e. schedule V.

7. A patient has been prescribed hydrocodone 5 mg and acetaminophen 500 mg (Vicodin), a schedule IV drug. Federal regulations regarding refills of this drug are that it:
   a. cannot be refilled.
   b. may be refilled two times within 3 months.
   c. may be refilled five times within 6 months.
   d. may be refilled as many times as the prescriber specifies within 12 months.

8. When there are different laws on the state and federal level regarding prescribing controlled substances the:
   a. most restrictive law takes precedence.
   b. least restrictive law takes precedence.
   c. federal law takes precedence.
   d. state law takes precedence.

## CASE STUDIES AND PATIENT TEACHING

*(Use a separate piece of paper for your responses.)*

### Case Study 1

*The nurse is working on a drug and alcohol detoxification unit. Describe how the nurse's expertise can be applied to address the following issues of drug abuse:*

1. Diagnosis and treatment of toxicity.

2. Diagnosis and treatment of secondary medical complications.

3. Facilitating withdrawal.

4. Educating and counseling drug abusers in hopes of maintaining long-term abstinence.

# 38 Drug Abuse II: Alcohol

## OBJECTIVES

See page 26 for the Objectives.

## CRITICAL THINKING AND STUDY QUESTIONS

1. The nurse is caring for a patient with a history of chronic alcohol abuse. The patient is prescribed thiamin to prevent Wernicke's encephalopathy. The nurse should assess for symptoms of this disorder including:
   a. abnormal ocular movements.
   b. confabulation.
   c. confusion.
   d. inability to convert short-term memory to long-term memory.
   e. nystagmus.
   f. polyneuropathy.

2. Research suggests consumption of one alcoholic drink per day has been associated with:
   a. atrophy of the cerebrum.
   b. lower levels of HDL.
   c. improving the quality of sleep.
   d. preservation of cognitive functioning in the elderly.

▸ 3. A patient who has been a heavy drinker for 30 years is admitted with constant severe midepigastric pain radiating to the flank. Which of the following laboratory test results should be reported immediately to the physician?
   a. Amylase 500 International Units /L
   b. BNP 33 pg/mL
   c. Bilirubin 1 mg/dL
   d. Protein 6.5 gm/dL

4. For the average person with normal liver functioning, alcohol levels in the blood will begin to increase if a person consumes in 1 hour: (Select all that apply.)
   a. one (1.5 ounces) shot of whiskey.
   b. 8-ounce glass of wine.
   c. two (12 ounces) beers.

5. Matching: Effect of substances when combined with alcohol

| | | |
|---|---|---|
| _____ | a. Acetaminophen | 1. Counteracts effects when alcohol dose is high |
| _____ | b. Antihypertensives | 2. Increases risk of injury to GI mucosa |
| _____ | c. Benzodiazepines | 3. Increases risk of liver damage |
| _____ | d. Disulfiram | 4. Intensifies CNS depression |
| _____ | e. NSAID | 5. Produces nausea and vomiting; can produce death |

6. Chronic alcohol consumption does not produce tolerance to:
   a. activation of the reward circuit.
   b. decreased alertness.
   c. diminished reflexes.
   d. respiratory depression.

7. Which of the following benzodiazepine regimens has been shown to protect against seizures and breakthrough symptoms of alcohol withdrawal while promoting speedier withdrawal?
   a. Administered as needed in response to symptoms
   b. Administered as needed in response to symptoms in combination with another drug to reduce withdrawal symptoms
   c. Administered around-the-clock on a fixed schedule
   d. Administered around-the-clock in declining doses on a fixed schedule

8. Disulfiram (Antabuse) reactions can occur if a patient is exposed to alcohol and takes which of the following antimicrobial medications?
   a. azithromycin (Zithromax)
   b. gentamicin (Garamycin)
   c. metronidazole (Flagyl)
   d. cefazolin (Ancef)

▶ 9. A patient is admitted with a fractured hip and scheduled for surgery. It is important to inform the surgeon of the patient's history of alcohol abuse and use of naltrexone (ReVia) to assist with abstinence because:
   a. there are specific analgesic drugs that the patient should not receive.
   b. the patient is at risk for addiction to opioids used for postoperative pain.
   c. the patient should not receive any opioid analgesics for postoperative pain.
   d. usual doses of opioid analgesics for postoperative pain may be ineffective.

10. It is important for the nurse to teach a patient who has been prescribed acamprosate (Campral) to support abstinence from alcohol because:
    a. full effects do not occur for about a week.
    b. he needs to increase fluid and fiber in the diet to prevent diarrhea.
    c. severe hypotension can occur if alcohol is used while taking this drug.
    d. the drug blocks craving for alcohol.

11. Dietary counseling for a patient with alcohol abuse should include adequate servings of what type of food to prevent thiamin deficiency?
    a. Fruit
    b. Green leafy vegetables
    c. Milk
    d. Pork

## CASE STUDIES AND PATIENT TEACHING

*(Use a separate piece of paper for your responses.)*

### Case Study 1

*The nurse is caring for 45-year-old man with a history of alcohol abuse and cirrhosis of the liver who is newly admitted with gastrointestinal bleeding from ulcers.*

1. What would be appropriate nursing diagnoses and related assessments for this patient?

2. The patient's blood alcohol level is 0.320%. Chlordiazepoxide (Librium), a drug that is believed to enhance the action of GABA transmission in the CNS, was ordered at 100 mg IM STAT. The drug is then ordered by mouth at high doses with the dose decreasing every 3 days. What is the rationale for this treatment regimen?

3. What would be an appropriate nursing outcome for this patient relating to the reason for administrating chlordiazepoxide (Librium)?

4. The patient has been admitted once before for detoxification. He was discharged at that time on a maintenance dose of chlordiazepoxide (Librium). Based on the believed effects of alcohol on the CNS, why would this patient revert back to alcohol abuse?

5. After detoxification the patient states he is motivated to quit. He asks for disulfiram (Antabuse) to help him refrain from drinking. What teaching should the nurse provide to the patient and family about this drug?

6. Shortly after discharge, the patient stops taking the drug and resumes drinking. One morning, his wife crushes the disulfiram and puts it in his breakfast. The patient drinks alcohol and goes into shock and dies. What are possible consequences for the wife?

## Case Study 2

*Senior-level student nurses have just finished clinical hours in a local hospital ED and are having a postconference. They are discussing a 17-year-old female patient who was brought in during their shift and was resuscitated in the ED after acute overdose of alcohol. An adolescent accompanying the patient reported that the girl had drunk four shots in 15 minutes while playing a drinking game. They had not eaten anything for over 3 hours before starting the game.*

1. The nursing students identify which of the following as a priority nursing problem for this patient at this time?
   a. Airway clearance
   b. Anxiety
   c. Knowledge deficit
   d. Sensory perceptual alterations

2. The parents of the patient arrived at the ED. The girl's father asked how this could happen. He has had more than five drinks in an evening and has been fine. What factors contributed to the adolescent's extreme intoxication?

3. Once awake the patient reveals to the nurse that she is sexually active. What fetal problems can be encountered if this patient is pregnant?

# 39 Drug Abuse III: Major Drugs of Abuse (Other Than Alcohol)

## OBJECTIVES

See page 26 for the Objectives.

## CRITICAL THINKING AND STUDY QUESTIONS

1. A priority concern of the nurse when caring for an opioid addict who is experiencing abstinence syndrome is:
   a. central nervous system depression.
   b. preventing respiratory arrest.
   c. relapse to opioid use.
   d. timing of doses of nalmefene (Revex).

▶ 2. A patient who has a history of heroin abuse is brought into the emergency department unresponsive with pinpoint pupils. The nurse assesses that the patient has stopped breathing. In addition to supporting respirations, the patient is prescribed intravenous naloxone HCl (Narcan). The nurse notes an improvement in level of consciousness, respiratory rate, and effort within minutes. The most important action by

the nurse 30 to 40 minutes after administration of the naloxone is:
a. assessing the patient for withdrawal symptoms.
b. identifying the abused opioid.
c. monitoring of pulse and blood pressure.
d. reassessing for respiratory depression.

▸ 3. Which of the following would be the most accurate indicator to the nurse that the dose of methadone prescribed to minimize abstinence syndrome is inadequate?
a. Nurse notes that the patient has difficulty arising in the morning.
b. Nurse notes that the patient is experiencing vomiting and diarrhea.
c. Patient is exhibiting kicking motions.
d. Patient states that the dose is inadequate.

4. Which of the following statements, if made by a patient who has been prescribed clonidine for withdrawal from addiction to oxycodone (OxyContin), would indicate a need for further teaching?
a. "I'm glad that I won't feel like I need the drug."
b. "I need to be careful not to jump up out of bed too quickly."
c. "I should have less muscle pain if I take this drug."
d. "The medication should help prevent vomiting and diarrhea."

5. Which of the following outcomes best reflects the goal of administering methadone for suppressive therapy?
a. The patient does not experience abstinence syndrome.
b. The patient does not experience euphoria when taking opioids.
c. The patient does not experience respiratory depression.
d. The patient will not crave opioids.

6. A patient has been prescribed sublingual buprenorphine-naloxone (Suboxone) for long-term management of heroin addiction. It is important for the nurse to teach the patient that the drug should not be crushed, dissolved, and injected intravenously because this could cause:
a. an overdose.
b. heroin-induced euphoria.
c. respiratory depression.
d. withdrawal symptoms.

7. Research suggests that maintenance therapy with opioids for addicts who have abused opioids has a substantial risk for which of the following effects?
a. Abstinence syndrome if doses are missed
b. Inability to form relationships with other people
c. Increased risk for COPD
d. Lack of productivity

8. A known drug user is admitted to the emergency department. Assessment findings include bradypnea, pinpoint pupils, and unresponsive to painful stimuli. Overdose of which of the following drugs is known to cause these symptoms? (Select all that apply.)
a. Cannabis (marijuana)
b. Cocaine
c. dexadrine (Adderall)
d. Heroin
e. LSD
f. methadone (Dolophine)
g. methylphenidate (Ritalin)
h. MDMA (Ecstasy)
i. nalmefene (Revex)
j. oxycodone (OxyContin)
k. temazepam (Restoril)

▸ 9. A suspected overdose patient is brought into the emergency department unresponsive with pinpoint pupils. A priority nursing intervention is:
a. administering an antidote.
b. administering phenobarbital.
c. maintaining respirations.
d. preventing shock.

▸ 10. When responding to acute overdose of cocaine, which of the following outcomes would best indicate that therapy has been successful?
a. Adequate cardiac output
b. Sensory perceptions normal
c. Effective breathing pattern
d. Temperature 98° F to 99° F

11. The nurse is caring for a patient who has been admitted for amphetamine abuse. Assessment findings include T 99.4°F, BP 178/102 mm Hg, P 110 beats/min, respirations 25 per minute, productive cough, rhinorrhea, and coryza. The nurse should consult the prescriber before administering which of the following medications for cold and allergy symptoms?
a. chlorpheniramine (Chlor-Trimeton)
b. dextromethorphan (Benylin)
c. guaifenesin (Humibid)
d. pseudoephedrine (Sudafed)

12. Intravenous dantrolene (Dantrium) is prescribed if needed for a patient who has been admitted with adverse effects of taking MDMA (Ecstasy). Which of the following assessment findings would warrant administration of the dantrolene?
   a. Extreme anxiety and confusion
   b. Hallucinations and delusions
   c. Spasmodic jerking and elevated temperature
   d. Suicidal thoughts and behavior

13. A patient who has taken phencyclidine (PCP) is brought to the emergency room exhibiting combative behavior and hallucinations. An appropriate nursing intervention is:
   a. inserting an NG tube.
   b. reducing external stimuli.
   c. sodium bicarbonate administration.
   d. talking down.

14. A 9-month-old child is admitted to the emergency department after eating cigarettes. Which of the following assessment findings would be of most concern to the nurse?
   a. Apical pulse 145 beats/min
   b. Blood pressure 66/48 mm Hg
   c. Respirations 15 per minute
   d. Temperature 37° C

15. The nurse would withhold which of the following smoking cessation aid drugs and contact the prescriber if the patient exhibited seizure activity?
   a. bupropion (Zyban, Wellbutrin)
   b. nicotine patch (Nicotrol, Nicoderm CQ)
   c. nicotine lozenge (Commit)
   d. nortriptyline (Aventyl, Pamelor)

## CASE STUDIES AND PATIENT TEACHING

*(Use a separate piece of paper for your responses.)*

### Case Study 1

*A student nurse is working with a clinical group in the drug abuse section of the healthcare facility. A 43-year-old woman shares her story of drug abuse. She began drinking in high school and by 10th grade was getting drunk several times a week. She married an alcoholic and drank with him for many years. She then began taking diazepam (Valium) with her alcohol. She says she had hangovers in the mornings so she would have a beer or two and some amphetamines to "get myself together." She would also take a few aspirins for the headache and go to work feeling sick. As a rule, she would leave work at 5:00 PM, stop by the liquor store, then go home to watch TV, drink, and take a few diazepam to calm down. After a few years of this, she began to get crack cocaine from the streets. She was unable to do her job because she was either high or was in need of a fix, so she was fired. She stayed home and drank and found she was having difficulty buying the drugs. She would get into violent arguments with her husband. He physically abused her, and she finally left him and sought help at a women's shelter. She tried to stop using drugs many times over the years, but could only stop for a few days before she began to feel ill. She started stealing to support her habit. After being arrested for stealing, she was required to enter a treatment program.*

1. How has tolerance and physical dependence contributed to this person's drug abuse?

2. What assessments should the nurse perform to assess for drug withdrawal?

3. What interventions might the nurse employ to decrease the adverse effects of withdrawal?

## Case Study 2

*A school nurse is developing a program relating to preventing use of marijuana for 12- to 14-year old students. Complete the following teaching plan.*

| Prevention of Marijuana Abuse | |
|---|---|
| Teaching approaches based on thinking of 12- to 14-year-old according to Piaget | |
| Teaching approaches based on psychosocial developmental stage according to Erikson | |
| Desired environment for teaching | |
| Desired outcomes | |
| Developmentally appropriate content | |
| Method of teaching | |

## Case Study 3

*Debate the pros and cons of legalizing marijuana.*

## Case Study 4

*The nurse is creating a plan to prevent and/or address tobacco abuse using the Nola Pender revised Health Promotion Model (see below).*

1. Complete the following charts relating to the developmental stage as it influences promoting abstinence. Consider the personal sociocultural factors of the age group to identify behavior-specific cognitions and affect influencing tobacco use.

## INDIVIDUAL CHARACTERISTICS AND EXPERIENCES

- Personal sociocultural factors
  - Characteristics of the workers including race, ethnicity, education, and sociocultural factors that influence beliefs, affect, and performance of a health-promoting behavior

| Developmental stage | Personal sociocultural factors that influence tobacco use | How these characteristics influence ability and willingness to attempt health-promoting behavioral change |
|---|---|---|
| Young adult | | |
| Adult | | |
| Older adult | | |

## BEHAVIOR-SPECIFIC COGNITIONS AND AFFECT

- Perceived benefits of action
  - Positive effects the person thinks they will experience from not smoking
- Perceived barriers to action
  - Negative effects the person thinks they will experience if they smoke
- Perceived self-efficacy
  - Belief that the person can be successful
- Activity related affect
  - Positive and negative effects experienced when smoking or when being encouraged to smoke
- Interpersonal influences
  - Behaviors, beliefs, or attitudes of others that can influence the person's decision to smoke or not smoke
- Situational influences
  - Environmental factors that can influence the person's decision to smoke or not smoke

## Reference

Pender, N, et al: *Health promotion in nursing practice,* 4th ed., Upper Saddle River, NJ, Prentice Hall, 2002.

| Behavior-specific cognitions and affect relating to substance abuse | Young adult | Nursing interventions |
|---|---|---|
| Perceived benefits of action | | |
| Perceived barriers to action | | |
| Perceived self-efficacy | | |
| Activity related affect | | |
| Interpersonal influences | | |
| Situational influences | | |

| Behavior-specific cognitions and affect relating to tobacco use | Adult | Nursing interventions |
|---|---|---|
| Perceived benefits of action | | |
| Perceived barriers to action | | |
| Perceived self-efficacy | | |
| Activity related affect | | |
| Interpersonal influences | | |
| Situational influences | | |

| Behavior-specific cognitions and affect relating to tobacco use | Older adult | Nursing interventions |
|---|---|---|
| Perceived benefits of action | | |
| Perceived barriers to action | | |
| Perceived self-efficacy | | |
| Activity related affect | | |
| Interpersonal influences | | |
| Situational influences | | |

# 40 Diuretics

## OBJECTIVES

See page 26 for the Objectives.

## CRITICAL THINKING AND STUDY QUESTIONS

1. Matching

| | | |
|---|---|---|
| _____ | a. Filtration | 1. Most significant regulator of urine composition |
| _____ | b. Reabsorption | 2. Moves passively following osmotic gradient |
| _____ | c. Active tubular secretion | 3. Filtered then reabsorbed by active transport |
| _____ | d. Solutes | 4. Nonselective |
| _____ | e. Water | 5. Uses pumps selective for organic acids and organic bases for active transport |

2. The kidney produces approximately 180 L (180,000 mL) of filtrate each day. How much is normally excreted as urine in a day?
   a. 0.9 L
   b. 1.8 L
   c. 3.6 L
   d. 4.5 L

3. Most diuretics work by:
   a. blocking synthesis of pumps responsible for sodium and potassium transport in the distal nephron.
   b. acting on the collecting duct to increase permeability to water.
   c. blocking sodium and chloride reabsorption.
   d. blocking reabsorption of sodium in the distal nephron and increasing potassium reabsorption.

4. Diuretics that produce the most significant diuresis affect reabsorption in the:
   a. thick segment of the ascending Loop of Henle.
   b. early distal convoluted tubule.
   c. late distal convoluted tubule.
   d. collecting ducts.

5. A patient in heart failure who weighs 176 lbs has been prescribed a high-ceiling diuretic with the goal of loss of 500 mL of additional urine output in the next 24 hours. If this goal is met, the nurse would expect the patient's weight to be:
   a. 172 lbs.
   b. 173 lbs.
   c. 174 lbs.
   d. 175 lbs.

6. A patient in chronic renal failure has been retaining fluid despite dialysis. Which diuretic would the nurse expect to administer?
   a. bumetanide (Bumex)
   b. hydrochlorothiazide (Oretic, HydroDIURIL)
   c. metolazone (Zaroxolyn)
   d. spironolactone (Aldactone)

7. Research the mechanism of action of the diuretics furosemide (Lasix) and spironolactone (Aldactone). Explain why a prescriber may prescribe a lower dose of each of these medications instead of a higher dose of one of the drugs.

8. A patient with heart failure has been prescribed a high-ceiling diuretic. The assessment that most accurately reflects a therapeutic effect of this drug is:
   a. drop in systolic blood pressure of 10 mm/Hg.
   b. normal heart sounds.
   c. clear lung sounds.
   d. pulse 80 and regular.

▶ 9. A patient who has been diagnosed with heart failure (HF) and type diabetes mellitus (DM) has been prescribed furosemide (Lasix) 20 mg by mouth once a day. Based on the effect of furosemide on the patient's DM, it is important for the nurse to assess this patient for:
   a. irritability, paresthesias, and muscle weakness.
   b. diaphoresis, shakiness, and tachycardia.
   c. increased thirst, confusion, and dry, hot skin.
   d. nausea, vomiting, and diarrhea.

▶ 10. A patient is receiving a diuretic. The nurse takes orthostatic BP readings before administering the diuretic. Which change in orthostatic BP should be reported to the prescriber?
   a. 150/90 mm Hg lying; 125/70 mm Hg sitting
   b. 140/82 mm Hg lying; 125/72 mm Hg sitting
   c. 130/90 mm Hg lying; 118/78 mm Hg sitting
   d. 116/70 mm Hg lying; 110/68 mm Hg sitting

11. A patient has been prescribed a high-ceiling diuretic. Which of the following foods are important to include in the diet to prevent hypokalemia? (Select all that apply.)
   a. Bananas
   b. Beans
   c. Cheese
   d. Red meat
   e. Oranges
   f. Pork
   g. Raisins
   h. Spinach
   i. Yogurt

12. A patient has been prescribed a high-ceiling diuretic. The nurse should monitor lab tests for: (Select all that apply.)
   a. hypocalcemia.
   b. hypochloremia.
   c. hypoglycemia.
   d. hypokalemia.
   e. hypomagnesemia.
   f. hyponatremia.
   g. increased HDL.
   h. decreased triglycerides.
   i. elevated LDL.
   j. elevated uric acid.

13. Over-the-counter medications that can counteract the effects of diuretics include:
   a. acetaminophen.
   b. ibuprofen.
   c. iron.
   d. multiple vitamins.

14. The recommended diuretic for initial therapy of essential hypertension is a(n):
   a. high ceiling (loop).
   b. osmotic.
   c. potassium sparing.
   d. thiazide.

15. It is important for the nurse to assess for ototoxicity when a patient has been prescribed a high-ceiling diuretic and a(n):
   a. aminoglycoside antibiotic.
   b. cephalosporin antibiotic.
   c. macrolide antibiotic.
   d. penicillin antibiotic.

▶ 16. The nurse is reviewing the lab values for a patient who has been prescribed lithium carbonate for bipolar disorder and furosemide for HF. Which of the following electrolyte results would be a reason for concern?
   a. Chloride 100 mEq/L
   b. Magnesium 1.8 mEq/L
   c. Potassium 4.1 mEq/L
   d. Sodium 128 mEq/L

▶ 17. Patients with hypertension often need more than one antihypertensive drug. The nurse is doing an admission history and assessment. The patient states that she is taking several drugs for "high blood pressure." The nurse would assess for what symptoms that suggest hyperkalemia if the patient has been prescribed spironolactone (Aldactone) and Enalapril (Vasotec) or Triamterene (Dyrenium)?
   a. Disorientation, psychosis, and seizures
   b. Muscle weakness, hypotension, and sedation
   c. Confusion, anxiety, heavy legs, and tall T waves on ECG
   d. Skeletal muscle weakness and absent bowel sounds

18. An 18-year-old female has been prescribed spironolactone (Aldactone) for primary hyperaldosteronism. Developmentally, what would be a priority nursing diagnosis?

19. The nurse is preparing to administer mannitol (Osmitrol) to a patient. The nurse notes crystals in a clear solution. The nurse should:
   a. administer the solution.
   b. discard the solution.
   c. use an in-line filter.
   d. warm the solution to dissolve the crystals, cool to body temperature, and use an in-line filter.

## CASE STUDIES AND PATIENT TEACHING

*(Use a separate piece of paper for your responses.)*

### Case Study 1

*An 80-year-old nonsmoking woman has been taking spironolactone (Aldactone) 100 mg/day for about 6 years to control her moderate hypertension and mild heart failure (HF). She comes to the emergency department with bilateral crackles (rales) in the lower and middle lobes and a blood pressure of 190/120 mm/Hg. She is short of breath, very anxious, tachycardic (HR 134), and diaphoretic. Her family assures you that she has been taking her medication. The family tells you she has been getting worse over the past 2 weeks since having friends bring her lunches of hot dogs and potato chips every day. The physician diagnoses pulmonary edema and orders STAT intravenous push furosemide (Lasix) 40 mg and morphine sulfate 2 mg, 3 L of oxygen via nasal cannula, electrolytes, and complete blood count, and an indwelling Foley catheter.*

1. How will furosemide (Lasix) help relieve this patient's symptoms?

2. What information must the nurse know about furosemide (Lasix) administration before administering the drug intravenous push?

3. The drug handbook states that 40 mg of furosemide (Lasix) can be administered undiluted over 1 to 2 minutes; do not exceed 4 mg/min in patients with renal impairment. The nurse is unsure of the patient's renal status and plans to administer the drug over 10 minutes (4mg/min). The furosemide (Lasix) vial states 40 mg/4 mL. The 5-mL syringe is marked with a line every 0.2 mL. The nurse will administer 0.2 mL (one line) of furosemide (Lasix) over what time period?

4. Why was the Foley catheter ordered?

5. It has been 45 minutes since the patient received her furosemide (Lasix). Her Foley catheter is in place. She says that she is very thirsty. What assessments should be made at this point?

6. Lab results, drawn before she received any medication, have returned. Her sodium is 140 (135 to 145 mEq/L), chloride is 110 (98 to 106 mEq/L), and potassium is 3.5 (3.5 to 5 mEq/L). Knowing that she received her furosemide (Lasix) after these lab values were drawn, what should be included in the nurse's plan of action?

7. The patient improves significantly within the first 6 hours. Her blood pressure is 138/90 mm/HG, pulse 102, respirations 20, and rales are heard only in her bases bilaterally. She asks you how this could have happened since she had been taking her medicine as her physician prescribed. What should the nurse discuss with the patient as possible reasons for her condition?

8. What nursing assessments would be made on at least a daily basis while she is in the hospital?

9. The patient continues to improve and is being discharged home on furosemide (Lasix) 20 mg twice a day and spironolactone (Aldactone) 50 mg daily. What teaching should be provided regarding dietary patterns, activity, and signs and symptoms of further problems?

10. What information should the nurse provide to prevent problems with drug interactions?

11. The patient will need to be started on digoxin. What must the nurse remember now that the patient is on digoxin and furosemide (Lasix)? What laboratory values need to be monitored?

### Case Study 2

*A 42-year-old female patient who has recently been diagnosed with essential hypertension has described to the nurse a recent concern of overactive bladder. The prescriber has just prescribed hydrochlorothiazide (HydroDIURIL) to treat the hypertension.*

1. List some nursing concerns and teachings.

# 41 Agents Affecting the Volume and Ion Content of Body Fluids

## OBJECTIVES

See page 26 for the Objectives.

## CRITICAL THINKING AND STUDY QUESTIONS

1. Matching

| | | |
|---|---|---|
| _____ | a. Hypertonic contraction | 1. Vomiting, diarrhea |
| _____ | b. Hypotonic contraction | 2. HF, cirrhosis |
| _____ | c. Isotonic contraction | 3. Extensive burns, older adult |
| _____ | d. Volume expansion | 4. Diuretics, chronic renal failure |

2. Total osmolality of plasma is equal to approximately:
   a. the osmolality of sodium.
   b. twice the osmolality of sodium.
   c. the osmolality of potassium.
   d. twice the osmolality of potassium.

3. Matching (Answers may be used more than once.)

| | | |
|---|---|---|
| _____ | a. Metabolic acidosis | 1. Can occur if ventilator set too high |
| _____ | b. Respiratory acidosis | 2. Lung changes from smoking are a risk for this condition |
| _____ | c. Metabolic alkalosis | 3. May be associated with severe diarrhea of *clostridium difficile* infection |
| _____ | d. Respiratory alkalosis | 4. Seen in uncontrolled diabetes mellitus |
| | | 5. Treat with rebreathing $CO_2$ |
| | | 6. Treat with $O_2$, deep exhalations, and sodium bicarbonate |
| | | 7. Treat NaCl plus KCl to increase excretion of bicarbonate |
| | | 8. Correct cause and administer $NaHCO_3$ |

▸ 4. A 15-year-old girl with bulimia abuses laxatives. She is admitted to the hospital after experiencing extreme leg weakness. Potassium chloride 40 mEq by mouth twice a day has been prescribed. The nurse reviews the most recent laboratory tests before administering the patient's medications. Results include Na 137 mEq/L, K 3.7 mEq/L, and Cl 100 mEq/L. The nurse should:
   a. page the physician STAT.
   b. administer the medication.
   c. hold the medication and contact the physician.
   d. administer the medication and contact the physician.

5. The nurse is administering furosemide (Lasix) and sustained-release potassium chloride (K-Dur) to a patient with HF. The nurse notes that the patient is chewing the potassium chloride. The patient states she cannot swallow the large pill. The nurse should:
   a. crush the pill and mix it with applesauce or pudding.
   b. instruct the patient to drink at least 8 ounces of water with the potassium pill.
   c. contact the physician.
   d. page the physician STAT.

6. A patient is admitted with serum glucose level of 750 mg/dL. Intravenous regular insulin is prescribed to lower the patient's blood sugar. When administering insulin the nurse needs to assess the patient for:
   a. skeletal muscle weakness and absent bowel sounds (hypokalemia).
   b. disorientation, psychosis, and seizures (hypomagnesemia).
   c. muscle weakness, hypotension, and sedation (hypermagnesemia).
   d. confusion, anxiety, heavy legs, and tall T waves on ECG (hyperkalemia).

7. Which of the following medications used to treat hypertension can increase the risk of hyperkalemia if prescribed with potassium or with each other?
   a. amlodipine (Norvasc)
   b. atenolol (Tenormin)
   c. carvedilol (Coreg)
   d. diltiazem (Cardizem)
   e. enalapril (Vasotec)
   f. hydrochlorothiazide (Oretic)
   g. ramipril (Altace)
   h. spironolactone (Aldactone)
   i. triamterene (Dyrenium)

8. The nurse is preparing to administer sodium polystyrene sulfonate (Kayexalate) to a patient in chronic renal failure. This medication needs to be used very cautiously in patients with what other chronic disorder?
   a. Asthma
   b. AV heart block
   c. HF
   d. Rheumatoid arthritis

9. Oral magnesium supplementation may not be effective if the patient:
   a. has impaired renal functioning.
   b. is a diabetic.
   c. has hypertension.
   d. experiences diarrhea.

10. The nurse is calling the physician to report a magnesium level of 1 mEq/L. It is most important for the nurse to inform the physician if the patient has a history of:
   a. asthma.
   b. AV heart block.
   c. HF.
   d. rheumatoid arthritis.

11. Because of the risk of neuromuscular blockade when administering magnesium, the nurse must have access to what intravenous medication?
   a. Calcium gluconate
   b. Potassium chloride
   c. Sodium chloride
   d. Sodium polystyrene sulfonate

## CASE STUDIES AND PATIENT TEACHING

*(Use a separate piece of paper for your responses.)*

### Case Study 1

*A patient is admitted with prolonged diarrhea. An intravenous solution of 0.45% sodium chloride with 40 mEq of potassium chloride is prescribed at 80 mL/hr.*

1. What laboratory tests does the nurse need to monitor when administering potassium supplements?

2. What assessments does the nurse need to perform to ensure safe infusion of the potassium solution?

3. What measures should the nurse take to ensure accurate infusion of the prescribed dose of fluid and electrolytes?

4. Which of the following findings would be a reason for the nurse to stop the intravenous infusion and notify the physician? (Select all that apply.)
   a. Blood pressure 100/65 mm/Hg
   b. Blood urea nitrogen (BUN) 28 mg/dL
   c. Creatinine 4.2 mg/dL
   d. Potassium 3.5 mEq/L
   e. Pulse 58 beats/min
   f. Serum glucose 220 mg/dL
   g. Sodium 140 mEq/L
   h. One-hour urine output of 10 mL

5. The nurse receives the electrolyte report for the sample drawn this morning. Results include pH 7.31, sodium 142 mEq/L, potassium 5.7 mEq/L, chloride 102 mEq/L, and magnesium 1.8 mEq/L. What treatments might the physician prescribe?

## Case Study 2

*A postoperative patient has been NPO for 4 days with a nasogastric tube set to low intermittent suction. The patient develops muscle cramping and disorientation. Serum Mg is 1.0 mEq/L. The physician prescribes intravenous solution of 10% magnesium sulfate to infuse at 100 mL/hr.*

1. What should the nurse do before initiating this intravenous therapy?

2. The prescriber changes the infusion rate to 90 mL/hr. What critical assessment should the nurse perform while administering magnesium?

# 42 Review of Hemodynamics

## OBJECTIVES

See page 26 for the Objectives.

## CRITICAL THINKING AND STUDY QUESTIONS

1. Which of the following statements about the circulatory system are true? (Select all that apply.)
   a. Arteries readily stretch in response to pressure changes.
   b. Arterioles determine blood flow to tissue.
   c. Conditions that decrease chest expansion with breathing decrease blood return to the heart.
   d. Conditions that cause an inability of skeletal muscle to contract (or severe weakness) can cause peripheral edema.
   e. Normal adult blood volume is 8 L.
   f. The heart of a normal adult pumps the entire blood volume in approximately 1 minute.
   g. The majority of the blood in the body is in the arteries and the heart.
   h. Vasodilation increases resistance to blood flow.

2. Individuals who have plaque occluding their arteries experience an increase in vessel resistance. The nurse should assess for which of the following that is the body's attempt to compensate?
   a. Decreased afterload
   b. Edema
   c. Rise in blood pressure
   d. Slowing of heart rate

3. Drugs that can be used to lower her blood pressure decrease venous resistance by:
   a. constricting veins.
   b. reducing blood volume.
   c. reducing right atrial pressure.
   d. stimulating auxiliary muscle pumps.

4. A patient with early heart failure has an average heart rate of 90 beats/min and a stroke volume of 55 mL. This patient's per minute cardiac output is:
   a. extremely low.
   b. low.
   c. normal.
   d. high.

5. A patient who experiences orthostatic (postural) hypotension gets up to go to the bathroom during the night to void. In addition to instructing him to change positions slowly, the nurse teaches him to try to void sitting down. What is the rationale for this teaching?
   a. Voiding can cause dehydration and hypotension.
   b. Voiding can cause tachycardia and hypertension.
   c. Voiding involves stimulation of beta-adrenergic receptors in the heart, and a rebound tachycardia can occur.
   d. Voiding involves stimulation of the vagus nerve, which can cause bradycardia and further hypotension.

▶ 6. The nurse is researching a drug. The handbook states that it decreases afterload. Before the nurse administers this medication to a patient, which of these assessments would be most critical to assess?
   a. Blood pressure for hypotension
   b. Pulse for bradycardia
   c. Respirations for tachypnea
   d. Temperature for fever

▶ 7. The nurse is assessing a patient who is receiving medication for acute heart failure. Which of the following assessments would be the most critical?
   a. Blood pressure 165/90 mm Hg
   b. Expiratory wheezes of bronchi and bronchioles
   c. Loud inspiratory and expiratory gurgling sounds throughout lung fields
   d. Pulse 100 beats/min

8. Drugs can cause vasodilation by:
   a. blocking parasympathetic receptors.
   b. blocking sympathetic receptors.
   c. stimulating parasympathetic receptors.
   d. stimulating sympathetic receptors.

▶ 9. The nurse is reassessing a patient 1 hour after administering a vasodilator to treat hypertension. Assessment findings include BP 130/70 mm Hg (down from 150/88 mm/Hg), pulse 98 (up from 84 beats/min), and respirations 22 (down from 20). The nurse should:
   a. document the findings.
   b. document the findings and continue to assess the patient.
   c. page the prescriber STAT and continue to assess the patient.
   d. prepare for a cardiac arrest.

▶ 10. A patient is receiving a vasodilator that has a high incidence of orthostatic hypotension. Before administering the medication and after the patient has rested supine for 10 minutes, the nurse assesses the blood pressure and pulse. Results are BP 145/80 mm Hg, P 68 beats/min. The nurse assists the patient to stand, providing safety and after 1 minute, reassess the BP and pulse. Which of the following readings would be a concern?
   a. BP 110/70 mm Hg, pulse 92 beats/min
   b. BP 120/70 mm Hg, pulse 78 beats/min
   c. BP 130/70 mm Hg, pulse 88 beats/min
   d. BP 140/82 mm Hg, pulse 70 beats/min

## CASE STUDIES AND PATIENT TEACHING

*(Use a separate piece of paper for your responses.)*

### Case Study 1

*A patient newly diagnosed with coronary artery disease (CAD) has been prescribed a nitroglycerin patch 12 hours on and 12 hours off. The nurse is explaining the medication to the patient and her daughter. Nitroglycerin is a drug that causes extensive venous vasodilation. The drug handbook states that the therapeutic effect is to decrease the workload of the heart. The patient wants to know how this helps her heart.*

1. How should the nurse explain this effect?

2. The patient verbalizes understanding of nitroglycerin, but states she is afraid to take off the patch because she might have a heart attack. The rationale for not using nitroglycerin patches continuously is:
   a. absorption is decreased if left on too long.
   b. skin irritation occurs.
   c. tolerance to the drug's effect develops.
   d. toxicity develops.

## Case Study 2

*The student nurse is caring for a patient in heart failure (HF). The heart is enlarged, weak, and its muscle fibers are stretch beyond the point of effective recoil. The student nurse must do a teaching project.*

1. Describe how the student nurse could use a balloon to demonstrate the pathophysiology of HF to the patient.

# 43 Drugs Acting on the Renin-Angiotensin-Aldosterone System

## OBJECTIVES

See page 26 for the Objectives.

## CRITICAL THINKING AND STUDY QUESTIONS

1. The nurse recognizes that the generic names of angiotensin II receptor blocker (ARB) drugs end in:
   a. -mycin.
   b. -olol.
   c. -pril.
   d. -sartan.

2. The nurse recognizes that the generic names of angiotensin-converting enzyme inhibitor (ACE inhibitor) drugs end in:
   a. -mycin.
   b. -olol.
   c. -pril.
   d. -sartan.

3. A nurse is teaching how drugs that block the effects of angiotensin II can be beneficial for heart failure patients. Which statement, if made by the patient, would indicate the need for further teaching?
   a. "The drug helps the heart function primarily by slowing the heart rate."
   b. "The drug can help heart function by preventing sodium and water retention by the kidneys, which would raise blood pressure."
   c. "The drug can decrease the formation of extra heart muscle mass."
   d. "The drug can help heart function by preventing thickening of the arterial wall and resultant hypertension."

4. Angiotensin-converting enzyme (ACE) is chemically the same as the enzyme kinase II, which stimulates the breakdown of bradykinin. A patient may experience which adverse effect from taking an ACE inhibitor reflecting accumulation of bradykinin?
   a. Dehydration
   b. Dry cough
   c. Hyperkalemia
   d. Hyponatremia

5. Drugs that block the renin-angiotensin-aldosterone system lower blood pressure by:
   a. constricting arteries.
   b. constricting veins.
   c. increasing excretion of potassium.
   d. increasing excretion of water.

▶ 6. When the nurse is scheduled to administer lisinopril to a patient, which of these lab values should be reviewed? (Select all that apply.)
   a. ALT
   b. BUN
   c. Calcium
   d. Creatinine
   e. CRP
   f. Fasting blood sugar
   g. Sodium
   h. Potassium
   i. Uric acid
   j. Urine protein

7. The nurse teaches the patient who is prescribed an ACE inhibitor that orthostatic blood pressure precautions are especially important when the:
   a. drug prescribed is lisinopril (Prinivil, Zestril).
   b. first dose or an increase in dose is taken.
   c. patient is taking a dose of an ACE inhibitor in the morning.
   d. potassium level is greater than 4.0 mEq/L.

▶ 8. Which of these ECG findings would suggest hyperkalemia in a patient who is prescribed an ACE inhibitor and was using a salt substitute?
   a. Flat T waves
   b. Prolonged QT interval
   c. Shortened QT interval
   d. Tall, peaked T waves

9. A patient who has been taking an ACE inhibitor for hypertension is concerned because she has just discovered that she is 7 weeks pregnant. The nurse knows that research suggests that if the patient stops taking the ACE inhibitor now, the risk for adverse effects on the fetus are:
   a. low.
   b. medium.
   c. high.

▶ 10. When a patient is prescribed enalapril (Vasotec), which of these assessment findings would warrant an immediate response by the nurse?
   a. Cough
   b. Neutrophil count 60%
   c. Swelling around the mouth
   d. Unilateral renal artery bruit

▶ 11. A patient is prescribed lithium for bipolar disorder and losartan (Cozaar) for hypertension. The nurse should assess for which electrolyte laboratory result that could increase the risk for lithium toxicity?
   a. Sodium greater than 145 mEq/L
   b. Sodium less than 135 mEq/L
   c. Potassium greater than 5.0 mEq/L
   d. Potassium less than 3.5 mEq/L

12. A patient who was previously prescribed an ACE inhibitor has now been prescribed an ARB. The nurse knows that research suggests this medication change will decrease the patient's risk of developing:
   a. angioedema.
   b. death from heart failure.
   c. death from kidney failure.
   d. hyperkalemia.

13. Spironolactone (Aldactone) is less selective than eplerenone (Inspra). The nurse knows that this means that spironolactone:
   a. causes more adverse effects.
   b. has less drug interactions.
   c. is less effective.
   d. produces therapeutic effects more rapidly.

14. The nurse assesses a hypertensive, diabetic patient who is prescribed eplerenone (Inspra) for common symptoms of the most likely electrolyte imbalance, which include:
   a. flushed, dry skin.
   b. hyperactive bowel sounds.
   c. spasm of facial muscles after tapping the facial nerve.
   d. spasm of the hand and wrist when the blood pressure cuff is inflated.

15. When taking a history from a patient who is prescribed an ACE inhibitor, ARB, or eplerenone (Inspra), which of the following questions would be most important for the nurse to ask?
    a. "Are you bothered by a frequent nonproductive cough?"
    b. "Do you eat 4 to 5 servings of fruits and vegetables each day?"
    c. "Have you ever been diagnosed with iron deficiency anemia?"
    d. "What spices do you use to season your food?"

16. A patient who has been prescribed quinapril (Accupril) for hypertension has not had the expected reduction in blood pressure. Regular use of which of the following over-the-counter medications may be contributing to lack of therapeutic effect of the ACE inhibitor?
    a. Aspirin
    b. Calcium carbonate
    c. Ibuprofen
    d. Milk of magnesia

## CASE STUDIES AND PATIENT TEACHING

*(Use a separate piece of paper for your responses.)*

### Case Study 1

*A 68-year-old male was admitted to the medical unit with complaints of a 10-lb weight gain over the past week, swollen ankles, and increasing shortness of breath. Although furosemide (Lasix) was partially effective, the physician chooses to add an ACE inhibitor. The patient is prescribed captopril (Capoten) 12.5 mg by mouth, three times a day. His blood pressure is currently 140/74 mm Hg. Significant history includes an anterior myocardial infarction 12 months ago and renal artery stenosis involving the right kidney.*

1. What question should the nurse ask when consulting the prescriber about this new medication order?

2. What teaching should the nurse provide about timing of the doses of captopril (Capoten)?

3. What assessments and actions should the nurse perform when administering the first dose of captopril (Capoten)?

4. What teaching should the nurse provide to the patient and family about reasons to contact the prescriber?

5. The patient's wife states that her sister used to take captopril (Capoten), but her sister's physician discontinued the ACE inhibitor and prescribed the newer drug valsartan (Diovan). She would like her husband to be prescribed valsartan because it is newer and better. How should the nurse respond?

# 44 Calcium Channel Blockers

## OBJECTIVES

See page 26 for the Objectives.

## CRITICAL THINKING AND STUDY QUESTIONS

1. The suffix of the generic name of most dihydropyridine calcium channel blockers is:
   a. (-azosin).
   b. (-lol).
   c. (-pine).
   d. (-sartan).

2. The drop in blood pressure produced by the calcium channel blockers (CCB) activates baroreceptors and stimulates the sympathetic nervous system. Which of these CCB is most likely to have the adverse effect of reflex tachycardia?
   a. diltiazem (Cardizem)
   b. nifedipine (Procardia)
   c. verapamil (Calan)

▸ 3. The nurse is caring for a patient who is scheduled to receive verapamil (Calan) and atenolol (Tenormin), a $beta_1$-adrenergic blocker at 0900. It is important for the nurse to assess for what critical adverse effects based on the combination of these two drugs before administration? (Select all that apply.)
   a. Bradycardia
   b. Crackles of pulmonary edema
   c. Muscle pain
   d. Shortness of breath
   e. Thrombocytopenia
   f. Urinary output of at least 45 mL/hr
   g. Weight gain of 3 lbs in 24 hours

▸ 4. A patient is prescribed diltiazem (Cardizem). Which of the following assessment findings would be a reason to hold the medication and contact the prescriber?
   a. Blood pressure 150/85 mm Hg
   b. Constipation
   c. Dizziness with position changes
   d. Pulse 50 beats/min

5. Which of the following is a contraindication for the use of nondihydropyridine calcium channel blockers, verapamil and diltiazem?
   a. Angina pectoris
   b. Atrial flutter
   c. Paroxysmal supraventricular tachycardia
   d. Sick sinus syndrome

6. The nurse is administering the Verelan PM form of verapamil. The patient states she takes all of her medications in the morning when she awakens. The nurse's response should be based on Verelan PM:
   a. produces maximal effects in the morning when most cardiac events occur.
   b. is given at night so it peaks during sleep to prevent orthostatic hypotension.
   c. should not be administered with any other medication.
   d. should be taken at night because it causes sedation.

▸ 7. A patient on a surgical unit has been prescribed intravenous diltiazem (Cardizem) for atrial fibrillation. The nurse should:
   a. move the resuscitation cart into the patient's room.
   b. arrange for the patient to be transferred to a unit where constant monitoring of blood pressure and electrocardiogram is possible.
   c. continuously monitor the patient's oxygen saturation and pulse during infusion.
   d. have another nurse check the calculated drip rate before hanging the medication by gravity feed.

8. A patient taking both verapamil (Calan) and digoxin (Lanoxin) is at greater risk for digitalis toxicity. The nurse should assess and monitor the patient for early symptoms of digitalis toxicity, which include:
   a. anorexia and nausea.
   b. confusion and slurred speech.
   c. hypertension and tachycardia.
   d. photophobia and halos around bright objects.

▶ 9. The nurse is administering medications on a medical-surgical unit in a hospital. The medication administration record states that the patient should receive Cardizem LA 120 mg once a day. The patient's drug supply includes Cardizem SR. The nurse should:
   a. administer the medication.
   b. administer the medication and notify the prescriber of the change.
   c. contact the pharmacy.
   d. hold the medication and contact the prescriber.

▶ 10. Diltiazem is prescribed for intravenous infusion for a patient in atrial fibrillation. The physician has prescribed a dose of 5 mg/hr. The pharmacy has supplied the drug in a concentration of 0.45 mg/mL. How many mL/hr will the nurse program into the intravenous infusion pump?

11. Which of the following drugs might be prescribed to counteract the reflex tachycardia associated with administration of dihydropyridine calcium channel blockers (CCB)?
   a. Digoxin (Lanoxin)
   b. Enalapril (Vasotec)
   c. Furosemide (Lasix)
   d. Metoprolol (Lopressor)

12. A patient who has experienced palpitations (reflex tachycardia) while taking nifedipine (Procardia) 20 mg three times a day has had his prescription changed to nifedipine (Procardia XL) 60 mg once a day. The patient asks the nurse how taking the same medication once a day instead of three times a day will help prevent palpitations. The nurse's response should include:
   a. rapid-acting formulas of nifedipine are more potent than sustained-release formulas.
   b. blood levels of rapid-acting formulas of nifedipine rise more rapidly than with sustained-release formulas.
   c. sustained-release formulas of nifedipine cause a more gradual drop in blood pressure.
   d. sustained-release formulas of nifedipine suppress the automaticity of the heart like verapamil.

13. Because of it's selectivity for blockade of calcium channels in cerebral blood vessels, which calcium channel blocker is used for prevention of cerebral artery spasm following subarachnoid hemorrhage and is being investigated for use with migraine headaches?
   a. nicardipine (Cardene)
   b. nimodipine (Nimotop)
   c. felodipine (Plendil)
   d. isradipine (DynaCirc)

14. A patient has been prescribed extended-release nifedipine (Procardia). Teaching regarding administration should include:
   a. administer 1 hour before or 2 hours after meals.
   b. do not crush or chew tablet.
   c. take with grapefruit juice to improve absorption.
   d. must be taken on an empty stomach.

▶ 15. The recommended initial dose of diltiazem (Cardizem) intravenous push is 0.25 mg/kg for adult patients. What is the recommended safe dose for a patient that weighs 178 lbs?

## CASE STUDIES AND PATIENT TEACHING

*(Use a separate piece of paper for your responses.)*

### Case Studies 1

*A 75-year-old female, nonsmoker, with a history of hypertension, esophageal cancer, and diabetes type 2 comes to the emergency department with fatigue and extreme shortness of breath. She is diagnosed with atrial fibrillation. The physician orders verapamil (Calan) 5 mg intravenous push.*

1. Verapamil is available as 5 mg/2 mL to be administered no faster than 2 minutes. The nurse administers 0.1 mL every 5 seconds. Is this a safe rate of administration?

2. The nurse is administering the verapamil (Calan) intravenous push. While administering the medication, the nurse notes a sudden reduction in heart rate and prolongation of the PR interval on the cardiac monitor. What should the nurse do?

3. Thirty minutes after injecting the intravenous verapamil, the patient requests assistance with getting up and using the toilet to void. The nurse should:
   a. assist the patient to the bathroom.
   b. secure a bedside commode.
   c. provide assistance with using a bedpan.
   d. get an order for a Foley catheter.

4. The patient is stabilized and the prescriber has prescribed verapamil (Calan) 120 mg three times a day. The nurse is reviewing the patient's laboratory tests. Which of the following laboratory values would require consultation with the prescriber regarding administration of verapamil? (Select all that apply and explain why.)
   a. Alanine aminotransferase (ALT) 250 units/L (7-56 units/L)
   b. Blood urea nitrogen (BUN) 28 mg/dL (10-20 mg/dL)
   c. Creatinine 3.2 mg/dL (0.5-1.2 mg/dL)
   d. Fasting glucose 250 mg/dL (70-100 mg/dL)
   e. Hemoglobin 10 mg/dL (14-18 gm/dL)
   f. International ration (INR) 1.8 (1 normal; 2-3.5 if on anticoagulants)
   g. Potassium 3.3 mEq/L (3.5-5 mEq/L)
   h. Sodium 146 mg/dL (135-145 mEq/dL)

5. The nurse is reviewing the patient's prescribed medications. In addition to verapamil 80 mg three times a day, the patient is taking nateglinide (Starlix) 120 mg, a medication that increases production of insulin by the pancreas and lowers the blood sugar to treat the patient's diabetes mellitus. Both verapamil and nateglinide are metabolized by the CYP3A4 hepatic enzyme. Verapamil inhibits the action of this enzyme. Because of this interaction, the nurse knows the patient is at increased risk for:
   a. hyperglycemia.
   b. hypoglycemia.

6. What teaching should the nurse provide that can prevent problems with common adverse effects of verapamil?

# 45 Vasodilators

## OBJECTIVES

See page 26 for the Objectives.

## CRITICAL THINKING AND STUDY QUESTIONS

1. Hydralazine, minoxidil, diltiazem, nifedipine, verapamil, and diazoxide: (Select all that apply.)
   a. decrease cardiac afterload.
   b. decrease tissue perfusion.
   c. have a high risk of postural hypotension.
   d. increase cardiac output.
   e. increase the force of cardiac contraction.
   f. reduce the force at which blood is returned to the heart.
   g. vasodilate arteries.
   h. vasodilate veins.

▸ 2. A priority nursing problem when the nurse is caring for a patient who is receiving an arterial vasodilator is:
   a. activity intolerance.
   b. decreased cardiac output.
   c. fluid volume excess.
   d. safety.

3. The adverse effect of minoxidil (Loniten) that decreases adherence to drug therapy in many women is:
   a. metrorrhagia.
   b. hypertrichosis.
   c. SLE syndrome.
   d. teratogenicity.

▸ 4. A patient with severe hypertension is prescribed minoxidil (Loniten). The nurse should not administer this drug if assessment findings include:
   a. distended neck veins, muffled heart sounds, and narrow pulse pressure.
   b. exertional dyspnea, 1+ ankle edema, and anxiety.
   c. headache, dizziness, and blurred vision.
   d. shift of PMI to left, bruits over carotid arteries, and wheezing.

▸ 5. The nurse is caring for a nonambulatory patient who is receiving hydralazine (Apresoline). When monitoring for adverse effects, the nurse would expect that edema would first appear:
   a. around the medial malleolus of the ankle.
   b. in the fingers.
   c. in the sacral area.
   d. on the dorsal aspect of the feet.

▸ 6. Laboratory test results on a patient receiving hydralazine (Apresoline) include elevated antinuclear antibodies (ANA). When notifying the prescriber of these lab results, which of the following assessment findings is most significant to also include in the report?
   a. Blood pressure 150/90 mm Hg
   b. Pulse 90 beats/min
   c. Respirations 22/min
   d. Temperature 101° F (38.3° C)

7. Which of the following elevated laboratory results is most likely to be related to administration of diazoxide (Hyperstat)? (Select all that apply.)
   a. Amylase
   b. Antinuclear antibody (ANA)
   c. Calcium
   d. Capillary blood sugar
   e. High-density lipoproteins
   f. Low-density lipoproteins
   g. Uric acid

▸ 8. What lab tests should be monitored in a patient who is receiving diazoxide (Hyperstat)? (Select all that apply.)
   a. Amylase and lipase
   b. Creatinine and creatinine clearance
   c. Fasting and postprandial glucose
   d. Uric acid and ESR

▸ 9. The nurse is administering nitroprusside (Nitropress) in a cardiac care unit. The physician also orders administration of oral antihypertensives. The patient's blood pressure is still elevated, but dropping slowly. The nurse should:
   a. administer both medications.
   b. hold both the nitroprusside and oral antihypertensives until the prescriber can be consulted.
   c. hold the nitroprusside and administer the oral antihypertensives until the prescriber can be consulted.
   d. hold the oral antihypertensives and administer the nitroprusside until the prescriber can be consulted.

▸ 10. A patient who weighs 110 lbs is receiving intravenous nitroprusside sodium (Nipride) 300 mcg/min. An important nursing assessment at this dose is for:
   a. adequate fluid intake and urinary output.
   b. anorexia, nausea, and vomiting.
   c. fever, flushing, and chills.
   d. palpitations, disorientation, and respiratory depression.

11. The nurse is preparing to administer nitroprusside sodium (Nipride). The solution has just been prepared in the pharmacy, but has a faint brown discoloration. The nurse should:
   a. administer the medication.
   b. consult the prescriber before administering the solution.
   c. discard the solution and get a new bag from the pharmacy.
   d. warm the intravenous bag and reassess to see if the brown color clears.

12. A patient who is receiving nitroprusside is receiving a concurrent dose of intravenous thiosulfate. The nurse knows that thiocyanate levels must be monitored and should not exceed what level?
   a. 0.01 mg/ml
   b. 0.1 mg/mL
   c. 1 mg/mL
   d. 10 mg/mL

## CASE STUDIES AND PATIENT TEACHING

*(Use a separate piece of paper for your responses.)*

### Case Study 1

*A 55-year-old patient has just been admitted to the intensive care unit in a hypertensive crisis. He is confused, lethargic, and his blood pressure is 240/160 mm/Hg. The healthcare providers are concerned that he may have a massive cerebrovascular accident (stroke or CVA) if his blood pressure is not brought down immediately. The physician orders an intravenous push of diazoxide (Hyperstat) 2 mg/kg. Recommended dose is 1 to 3 mg/kg up to a maximum of 150 mg per dose. The patient weighs 220 lbs.*

1. What dose of diazoxide is safe and therapeutic?

2. The drug comes in a concentration of 15 mg/mL and should be administered by rapid IV push over 3 minutes. How many milliliters should the nurse administer per 5 seconds if 100 mg is ordered?

3. What assessments does the nurse need to perform and how frequently should these assessments occur?

4. The patient's wife informs the nurse that her husband is a "brittle" diabetic. Why is it important to share this information with the prescriber?

5. Why must a patient on diazoxide (Hyperstat) stay recumbent for at least 30 minutes after discontinuing diazoxide injection, but only normal postural hypotension precautions are needed with nitroprusside?

### Case Study 2

*A 78-year-old woman is being seen in the ED in hypertensive crisis. She is 5 feet 2 inches and weighs 125 lbs. Her BP is 230/130 mm/Hg, and she is very edematous. She has a history of alcohol abuse. The physician orders intravenous nitroprusside sodium (Nipride) at 0.3 mcg/kg/min.*

1. What assessments of the solution and precautions should the nurse take when administering this medication?

2. Knowing that nitroprusside sodium (Nipride) creates a rapid response (within 1 to 2 minutes), what and how often should the nurse assess to follow the results of the drugs and the patient's response?

3. The patient suddenly becomes diaphoretic and complains of nausea, palpitations, and headache. What should the nurse do?

4. The patient has improved significantly. The physician has decided to prescribe hydralazine, metoprolol, and hydrochlorothiazide on a long-term basis to control her blood pressure. Explain the rationale for this combination of medications.

5. The nurse checks the drug handbook, and the dose recommendation for adults for hydralazine is listed as 10 to 50 mg 4 times a day or 100 mg 3 times a day. What are possible reasons for the low dose being extended to every 8 hours?

# 46 Drugs for Hypertension

## OBJECTIVES

See page 26 for the Objectives.

## CRITICAL THINKING AND STUDY QUESTIONS

1. The nurse knows it is important to teach lifestyle modifications to patients at risk for hypertension. Which of the following blood pressure findings, if identified in three or more separate readings, would be classified by JNC 7 as prehypertension? (Select all that apply.)
   a. 110/70 mm Hg
   b. 118/86 mm Hg
   c. 120/80 mm Hg
   d. 128/92 mm Hg
   e. 130/85 mm Hg
   f. 137/74 mm Hg
   g. 138/92 mm Hg
   h. 146/76 mm Hg

2. When possible, the nurse should assess the patient's blood pressure with the patient:
   a. lying flat in bed.
   b. lying in bed with the head elevated at least 45°.
   c. sitting, with feet dangling.
   d. sitting, with feet on the floor.

3. The nurse is reviewing a patient's history and notes "essential hypertension." This older term is synonymous with:
   a. isolated systolic hypertension.
   b. prehypertension.
   c. primary hypertension.
   d. secondary hypertension.

4. Pheochromocytoma causes hypertension because a tumor of the adrenal gland secretes excessive amounts of:
   a. dopamine.
   b. epinephrine.
   c. GABA.
   d. serotonin.

5. It is important for the nurse to discuss adverse effects of the antihypertensive drugs which are prescribed because adverse effects often:
   a. affect compliance.
   b. are life threatening.
   c. are necessary if the antihypertensive is at a dose that is effective.
   d. indicate the cause of hypertension.

6. The teaching plan for a patient taking antihypertensive drugs should include:
   a. cigarette smoking will cause antihypertensive drugs to be ineffective.
   b. following dietary and exercise recommendations will prevent the need for antihypertensive drugs.
   c. symptoms of hypertension usually do not occur until organ damage has occurred.
   d. treatment with antihypertensive drugs can cure hypertension.

7. When administering an antihypertensive drug to a patient who has a history of hypertension and type 2 diabetes mellitus, what would be an appropriate outcome for therapy?
   a. BP 100/60 to 110/70 mm Hg
   b. BP 110/70 to 130/80 mm Hg
   c. BP 120/80 to 130/85 mm Hg
   d. BP 128/80 to 138/90 mm Hg

8. Match the action of the following antihypertensives with the logical adverse effects for which the nurse should assess.

| | | |
|---|---|---|
| _____ | a. Arterial dilators | 1. Dizziness |
| _____ | b. Beta blockers | 2. Peripheral edema |
| _____ | c. Diuretics | 3. Slow heart rate |
| _____ | d. Venodilators | 4. Urinary output, electrolyte levels, and dehydration |

9. A patient is hypertensive and receiving drug therapy. When would the nurse expect reflex tachycardia to be most likely to occur?

10. Matching: Drugs affecting the renin-angiotensin-aldosterone system (RAAS)

| | | |
|---|---|---|
| ______ | a. ACE inhibitors | 1. Suppress renin release by the kidneys |
| ______ | b. Aldosterone | 2. Prevent activation of angiotensin blockers |
| ______ | c. ARBs | 3. Prevent activation of angiotensin receptors |
| ______ | d. Beta blockers | 4. Block receptors in kidney that alter excretion of water, sodium, and potassium |

11. Which of the following laboratory results should be reported to the prescriber if a patient is receiving a thiazide or loop diuretic?
    a. Blood urea nitrogen (BUN) 20 mg/dL
    b. Hemoglobin $A_{1C}$ 5.5%
    c. Potassium ($K^+$) 3.2 mEq/L
    d. Uric acid 20 mg/dL

12. The nurse would teach a patient who is on which of the following diuretics to avoid use of potassium-containing salt substitutes and excessive consumption of bananas and orange juice?
    a. ethacrynic acid (Edecrin)
    b. furosemide (Lasix)
    c. hydrochlorothiazide (HydroDiuril)
    d. triameterene (Dyrenium)

13. Acebutolol (Sectral), carteolol (Cartrol), penbutolol (Levatol), and pindolol (Visken) are beta blockers that have intrinsic sympathomimetic activity. This results in less:
    a. bradycardia at rest.
    b. bronchoconstriction.
    c. heart block.
    d. hypoglycemia.

14. When a patient has been prescribed an $alpha_1$ blocker, including doxazosin (Cardura), it is most important for the nurse to teach the patient to:
    a. change positions slowly.
    b. include adequate potassium in the diet.
    c. monitor urinary output.
    d. seek medical care if chest pain occurs.

15. A patient would most likely experience reflex tachycardia if receiving which of the following antihypertensive drugs?
    a. Alpha and/or beta blockers
    b. Beta blockers
    c. Direct-acting vasodilators
    d. Nondihydropine calcium channel blockers

▶ 16. Nurses can make a significant contribution toward assisting a patient with controlling blood pressure by:
   a. identifying obstacles to adherence to therapy.
   b. suggesting drugs that can be effective.
   c. teaching the patient to assess their blood pressure sitting and standing.
   d. telling the patient to exercise at least 30 minutes a day.

17. The intervention that is most likely to decrease adverse effects of hypertension in African American adults is:
   a. explaining measures to respond to adverse effects of antihypertensive drugs.
   b. identifying adverse effects of antihypertensive drugs.
   c. prescribing of the appropriate drug for hypertension.
   d. promoting regular screening of blood pressure.

18. The nurse would expect pharmacotherapy for an African American patient with hypertension to include a(n):
   a. ACE inhibitor.
   b. calcium channel blocker.
   c. diuretic.
   d. vasodilator.

19. The nurse would report the onset of menses (menarche) if an adolescent with hypertension was prescribed:
   a. captopril (Capoten).
   b. hydrochlorothiazide (HydroDiuril).
   c. prazosin (Minipress).
   d. propranolol (Inderal).

20. Research suggests that it is important to use pharmacotherapy to treat hypertension that was present before pregnancy in a pregnant woman if her blood pressure is greater than:
   a. 130/85 mm Hg.
   b. 140/90 mm Hg.
   c. 160/100 mm Hg.
   d. 180/110 mm Hg.

21. The best treatment for severe preeclampsia is:
   a. delivery of the fetus.
   b. labetalol (Normodyne).
   c. lisinopril (Zestril).
   d. methyldopa (Aldomet).

▶ 22. A nurse has been administering magnesium sulfate to an eclamptic patient. The nurse would notify the obstetrician if the magnesium level is:
   a. 4 mEq/L.
   b. 5.5 mEq/L.
   c. 7 mEq/L.
   d. 8.5 mEq/L.

## CASE STUDIES AND PATIENT TEACHING

*(Use a separate piece of paper for your responses.)*

### Case Study 1

*A 5 feet 9 inches 220-lbs 48-year-old black male with a history of type 2 diabetes mellitus comes to the emergency department (ED) with a frontal headache and generalized complaints of "not feeling well." Upon examination, his blood pressure is 210/120 mm/Hg, pulse is 98, and respirations are 24 and labored.*

1. What risk factors does this patient have for a cardiovascular event?

2. When is it important to lower this patient's blood pressure within 1 hour rather than slowly as for most hypertensive patients?

3. The ED resident writes an order for intravenous nitroprusside 80 mg/min. Is this dose within the recommended dose?

4. The resident changes the order to 80 mcg/min. What precautions should the nurse take while administering this medication?

5. The patient is stabilized and discharged on hydrochlorothiazide (HydroDiuril) and diltiazem (Cardizem). On the follow-up visit, the patient's blood pressure is 160/90 mm/Hg. The patient asks why the physician does not just give him a high enough dose to bring his blood pressure down to normal. How should the nurse respond?

### Case Study 2

*The industrial nurse is creating a health promotion plan for factory workers relating to lifestyle changes that can prevent or minimize hypertension. Most workers are 25 to 55 years old. Based on developmental knowledge of the target population, use the Nola Pender revised Health Promotion Model (see below) to complete the following charts.*

*Consider the personal sociocultural factors of the age group to identify behavior-specific cognitions and affect influencing tobacco use.*

## INDIVIDUAL CHARACTERISTICS AND EXPERIENCES

- Personal sociocultural factors
  - Characteristics of the workers, including race, ethnicity, education, and sociocultural factors, which influence beliefs, affect, and performance of a health-promoting behavior

| Characteristics of 25- to 55-year-old factory workers who are regularly employed, but are struggling to pay all home expenses | How these characteristics influence ability and willingness to attempt health-promoting behavioral change |
|---|---|
| | |

## BEHAVIOR-SPECIFIC COGNITIONS AND AFFECT

- Perceived benefits of action
  - Positive effects the person thinks they will experience from the lifestyle changes
- Perceived barriers to action
  - Negative effects the person thinks they will experience if they do not implement positive lifestyle changes
- Perceived self-efficacy
  - Belief that the person can be successful with lifestyle changes
- Activity-related affect
  - Positive and negative effects experienced when trying to change a behavior
- Interpersonal influences
  - Behaviors, beliefs, or attitudes of others that can influence the person's decision to change a behavior
- Situational influences
  - Environmental factors that can influence the person's decision to change a behavior

## Reference

Pender, N, et al: *Health promotion in nursing practice,* 4th ed., Upper Saddle River, NJ, Prentice Hall, 2002.

| Behavior-specific cognitions and affect | Recommended dietary changes | Developmentally appropriate plans to institute change |
|---|---|---|
| Perceived benefits of action | | |
| Perceived barriers to action | | |
| Perceived self-efficacy | | |
| Activity-related affect | | |
| Interpersonal influences | | |
| Situational influences | | |

| Behavior-specific cognitions and affect | Regular aerobic exercise | Nursing Interventions |
|---|---|---|
| Perceived benefits of action | | |
| Perceived barriers to action | | |
| Perceived self-efficacy | | |
| Activity-related affect | | |
| Interpersonal influences | | |
| Situational influences | | |

# 47 Drugs for Heart Failure

## OBJECTIVES

See page 26 for the Objectives.

## CRITICAL THINKING AND STUDY QUESTIONS

1. Which of the following statements, if made by a patient with heart failure, would indicate a need for further teaching?
   a. "If blood cannot get through my heart the backup of fluid will make it hard for me to breathe."
   b. "My heart is stretching so much it is loosing the ability to squeeze out the blood."
   c. "The changes in my heart started when I began to feel tired and short of breath."
   d. "When my heart beats too fast, it cannot fill properly."

2. Elevation of B-natriuretic peptide (BNP) suggests heart failure because BNP is released when the heart:
   a. beats faster.
   b. chambers stretch.
   c. does not get enough oxygen.
   d. muscle thickens.

▸ 3. The nurse would be most concerned if a patient with heart failure exhibits which of the following symptoms?
   a. Peripheral edema
   b. Urine output of 700 mL in 24 hours
   c. Visible distention of the jugular veins when the patient is supine
   d. Weight gain of 2 lbs in 24 hours

4. Loop diuretics are the type of diuretic most commonly administered to hospitalized patients in heart failure because they:
   a. are effective when kidney function declines.
   b. block receptors for aldosterone.
   c. do not increase the risk of digitalis toxicity.
   d. seldom cause hypotension.

5. Benefits of ACE inhibitors in heart failure include: (Select all that apply.)
   a. improving renal blood flow.
   b. increasing renal excretion of sodium, potassium, and water.
   c. promoting proper functioning of baroreceptors.
   d. reducing peripheral vascular resistance.
   e. reducing venous congestion and edema.
   f. stimulating the release of aldosterone.

▶ 6. A heart failure patient is prescribed eplerenone (Inspra) and enalapril (Vasotec). Which of the following symptoms, if exhibited by the patient, would warrant consultation with the prescriber regarding evaluation of the patient's potassium levels?
   a. Abdominal and muscle cramps
   b. Abdominal distention
   c. Diminished deep tendon reflexes
   d. Weakness and fatigue

7. Beta blockers differ from cardiac glycosides in that beta blockers:
   a. decrease the rate of cardiac contraction.
   b. decrease the force of cardiac contraction.
   c. decrease the conduction of impulses through the heart.
   d. do not prolong life.

▶ 8. A maintenance intravenous infusion of inamrinone is prescribed for a patient who has a current infusion of 5% dextrose and 0.45% NaCl running at 45 mL/hr. The nurse should administer the imanrinone:
   a. after flushing the primary line.
   b. as a secondary infusion through the primary line.
   c. over 2 to 3 minutes.
   d. via a second intravenous site or port.

9. Nitrates, including nitroglycerin and isosorbide, reduce the workload of the myocardium by:
   a. decreasing the amount of blood returning to the heart.
   b. decreasing conduction of impulses through the heart.
   c. decreasing the volume of blood in the vascular system.
   d. increasing myocardial remodeling.

10. When a patient is receiving isosorbide or nitroglycerin for heart failure, the nurse should carefully assess the patient for the adverse effects of:
   a. bradycardia and hypotension.
   b. bradycardia and hypertension.
   c. tachycardia and hypotension.
   d. tachycardia and hypertension.

11. A possible explanation for why digoxin has not demonstrated an improvement in mortality is that the drug does not:
   a. decrease heart rate.
   b. improve heart remodeling.
   c. increase cardiac output.
   d. increase urine production.

▶ 12. When a heart failure patient is prescribed digoxin and furosemide, the nurse should carefully assess the patient for early symptoms of the most likely electrolyte disturbance including:
   a. anorexia and nausea.
   b. anxiety and abdominal cramps.
   c. bone pain and constipation.
   d. muscle spasms and convulsions.

▶ 13. What findings would warrant that the nurse not administer digoxin and notifying the prescriber?
   a. Blood pressure 100/76 mm Hg
   b. Digoxin 2.4 ng/mL
   c. Heart rate 100 beats/min
   d. Potassium 5.3 mEq/L

14. Research suggests that a significant modifiable cause of heart muscle disease is:
   a. excessive chronic consumption of alcohol.
   b. high-fat diet.
   c. obesity.
   d. smoking two packs/day.

15. The nurse would consult the prescriber if a patient with heart failure is prescribed:
   a. acetaminophen.
   b. aspirin.
   c. celecoxib.
   d. morphine.

16. A fixed dose of hydralazine and isosorbide (BiDil) has been approved to treat heart failure in:
   a. African Americans.
   b. diabetics.
   c. men.
   d. women.

## CASE STUDIES AND PATIENT TEACHING

*(Use a separate piece of paper for your responses.)*

### Case Study 1

*A 78-year-old female has been admitted to the nursing unit from the emergency department on a Sunday evening with a diagnosis of right intratrochanteric femur fracture. Open reduction and internal fixation of the fracture is planned for Monday morning pending medical clearance for surgery. The patient is placed in Buck's traction to relieve muscle spasm and maintain reduction of the fracture and has a Foley catheter inserted.*

*The patient has a history of chronic heart failure, hypertension, type 2 diabetes mellitus, and chronic obstructive pulmonary disease. Current medication orders include aspirin 81 mg once a day, hydrochlorothiazide 25 mg once a day, atenolol (Tenormin) 50 mg once a day, ramipril (Altace) 5 mg once a day, glipizide/metformin (Metaglip) 2.5 mg 500 mg once a day, tiotropium (Spiriva) one inhalation per day, intravenous methylprednisolone 40 mg every 6 hours, and intravenous morphine 1 mg every 4-6 hours as needed. An intravenous solution of 5% dextrose in water is infusing at a rate of 83 mL per hour. Oxygen is being provided via nasal cannula at 2 L. The patient's daughter is very upset and tells the nurse that she thinks her mother fell because the doctor is drugging her with so many medications.*

1. How should the nurse respond?

2. The 3-11 (1500-2300) nurse is making initial patient rounds. What assessments are a priority for the nurse to obtain at this time relating to the patient's cardiovascular status?

3. What problem may the nurse encounter in maintaining traction relating to the patient's history of heart failure?

## Case Study 2

*An 81-year-old male with chronic heart failure (HF), who resides in a long term care facility, has been treated with digoxin (Lanoxin) 0.25 mg, furosemide 80 mg, and potassium chloride (K-Dur) 20 mEq once a day by mouth for a long time. Recently, the prescriber added eplerenone (Inspra) 50 mg orally once a day to the medication regimen.*

1. When consulting the prescriber about this patient, what questions might the nurse ask?

2. Why is it important for the nurse to monitor electrolyte and digoxin levels on this patient?

*The long term care nurse notes during report from the night shift that the patient has become increasingly restless, "coughs all night", and seems very fatigued when the staff is providing care. His appetite has been poor, even for things he normally enjoys. Assessment findings include BP 90/70 mm Hg; alternating weak and strong pulse at a rate of 118 BPM, S3 ventricular gallop, rales throughout lung fields, and five pound weight gain in the last week.*

3. What action should the nurse take at this time?

4. The patient is admitted to an acute care facility. Based on the knowledge of digoxin and its relationship to potassium, how could these blood levels have contributed to the patient's decompensation?

## Case Study 3

*A 64-year-old male patient is a direct admission to the nursing unit with the complaint of abdominal pain, nausea, and extreme weakness. The patient has a history of diabetes, chronic renal failure, and sleep apnea. Admission nursing assessment findings include temperature 99.3°F, BP 174/110 mm Hg, pulse 96 and irregular, PMI shifted to the left, JVD 4.5 cm above the angle of Louis, 3+ pitting edema in the lower extremities, and tenderness in the RUQ with abdominal palpation.*

1. What nursing diagnosis is most appropriate for this patient?

2. The nurse obtains laboratory results from tests drawn on admission including BNP 1275 pg/mL; K+ 5.4 mEq/L, creatinine 2.7 mg/dL, BUN 42 mg/dL. The nurse contacts the physician who orders a stat electrocardiogram which shows S-T changes. What action should the nurse take at this point?

3. The patient is transferred to the coronary care unit. Oxygen is administered along with furosemide (Lasix), morphine, nitroglycerin, and enalapril (Vasotec). What is the rationale for administration of these drugs?

4. The patient is stabilized and is transferred to the nursing unit. Prescribed drugs include carvedilol, enalapril, and furosemide. What laboratory values does the nurse need to monitor when a patient is receiving these drugs?

5. What teaching should the nurse provide to prepare this patient for discharge?

6. The patient lives in an apartment building with 12 stairs to climb to his apartment. After climbing the stairs, he needs to rest because he is short of breath. He can, however, perform most activities of daily living. According to the New York Heart Association (NYHA), what is this patient's heart failure classification?

# 48 Antidysrhythmic Drugs

## OBJECTIVES

See page 26 for the Objectives.

## CRITICAL THINKING AND STUDY QUESTIONS

▶ 1. The priority nursing concern for a patient with a dysrhythmia is:
   a. alteration in cardiac output.
   b. imbalance of fluid and electrolytes.
   c. inadequate peripheral tissue perfusion.
   d. ineffective breathing pattern.

2. Cells other than the sinoatrial node (ectopic) can dominate the pace of the heart if the discharges of the ectopic stimuli are:
   a. atrial in origin.
   b. faster than the SA node.
   c. from the ventricles.
   d. slower than the SA node.

▶ 3. When caring for a patient with a dysrhythmia, it is important for the nurse to monitor which of the following laboratory values because abnormalities are very likely to affect depolarization and repolarization of cardiac cells?
   a. ALT, AST, and bilirubin
   b. BUN, creatinine, and FBS
   c. Hematocrit, hemoglobin, and RBC count
   d. Sodium, calcium, and potassium

▶ 4. The nurse should teach a patient who has been prescribed a class IA or IV antidysrhythmic drug the importance of reporting which of the following symptoms suggests that torsades de pointes, a potentially fatal prodysrhythmic adverse effect of the prescribed drugs, may be occurring?
   a. Ankle edema
   b. Headache
   c. Near syncope
   d. Shortness of breath

5. A patient asks the nurse why she is receiving a different treatment for her dysrhythmia than her husband. The nurse's response should be based on the fact that selection of antidysrhythmic drug therapy selection is based on the patient's:
   a. age.
   b. family history of dysrhythmia.
   c. response to drug therapy.
   d. sex.

▶ 6. An action that can slow an acute supraventricular dysrhythmia is instructing the patient to:
   a. bear down as if having a bowel movement.
   b. breathe through pursed lips.
   c. pant like a dog.
   d. perform Kegel exercises.

▶ 7. A focused nursing assessment of a patient with atrial fibrillation should always include assessment of changes in:
   a. appetite.
   b. deep tendon reflexes.
   c. kidney functioning.
   d. mental status.

▶ 8. Which of these laboratory results for international normalized ratio (INR), if identified in an atrial fibrillation patient who is receiving warfarin (Coumadin), would indicate that therapy has achieved the desired effect?
   a. INR 1
   b. INR 3
   c. INR 5
   d. INR 7

9. The nurse responds quickly when a ventricular tachydysrhythmia is identified because this type of dysrhythmia impairs the ability of the heart:
   a. to contract rapidly enough to meet body needs.
   b. to eject an adequate amount of blood.
   c. valves to close properly.
   d. valves to open properly.

▶ 10. It would be most important for the nurse to promptly consult the physician if premature ventricular beats were noted during cardiac monitoring of a patient who has been admitted with the diagnosis of:
a. acute renal failure.
b. chronic obstructive pulmonary disease.
c. myocardial infarction.
d. systemic lupus erythematosus.

11. Matching: Antidysrhythmic drugs and action

| | | |
|---|---|---|
| ______ | a. Class I | 1. Delay repolarization of fast potentials by blocking potassium ($K^+$) channels. |
| ______ | b. Class II | 2. Reduce calcium ($Ca^{++}$) entry during fast and slow depolarization and depress phase 4 repolarization of slow potentials. |
| ______ | c. Class III | 3. Slow impulse conduction in atria and ventricles by blocking sodium ($Na^+$) channels. |
| ______ | d. Class IV | |

▶ 12. A patient with a dysrhythmia, type 2 diabetes mellitus (DM), and heart failure (HF) is prescribed quinidine, metformin, furosemide, and digoxin. The nurse should be vigilant in monitoring for early adverse effects of common interactions of these drugs including:
a. anorexia and nausea.
b. cool, clammy skin.
c. excessive urination and thirst.
d. yellow tinted blurred vision.

13. A patient has received instructions regarding administration of quinidine. Which of these statements made by the client would indicate the patient understood the directions?
a. "I should take this medication 1 hour before or 2 hours after I eat food."
b. "I should take this medication at bedtime."
c. "I should take this medication first thing in the morning, 30 minutes before I eat or drink anything, and I should not lie down for at least 30 minutes after taking the drug."
d. "I should take this medication with food."

▶ 14. Which of these assessment findings, if identified in a patient who is receiving quinidine, should the nurse report to the prescriber immediately?
a. BP 150/88 mm Hg
b. Ringing in the ears
c. Three soft stools in 8 hours
d. Wheezing at the end of expiration

15. A patient asks the nurse why he was instructed to take quinidine with food. An appropriate response by the nurse is that taking the drug with food:
a. decreases the incidence of diarrhea.
b. increases absorption.
c. prevents cinchonism.
d. prevents ventricular tachycardia.

▶ 16. The nurse is monitoring the ECG of a patient who received the first dose of quinidine 45 minutes ago. The nurse notes that the QRS complex was widened 10% from predrug therapy findings. The nurse should:
a. administer a beta blocker.
b. continue to assess.
c. discontinue monitoring the ECG.
d. notify the prescriber immediately.

17. The nurse should assess patients receiving long-term therapy with procainamide for which of the following adverse effects? (Select all that apply.)
a. Chest pain and dyspnea
b. Elevated ANA and painful joint swelling
c. Elevated platelet levels and increased thrombi formation
d. Enlarged liver and elevated liver enzymes
e. Sore throat, fever, and chills
f. Ventricular tachycardia

▶ 18. The prescriber wrote an order to switch a patient from intravenous (IV) to oral procainamide. The IV drug was discontinued at 11:30 AM. When should the nurse administer the first dose of oral procainamide?
a. Immediately
b. 1:00 PM
c. 2:30 PM
d. 4:00 PM

19. When administering disopyramide (Norpace), the nurse should assess for which of the following anticholinergic adverse effects of the drug?
    a. Chest pain and palpitations
    b. Nausea, vomiting, and diarrhea
    c. Isolated systolic hypertension
    d. Postvoid residual greater than 100 mL of urine

20. Because of extensive first pass effect, the nurse expects to administer lidocaine:
    a. in a sustained-release formula.
    b. intravenously.
    c. orally, on an empty stomach.
    d. with a full glass of water.

▶ 21. The nurse is preparing to administer the cardioselective beta blocker acebutolol (Sectral). Which of the following assessments would indicate the need for immediate consultation with the prescriber?
    a. Apical pulse 155 beats/min
    b. Bronchial wheezes
    c. Capillary blood glucose 220 mg/dL
    d. One plus pitting edema of the dorsal aspect of the foot

22. In addition to monitoring the heart rate and rhythm, what must the nurse continuously monitor when administering the potassium channel blockers, bretylium, or amiodarone?
    a. Blood pressure
    b. Level of consciousness
    c. Intravenous site
    d. Respiratory effort

23. The patient must be informed of possible damage to the lungs when prescribed oral therapy with which of the following drugs?
    a. amiodarone (Cordarone)
    b. dofetilide (Tikosyn)
    c. propafenone (Rhythmol)
    d. propranolol (Inderal)

▶ 24. What teaching should the nurse provide relating to blockade of calcium channels in vascular smooth muscle when a patient is prescribed verapamil (Calan)?
    a. Drink 2500 mL of fluid each day, especially water.
    b. Increase fiber in diet.
    c. Take orthostatic BP precautions.
    d. Report bruising.

▶ 25. A patient who weighs 165 lbs is prescribed intravenous diltiazem. The recommended initial bolus dose is 0.25 mg/kg. What is the recommended dose for this patient?

▶ 26. When a patient who is receiving adenosine exhibits facial flushing and chest pain, which action should the nurse take first?
    a. Administer oxygen.
    b. Assess vital signs.
    c. Discontinue the infusion.
    d. Initiate CPR.

27. In most cases the need for antidysrhythmic drugs exceeds the risks of adverse effects when:
    a. the dysrhythmia is prolonged.
    b. the QT interval is excessively long.
    c. ventricular pumping is ineffective.
    d. when the sinoatrial node discharges at a rate exceeding 160 beats/min.

▶ 28. A patient with a dysrhythmia, type 2 diabetes mellitus (DM), and heart failure (HF) is prescribed quinidine, metformin, furosemide, and digoxin. The patient complains of nausea, and the nurse notes that the patient has only consumed 10% to 25% of his meals over the past 48 hours. The nurse should review the most recent laboratory results for:
    a. digoxin levels less than 0.8 ng/mL.
    b. fasting blood glucose less than 60 mg/dL.
    c. potassium levels less than 3.5 mEq/L.
    d. sodium levels less than 140 mEq/L.

## CASE STUDIES AND PATIENT TEACHING

*(Use a separate piece of paper for your responses.)*

### Case Study 1

*An overweight 75-year-old retiree underwent open-heart surgery 5 days ago and postoperatively developed a cerebrovascular accident (CVA). His history includes hypertension, renal insufficiency, alcohol abuse, and a 2-pack-per-day smoking habit. He was progressing well postoperatively without any further complications. A physical therapist and nurse assisted the patient to transfer to a chair. Following transfer to a recliner, the patient complained to the physical therapist that his "heart felt like it was racing."*

1. What assessments should the nurse perform at this time?

*The monitor nurse walks in to check on the patient because the monitor revealed to heart rate of 185 BPM. The nurse asks the patient to bear down to stimulate the vagus nerve and slow the heart rate. After obtaining a full set of vital signs, the nurse places a call to the attending physician. The physician orders a STAT 12 lead ECG. The attending physician arrives on the unit, examines the 12-lead ECG, and diagnoses ventricular tachycardia (v-tach). A bolus dose of lidocaine 100 mg is ordered.*

2. What elements of the patient's history are important when the prescriber is determining the dose of lidocaine to be infused?

3. What precautions must the nurse take when administering this bolus dose?

4. The bolus dose is followed by an infusion of a solution of lidocaine. What patient data can the nurse provide to assist the prescriber with determining the amount of fluid in which to dilute the lidocaine?

5. Prescribed is 1 gram of lidocaine in 250 mL of 5% dextrose in water at a rate of mg/minute. The intravenous pump is calibrated in mL per hour. What rate should be programmed into the pump?

6. Before infusing the drug, the nurse should examine the intravenous solution and not administer the drug if the solution contains what additives?

0.5% LIDOCAINE HCl
Injection, USP
5 mg/mL

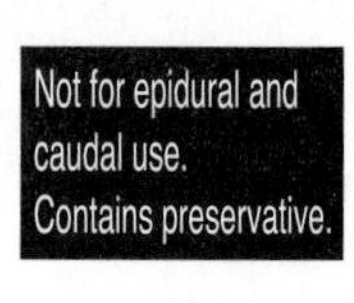


A

Lidocaine 4 mg/mL

0.4% Lidocaine Hydrocloride
and 5% Dextrose Injection USP

B

50 mL MULTIPLE-DOSE Fliptop Vial

LIDOCAINE HCl 0.5% and
EPINEPHRINE 1:200,000
Injection, USP

C

7. What should be included when the nurse reports to the prescriber the patient's response to lidocaine?

# 49 Prophylaxis of Coronary Heart Disease: Drugs That Lower LDL Cholestrol Levels

## OBJECTIVES

See page 26 for the Objectives.

## CRITICAL THINKING AND STUDY QUESTIONS

1. A 45-year-old female smoker with a family history of coronary heart disease has been prescribed a lipid-lowering medication. Which of these outcomes would be most important for this patient?
   a. Cholesterol, total 170 mg/dL
   b. HDL 50 mg/dL
   c. LDL 90 mg/dL
   d. Triglycerides 120 mg/dL

2. A patient has received instructions regarding cholesterol and the body. Which of these statements made by the client would indicate the patient needs further teaching?
   a. "Drugs that decrease the liver's ability to produce cholesterol should be taken so that they peak during the night."
   b. "Drugs that prevent the absorption of cholesterol from food are more effective than drugs that limit the making of cholesterol by the liver."
   c. "It is more important to limit the amount of saturated fat in my diet than the total amount of cholesterol."
   d. "My cholesterol can be high even if I eat a low fat diet and exercise regularly."

▶ 3. Recent laboratory results for a patient include HDL 85 mg/dL, LDL 145 mg/dL, and triglycerides 530 mg/dL. The nurse should assess the patient for:
   a. abdominal pain and nausea.
   b. chest pain and shortness of breath.
   c. rash and pruritus.
   d. tachycardia and diaphoresis.

4. The nurse is preparing a teaching for a community health fair. Which of the following risk factors for coronary heart disease (CHD) should be stressed because they correlate to the greatest risk of a major coronary event within 10 years? (Select all that apply.)
   a. Abdominal aortic aneurysm
   b. Diabetes insipidus
   c. Diabetes mellitus
   d. HDL cholesterol less than 50 mg/dL
   e. Older than 44 years of age
   f. Peripheral artery disease
   g. Smoker
   h. Systolic blood pressure greater than 120 mm/Hg

5. The nurse is caring for a 68-year-old man who has been admitted for a left below the knee amputation because of peripheral vascular disease associated with type 2 diabetes mellitus. He is receiving a lipid-lowering drug. Which of these levels of LDL would be an appropriate outcome for pharmacotherapy?
   a. LDL 35 mg/dL
   b. LDL 50 mg/dL
   c. LDL 75 mg/dL
   d. LDL 90 mg/dL

6. Clinical trials suggest that HMG-CoA reductase inhibitors (statins) benefit patients with atherosclerosis by:
   a. increasing serum LDL.
   b. promoting the production of thrombin.
   c. reducing serum HDL.
   d. stabilizing endothelial plaque.

7. The nurse has reviewed the laboratory results for a patient who is scheduled to receive lovastatin (Mevacor) 40 mg. Results include AST 78 International Units/L, CK 100 units/L, HDL 45 mg/dL, and LDL 245 mg/dL. The nurse should:
   a. administer the drug and continue nursing care.
   b. hold the drug and assess for chest pain.
   c. hold the drug and assess for abdominal pain.
   d. hold the drug and notify the prescriber of the laboratory results.

8. A 38-year-old female has been diagnosed with hypercholesterolemia. The prescriber has ordered simvastatin (Zocor) 20 mg, once a day at hour of sleep, to be started after laboratory results are obtained. Which of the following laboratory results would be a reason to withhold the drug?
   a. ALT 7 International Units/L
   b. Creatinine 1 mg/dL
   c. CRP 3.0 mg/dL
   d. HCG 287 International Units/L

9. A patient who is receiving lovastatin experiences chest pain. CK level is 580 units/mL (CK-MM 99%) and troponin T 0.02 g/mL. It is most important for the nurse to monitor functioning of which organ?
   a. Brain
   b. Heart
   c. Kidneys
   d. Lungs

10. A patient who is receiving nicotinic acid to elevate HDL and reduce triglycerides exhibits dry, hot, and flushed skin; thirst; hunger; and confusion. The nurse should:
   a. administer the drug and continue nursing care.
   b. hold the drug and assess for chest pain.
   c. hold the drug and assess for abdominal pain.
   d. hold the drug and notify the prescriber.

11. A patient who has been taking cholestyramine (Questran) complains of nausea. Which of the following assessment findings would be of most concern to the nurse?
   a. Bloating after medication administration
   b. Flatulence
   c. Increase in bowel sounds and "hush" sounds
   d. Indigestion

12. A patient has been prescribed cholestyramine in addition to other drugs for diabetes mellitus and hypertension. The cholestyramine should be administered:
   a. one hour before other drugs.
   b. two hours before other drugs.
   c. three hours before other drugs.
   d. four hours before other drugs.

13. The nurse should teach a patient who has been prescribed colestipol (Colestid) to prevent the most common adverse effect by:
   a. avoiding gas-producing vegetables.
   b. consuming 2500 mL of fluid each day.
   c. decreasing fat in the diet.
   d. taking the medication with milk.

14. The nurse would be most concerned about which of the following patients?
   a. A patient receiving lovastatin and experiencing a rash
   b. A patient receiving nicotinic acid and experiencing hot flashes with facial flushing
   c. A patient receiving colesevelam and experiencing nausea
   d. A patient receiving gemfibrozil and experiencing right upper quadrant pain

## CASE STUDIES AND PATIENT TEACHING

*(Use a separate piece of paper for your responses.)*

### Case Study 1

*A 52-year-old white female underwent a thorough physical examination. She smokes one pack of cigarettes each day and leads a sedentary lifestyle because of knee pain from osteoarthritis. She takes acetaminophen every day for joint pain, but does not take any prescription medications. Her examination was unremarkable except for being overweight. BP 140/80 mm/Hg, pulse 78 beats/min, respirations 22 and regular. Her family history is negative for coronary artery disease (CAD), myocardial infarction (MI), and cerebrovascular accident (CVA). Her diet is high in fat because of her intake of fast foods. Her laboratory results include cholesterol 285 mg/dL, HDL 33 mg/dL, and LDL 129 mg/dL.*

1. What is her 10-year risk for CHD according to the Framingham Risk Prediction Score?

2. Because of the elevated cholesterol in addition to a low HDL, the patient is considered to be at an increased risk for coronary artery disease. The physician has placed her on a restricted diet in an attempt to lower serum cholesterol and has mentioned that if this does not correct the problem, he may need to place her on medication. She asks the nurse about nondrug therapies that she can implement in an attempt to lower her cholesterol. What should be included in the nurse's response?

3. The patient returns 3 months later and has shown no improvement in lipid levels despite therapeutic lifestyle changes. Atorvastatin 10 mg at bedtime is prescribed. When the patient gets to the pharmacy, the pharmacist informs her that her prescription plan does not cover atorvastatin, but he has called the prescriber and received an order to dispense lovastatin 20 mg once a day, to be taken with the evening meal. After going home, the patient calls the prescriber's office and asks to speak with the nurse. She is upset about the change in medication and asks why she has been given a different drug with a higher dose, to be taken at a different time of the day. How should the nurse respond?

## Case Study 2

*The middle school nurse is concerned about the incidence of obesity in the fifth and sixth grade population of the inner city school. The physical education faculty have collaborated with the nurse and identified that many of the children do not get outside for active play because of danger in the neighborhood. They are planning an activity to help the children make healthier choices.*

1. What are possible developmentally appropriate health promotion strategies that could be included?

# 50 Drugs for Angina Pectoris

## OBJECTIVES

See page 26 for the Objectives.

## CRITICAL THINKING AND STUDY QUESTIONS

▶ 1. A priority nursing concern for a patient with angina pectoris is:
   a. alteration in cardiac output.
   b. impaired gas exchange.
   c. inadequate myocardial tissue perfusion.
   d. ineffective breathing pattern.

2. The goal of drug therapy for chronic stable angina is to:
   a. constrict coronary arteries to increase blood pressure during stress.
   b. decrease myocardial need for oxygen during stress.
   c. increase myocardial blood flow during systole.
   d. prevent coronary artery spasms.

3. Match drugs for unstable angina pectoris with therapeutic effect.

_____ a. ACE inhibitor
_____ b. Anticoagulant
_____ c. Antiplatelet
_____ d. Beta blocker
_____ e. Morphine
_____ f. Nitroglycerin

1. Decrease venous thrombus formation.
2. Prevent thrombocytes from sticking to plaque in arteries.
3. Reduce blood returning to heart by venous dilation, decreasing workload of heart.
4. Relieve pain, which decreases sympathetic stimulation and myocardial workload.
5. Slow heart rate, decreasing myocardial need for oxygen.
6. Vasodilate and increase fluid excretion, decreasing blood pressure.

4. A patient asks the nurse why nitroglycerin can be administered in so many ways. The basis of the nurse's response is that nitroglycerin:
   a. does not undergo first-pass effect in the liver.
   b. has few adverse effects, so varying doses can be administered via different routes.
   c. is an inactive compound, so it does not matter which route it is administered.
   d. is lipid soluble, so it is readily absorbed via different routes.

5. Nitroglycerin has myocardial vasodilation effects in variant (Prinzmetal's) angina but not in chronic stable angina because in chronic stable angina myocardial arterioles are:
   a. already maximally dilated.
   b. experiencing spastic vasoconstriction.
   c. occluded with thrombi.
   d. unable to diffuse oxygen into the cell.

6. A patient who has been using a nitroglycerin patch for angina has recently been prescribed diltiazem (Cardizem). Which statement, if made by this patient, would suggest that the patient understood teaching about the new drug?
   a. "I need to take this drug because nitroglycerin causes my blood pressure to go up."
   b. "If I take both of these drugs, I can use sildenafil (Viagra) if I experience erectile dysfunction."
   c. "This drug prevents my heart from racing, which can happen when people take nitroglycerin."
   d. "This drug will make the nitroglycerin work better."

▸ 7. A patient is prescribed a nitroglycerin patch that is to be applied at 0900 (9:00 AM) and removed at 2100 (9:00 PM). When preparing to administer the 0900 patch, the nurse notes that a nitroglycerin patch is still in place. The nurse should:
   a. apply the new patch to a different site, but leave the old patch on until the nursing supervisor is contacted.
   b. consult with the prescriber.
   c. remove the old patch and apply the new patch to a different site.
   d. remove the old patch and change the timing of the medication so that the patch is removed at 0900 and applied at 2100.

8. During data collection from a patient who is not obtaining relief from nitroglycerin tablets, the nurse should ask the patient if she allows that tablet to completely dissolve while in her mouth because swallowing sublingual nitroglycerin tablets:
   a. inactivates the drug.
   b. increases tolerance.
   c. prevents absorption.
   d. speeds excretion.

9. It is important for the nurse to teach a patient who has been prescribed nitroglycerin (NitroQuick) on an as needed basis to:
   a. discard unused tablets after 24 months.
   b. store the tablets in a locked medicine cabinet in the bathroom.
   c. take a few tablets from the bottle and keep them in a plastic bottle in your purse or pocket.
   d. write the date that the tablets are opened on the outside of the bottle.

▶ 10. When assessing a patient who is scheduled to receive the second dose of newly prescribed sustained-release nitroglycerin, the patient complains of a headache. The nurse should:
   a. administer as needed acetaminophen, if ordered, within the time constraints.
   b. crush the medication to speed absorption through the oral mucosa.
   c. notify the prescriber of the headache STAT.
   d. withhold the drug and consult the prescriber.

11. The nurse is aware that which of the following nitroglycerin preparations has a rapid onset and sustained effect?
   a. Sublingual tablets
   b. Sustained-release capsule
   c. Topical ointment
   d. Transdermal patch
   e. Translingual spray
   f. Transmucosal tablet

12. It would be most important for the nurse to report to the prescriber that a family member smokes cigarettes in the home if a patient is prescribed which of the following medications for angina?
   a. Amyl nitrate
   b. Beta blocker
   c. Diltiazem or verapamil
   d. Isosorbide
   e. Nitroglycerin

13. The nurse recognizes that a drug is a beta blocker if the generic name of the drug ends in:
   a. -cillin.
   b. -lol.
   c. -pril.
   d. -sartan.

14. Beta blockers are useful to improve myocardial oxygen supply in angina because they:
   a. dilate coronary arteries.
   b. dilate veins.
   c. lengthen diastole.
   d. reduce cardiac preload.

▶ 15. When administering a beta blocker for angina, which of the following pulse assessments would indicate that therapy has achieved the desired effect?
   a. 50 beats/min at rest; 100 beats/min immediately after physical therapy
   b. 60 beats/min at rest; 80 beats/min immediately after physical therapy
   c. 70 beats/min at rest; 90 beats/min immediately after physical therapy
   d. 80 beats/min at rest; 100 beats/min immediately after physical therapy

16. The nurse would withhold a beta blocker and immediately contact the prescriber if it was discovered that the patient has a history of :
   a. asthma.
   b. first degree heart block.
   c. hyperglycemia.
   d. sick sinus syndrome.

17. The nurse would assess for bradycardia when an anginal patient is receiving which of the following drugs for angina?
   a. Diltiazem
   b. Isosorbide
   c. Metoprolol
   d. Nifedipine
   e. Nitroglycerin
   f. Verapamil

## CASE STUDIES AND PATIENT TEACHING

*(Use a separate piece of paper for your responses.)*

### Case Study 1

*A 75-year-old male with a history of stable angina, asthma, and hypertension is admitted to the hospital with substernal chest pain that was not relieved by 3 sublingual nitroglycerin (NTG) tablets. In the emergency room, the patient is prescribed diltiazem and an intravenous nitroglycerin drip.*

1. What actions must the nurse take when administering intravenous nitroglycerin?

2. The patient's pain is relieved after receiving a dosage of 330 mcg/hr. He is admitted to the coronary care unit. His vital signs are stable, and he is currently without pain. Cardiac enzyme levels do not suggest myocardial cell death. The ECG shows normal sinus rhythm. The physicians believe that the patient is having classic angina and not a myocardial infarction (MI). The attending physician orders that the patient be weaned from the NTG drip and that NTG transdermal patches 10 mg/24 hr be started. He is also prescribed aspirin 81 mg, diltiazem-CD (30 mg) and ramipril (Altace) 2.5 mg, which he is to receive once a day. If the prescriber wants a continuous administration of nitroglycerin when changing the patient from the NTG drip to the patch, when, in relation to discontinuing the intravenous NTG, should the nurse apply the nitroglycerin patch?

3. What teaching should the nurse provide about administration of the nitroglycerin patch?

4. The patient has the NTG drip turned off, the NTG patch is applied, and the diltiazem-CD is administered. He asks the nurse what may have been the reason that his NTG sublingual tablets did not work. Based on knowledge of NTG sublingual tablets, what factors may have contributed to why the NTG tablets may not have relieved his anginal pain?

5. The nurse asks the patient's wife to bring his supply of sublingual NTG tablets in to the hospital. The wife pulls out a small plastic pill container from her purse. "Heart pills" is handwritten on a masking tape label. What teaching does the nurse need to provide?

6. The patient states that he guesses he will not need to get any more NTG sublingual tablets now that he is using the NTG patches. How should the nurse respond?

7. The nurse is reviewing medications during discharge instructions. The patient admits to adherence issues with taking his antihypertensive drug therapy because of experiencing erectile dysfunction. He asks what the nurse thinks about sildenafil (Viagra). What information should the nurse provide?

## Case Study 2

*A farmer who lives in a remote area was admitted with chest pain. He has been diagnosed with angina and is being discharged with a prescription for sublingual nitroglycerin tablets.*

1. What teaching should the nurse provide about administration and storage of this drug?

2. The prescriber has written instructions that this patient should take the nitroglycerin before participating in stressful activity. What teaching should the nurse provide, considering farm work includes operation of potentially dangerous equipment?

3. The prescriber has instructed this patient to continue to take nitroglycerin up to 3 tablets 5 minutes apart, take an aspirin, and to seek emergency medical care if relief is not obtained after administration of the first sublingual nitroglycerin tablet. The patient's wife states that her mother took nitroglycerin and had been instructed to seek medical care if not obtaining relief after taking 3 tablets. Why are the prescriber's instructions logical for this patient?

4. The patient has been instructed to take 1 baby aspirin tablet per day. The patient verbalizes that this seems silly as 1 baby aspirin tablet will not do much to relieve his chest pain. How should the nurse respond?

## Case Study 3

*The occupational nurse is preparing for a health promotion fair at the manufacturing plant. Coronary artery disease has been identified at a level higher than the national and state level in the community where the plant is located. The nurse wants to develop a teaching plan, including realistic interventions to help employees and their families prevent the incidence and adverse effects of coronary artery disease.*

1. Complete this chart that could be used by the nurse as the basis of developing a presentation appropriate for this setting.

| Coronary Artery Disease | | |
|---|---|---|
| **Risk factors for CAD** | **How this factor increases risk of CAD** | **Interventions to prevent, reverse, or minimize negative effects on heart** |
| Smoking | | |
| High cholesterol | | |
| Hypertension | | |
| Diabetes | | |
| Obesity | | |
| Physical inactivity | | |

# 51 Anticoagulant, Antiplatelet, and Thrombolytic Drugs

## OBJECTIVES

See page 26 for the Objectives.

## CRITICAL THINKING AND STUDY QUESTIONS

1. A patient asks why heparin cannot be administered orally. The basis of the nurse's response is heparin:
   a. has a prolonged half-life when administered orally.
   b. can only be prepared as an oral solution and is bitter tasting.
   c. is destroyed by proteases in the gastrointestinal tract.
   d. is large and negatively charged limiting absorption.

▸ 2. Which of these laboratory test results (which are flagged on the laboratory sheet as abnormal), if identified in a patient who is receiving heparin, should the nurse report to the prescriber immediately?
   a. aPTT 75 seconds
   b. BUN 22 mg/dL
   c. Platelet count 80,000/$mm^3$
   d. WBC 11,000/$mm^3$

▸ 3. A patient who has been receiving heparin tells the nurse that she thinks she could be pregnant. The nurse should:
   a. administer the heparin as ordered and notify the physician of the possible pregnancy status.
   b. withhold the heparin.
   c. withhold the heparin until pregnancy status can be confirmed.
   d. withhold the heparin and consult the prescriber regarding administration of the antidote protamine sulfate.

▸ 4. A patient has been receiving long-term high-dose heparin therapy. What nursing teaching would be best to prevent a common adverse effect of this type of therapy?
   a. Avoid crowds
   b. Develop a plan for weight-bearing exercise as approved by physician
   c. Increase fluid and fiber in diet
   d. Regular use of any over-the-counter antacid

5. Protamine sulfate acts as an antidote to heparin by:
   a. activating clotting factor Xa.
   b. activating thrombin.
   c. binding with the negatively charged groups on the heparin molecule.
   d. suppressing antithrombin activity.

▸ 6. A patient is scheduled for a below-knee amputation at 1000 (10:00 AM) the next day. Heparin 5000 units are scheduled to be administered subcutaneously at 2100 (9:00 PM) today. The nurse should:
   a. administer the medication.
   b. withhold the medication and contact the prescriber.

▸ 7. A patient who received 5000 units of heparin subcutaneously at 0900 develops hematemesis at 1030. The physician orders 50 mg of protamine sulfate via slow intravenous push injection. Protamine sulfate is available as 10 mg/mL. If the nurse administers this dose over 5 minutes, how much will be administered every 15 seconds?

8. Heparin therapy is considered therapeutic when the results of the aPTT are:
   a. 30 to 40 seconds (normal).
   b. 40 to 50 seconds (1 to 1.5 times normal).
   c. 60 to 80 seconds (2 times normal).
   d. 90 to 120 seconds (3 times normal).

9. One unit of heparin will prevent 1 mL of sheep plasma from coagulating for what period of time?
   a. 1 hour
   b. 2 hours
   c. 4 hours
   d. 12 hours

10. It is important for the nurse to distinguish between concentrations of heparin used for intravenous flushing from concentrations used for subcutaneous injection because the concentration for subcutaneous use is how much greater than that for intravenous flushing?
    a. 1 to 25 times greater
    b. 10 to 100 times greater
    c. 25 to 400 times greater
    d. 100 to 2500 times greater

11. The nurse would consult the prescriber if which of the following drugs was prescribed, but there was no order for monitoring of aPTT?
    a. Fragmin
    b. Heparin
    c. Innohep
    d. Lovenox

▸ 12. A patient who weighs 176 lbs has been prescribed intravenous lepirudin (Refludan) 12 mg/hr after experiencing heparin-induced thrombocytopenia. Before the first dose, the nurse reviews the patient's laboratory results, which include patient aPTT 47 seconds, reference aPTT 40 seconds, creatinine clearance 42 mL/min/1.73 $m^2$, AST 35 units/L, and ALT 22 International Units/L. Which of the following is a possible concern to the nurse that should be communicated to the prescriber?
    a. Abnormal aPTT
    b. Dose too high for weight
    c. Liver dysfunction
    d. Renal insufficiency

▸ 13. The nurse should teach patients who are prescribed warfarin (Coumadin) to eat consistent amounts of which of the following foods? (Select all that apply.)
    a. Cabbage
    b. Citrus fruits
    c. Dairy products
    d. Green vegetables
    e. Liver
    f. Red meat

14. Which of the following should the nurse teach a patient about precautions before dental surgery when the patient is prescribed long-term warfarin therapy?
    a. No action is needed.
    b. Inform the dentist of the most recent INR results.
    c. Stop warfarin 3 days before dental surgery.
    d. Take half of the normal dose of warfarin for 3 days before dental surgery.

▸ 15. A patient is diagnosed with GI bleeding during warfarin therapy. The nurse is preparing to administer intravenous phytonadione (Vitamin $K_1$). Assessment findings include INR 5.8, blood pressure 98/54 mm Hg, oxygen saturation 96%, respirations 25 per minute, and temperature 102.8° F. The nurse should:
    a. administer acetaminophen to reduce fever.
    b. administer aspirin to reduce fever.
    c. administer the intravenous phytonadione (Vitamin $K_1$) very slowly.
    d. withhold the intravenous phytonadione (Vitamin $K_1$) and contact the prescriber.

16. For what period of time should the nurse take precautions to prevent bleeding, including applying pressure to puncture sites for 5 minutes, after warfarin (Coumadin) therapy has been discontinued?
    a. 6 hours
    b. 8 to 12 hours
    c. 2.5 days
    d. 5 days

17. Which of the following statements, if made by a patient who has been prescribed low-dose aspirin therapy, would indicate a need for further teaching?
    a. "I need to inform my pharmacist that I am taking aspirin therapy."
    b. "I should quit smoking."
    c. "I should not use a drug that reduces stomach acid while on aspirin therapy."
    d. "If I use an enteric-coated aspirin, I don't need to worry about bleeding."

▶ 18. Which of the following adverse effects, if noted in a patient who has recently been prescribed ticlopidine (Ticlid), would be a reason for the nurse to contact the prescriber immediately?
    a. Change in level of consciousness
    b. Diarrhea
    c. Dyspepsia
    d. Itchy rash

▶ 19. The nurse is reviewing the laboratory tests of a patient who has been prescribed ticlopidine (Ticlid) for the past week. The WBC count is 3000/mm$^3$, and the neutrophil count is 30%. A nursing priority for this patient is:
    a. adequate cardiac output.
    b. effective airway clearance.
    c. maintaining skin integrity.
    d. preventing infection.

▶ 20. Which of the following laboratory tests, if not ordered for a patient who has been recently prescribed clopidogrel (Plavix), would be a reason for the nurse to consult with the prescriber?
    a. aPTT
    b. INR
    c. Platelets
    d. PT

▶ 21. The nurse calculates the safe dose of tirofiban (Aggrastat) for a 220-lb patient undergoing balloon angioplasty per table 51-7. The drug comes in a solution of 12.5 mg/250 mL. The intravenous pump is calibrated in milliliters per hour. What rate will the nurse enter into the intravenous pump per hour?
    a. 24 mL/hr
    b. 48 mL/hr
    c. 72 mL/hr
    d. 96 mL/hr

▶ 22. The nurse teaches a patient who has been prescribed cilostazol (Pletal) that risk of the adverse effect of bleeding is increased if the patient includes in the diet which of the following foods?
    a. Cabbage
    b. Dairy products
    c. Grapefruit juice
    d. Green vegetables

23. The nurse should have available which of the following drugs when streptokinase is being administered?
    a. Aminocaproic acid (Amicar)
    b. Phytonadione (Vitamin $K_1$)
    c. Protamine sulfate

24. The critical care nurse monitors for the adverse effects of hypotension and fever in a patient who is receiving which of the following thrombolytic drugs?
    a. Alteplase
    b. Reteplase
    c. Streptokinase
    d. Tenecteplase

## CASE STUDIES AND PATIENT TEACHING

*(Use a separate piece of paper for your responses.)*

### Case Study 1

*A 185-lb patient with a history of osteoarthritis, type 2 diabetes mellitus, hypertension, hyperlipidemia, and benign prostatic hyperplasia experiences a pulmonary emboli after right total hip replacement surgery.*

*The physician orders include:*

- *STAT baseline CBC, INR, aPTT, and platelets*
- *If baseline laboratory results are within normal limits:*
    - *One dose of heparin 100 units/kg intravenous push (round to nearest 100 units)*
    - *Heparin 25,000 units/250 mL 5% dextrose in water to infuse at 12 units/kg/hr*
    - *STAT aPTT 6 hours after start of heparin infusion*

1. Baseline laboratory results are within normal limits. How much heparin will the nurse administer as the initial intravenous push dose in units?

2. Heparin is available in concentrations of 100 units/mL and 5000 units/mL. Which concentration of heparin should the nurse use, and how many milliliters should the nurse administer intravenous push for the initial dose?

3. What is the initial dose and infusion rate of heparin based on the above orders?

Further heparin orders are by the following protocol (round to nearest 100 units):

| aPTT (sec) | IV Bolus (units) | Hold Heparin (min) | IV Heparin Rate Change | Repeat aPTT and INR |
|---|---|---|---|---|
| Less than 50 sec | 5000 | 0 | + 3 units/hr | 4 hr |
| 50–59 sec | 0 | 0 | + 2 units/hr | 6 hr |
| 60–80 sec | 0 | 0 | none | Next AM |
| 80–95 sec | 0 | 0 | – 2 units/hr | 6 hr |
| 96–120 sec | 0 | 30 | – 3 units/hr | 4 hr |
| Greater than 120 sec | 0 | 60 | Contact prescriber | 4 hr |

4. The patient's aPTT results after 6 hours of heparin therapy is 30 seconds. Based on the protocol, the nurse should set the infusion pump to what rate?

5. After 12 hours, the patient's aPTT results are 75 seconds. What actions should the nurse take?

6. What precautions should the nurse take to prevent accidentally infusing too much intravenous heparin?

7. The hospital has a policy that heparin must be infused using a separate intravenous site and separate pump. Piggyback medication can never be added to the heparin line. The patient asks why she must have two intravenous sites. What would the nurse include in her explanation?

8. After 4 days, the intravenous heparin is discontinued, and the patient is ordered subcutaneous heparin. How soon after discontinuation of the intravenous heparin do anticoagulant effects diminish and end?

9. Describe the technique for nursing administration of subcutaneous heparin, including the rationale for each step.

10. What antidote should be available to the nurse when a patient is receiving heparin? How long does this antidote effect last?

## Case Study 2

*A 36-year-old, 132-lb female whose job requires frequent long airplane trips is admitted for treatment of a deep venous thrombosis (DVT) in the right thigh. The patient's husband asks why her primary care provider did not prescribe low-dose aspirin to prevent DVTs.*

1. How should the nurse respond?

2. The patient is initially ordered a heparin drip by the emergency department physician. What is the most common adverse effect of heparin, and what symptoms of this adverse effect should be monitored by the nurse?

3. Heparin is pregnancy category C, which means that research studies suggest that risk to the developing fetus cannot be ruled out. If heparin does not cross the placenta, why is it not categorized as pregnancy class B?

4. The patient's primary care practitioner discontinues the intravenous heparin and orders enoxaparin 60 mg every 12 hours. How much time should elapse between the nurse discontinuing the heparin drip and starting the subcutaneous enoxaparin (Lovenox)? Why?

## Case Study 3

*A patient is admitted with atrial fibrillation and is initially prescribed subcutaneous heparin and warfarin.*

1. Why is this patient ordered both anticoagulant drugs?

2. Daily INR is ordered. What information does the nurse have to provide to the phlebotomist who will be collecting the blood sample for this test?

3. The patient asks what the INR measures. How should the nurse explain the results of this test?

4. After 4 days of both drugs, the patient is to be discharged with a prescription for warfarin (Coumadin). What is the antidote and dosing for an overdose of warfarin?

5. What patient information does the nurse need to provide the patient before he is discharged home on warfarin?

# 52 Management of ST-Elevation Myocardial Infarction

## OBJECTIVES

See page 26 for the Objectives.

## CRITICAL THINKING AND STUDY QUESTIONS

1. A protocol in the emergency department is to administer 4 81-mg chewable aspirin tablets (total 324 mg) to patients with suspected myocardial infarction. A student nurse asks the nurse why 4 chewable aspirin tablets are administered instead of 2 regular aspirin tablets (650 mg). Which of the following would not be included in the nurse's explanation?
   a. Aspirin is an acid, and acids are more readily absorbed in the acid environment of the stomach.
   b. Chewable forms of aspirin are absorbed through the buccal mucosa bypassing hepatic first pass.
   c. Chewing breaks the tablet into smaller particles, which are more readily absorbed.
   d. Exceeding 325-mg doses can offset the vasodilation and antiplatelet effects of lower doses.

▸ 2. A patient who is undergoing an acute STEMI is prescribed metoprolol 50 mg by mouth every 6 hours. Which of the following assessment findings would be a reason to withhold the medication and immediately contact the prescriber?
   a. Altered taste
   b. Insomnia
   c. Rhinorrhea
   d. Wheezing

3. Which of the following drugs prescribed for acute STEMI should be withheld and the prescriber consulted immediately if the patient's pulse is 118 beats/min?
   a. Aspirin
   b. Atenolol
   c. Morphine
   d. Nitroglycerin

4. The nurse knows that nitroglycerin decreases the workload of the heart by:
   a. decreasing venous return to the heart.
   b. dissolving existing clots.
   c. preventing clot formation.
   d. slowing the heart rate.

5. Which of the following drugs would inhibit angiotensin II–mediated ventricular remodeling in the STEMI patient's myocardium?
   a. Captopril (Capoten)
   b. Clopidogrel (Plavix)
   c. Diltiazem (Cardizem)
   d. Verapamil (Calan)

## CASE STUDIES AND PATIENT TEACHING

*(Use a separate piece of paper for your responses.)*

### Case Study 1

*A 57-year-old male who is vacationing locally is admitted to the emergency room with severe, crushing chest pain. The pain radiates into his left arm, and he is experiencing diaphoresis, weakness, and nausea. The ECG shows elevated ST segments in the inferior leads. Troponin T (TnT) is elevated 3 times above lower limits, and the total creatine kinase (CK) and the CK-MB isoenzyme are slightly elevated. The physician diagnoses STEMI. The physician deicdes to start thrombolytic therapy with alteplase (tPA).*

1. What assessments should the nurse monitor relating to the risk of intracranial bleed?

2. The nurse is directed to interview the patient's wife. What information does the nurse need to obtain to assist the physician with deciding if thrombocytic therapy is appropriate?

3. The following medications are ordered. What is the purpose of these drugs, and what assessment should the nurse perform relating to administration of these drugs?
   a. Aspirin (ASA) 81 mg chewable tablets, 4 tablets STAT
   b. Intravenous morphine 4 mg followed by 2 mg every 10 minutes as needed to control pain
   c. Metoprolol 5 mg intravenous every 2 minutes for 3 doses then 50 mg orally every 6 hours × 48 hours
   d. Nitroglycerin intravenous drip 10 mcg per minute

4. Why is it important for the nurse to assess if this patient has taken sildenafil in the past 24 hours?

5. The patient is being discharged with prescriptions for metoprolol (Lopressor) 100 mg once a day, captopril (Capoten) 25 mg every 8 hours, aspirin 81 mg once a day, and warfarin (Coumadin) 5 mg once a day. The patient's wife asks why he must have blood work done every week. How should the nurse respond?

6. When explaining warfarin therapy, the nurse shares the patient's INR results, which most recently were 1.8. The laboratory result from lists the normal INR as 0.85-1.2. How can the nurse explain that the target INR is 3, which appears to be abnormal?

### Case Study 2

*A nurse is leading an educational program for patients in a cardiac rehabilitation program.*

1. What teaching regarding drugs and non-pharmacologic interventions can the nurse provide to decrease these risk factors for reinfarction?
   a. Diabetes
   b. Hyperlipidemia
   c. Hypertension
   d. Obesity and sedentary lifestyle
   e. Smoking cessation

2. What are reasons why the nurse should teach pateints to seek medical care immediately if experiencing chest pain?

# 53 Drugs for Hemophilia

## OBJECTIVES

See page 26 for the Objectives.

## CRITICAL THINKING AND STUDY QUESTIONS

1. Hemophilia: (Select all that apply.)
   a. always produces a severe bleeding disorder.
   b. can result from a spontaneous gene mutation.
   c. has a carrier risk of 100% for daughters of a hemophiliac.
   d. interferes with the formation of a platelet plug.
   e. is inherited on the Y chromosome.
   f. has a risk factor of 50% for every boy born to a mother who is a carrier for the defective gene, no matter how many brothers have the disease.
   g. has a risk factor of 50% for all sons of a hemophiliac.
   h. treatment with clotting factor replacement is highly effective.

2. A male with 10% normal and 90% abnormal levels of clotting factor IX is classified as having:
   a. mild hemophilia A.
   b. moderate hemophilia A.
   c. severe hemophilia A.
   d. mild hemophilia B.
   e. moderate hemophilia B.
   f. severe hemophilia B.

▸ 3. The nurse is teaching a patient with severe hemophilia and his family the importance of protecting joints from injury. The nurse teaches that it is most critical to prevent injury to the:
   a. ankle.
   b. elbow.
   c. knee.
   d. skull.

▸ 4. The nurse needs to give an immunization to a patient with a history of mild hemophilia B. The nurse should:
   a. administer the immunization as usual.
   b. administer the immunization subcutaneously.
   c. ask the pediatrician to administer the immunization.
   d. only administer with an oral or nasal route.

5. The mother of a child with hemophilia calls the pediatrician's office. She has forgotten which medication she can give her son for mild pain and fever. The telephone triage nurse follows protocol and explains that the safest choice for hemophiliacs is:
   a. acetaminophen (Tylenol)
   b. acetylsalicylic acid (aspirin)
   c. celecoxib (Celebrex)
   d. ibuprofen (Motrin)

▸ 6. A priority nursing diagnosis for a 9-year-old boy with hemophilia is:
   a. anxiety.
   b. impaired parenting.
   c. ineffective coping.
   d. risk for injury.

7. The parents of a boy newly diagnosed with hemophilia express concern that their son will contract HIV, other infections, or have an allergic reaction from factor concentrates. The basis of the nurse's response is:
   a. no case of virus transmission has been reported with any of the products now used in the United States.
   b. recombinant factor concentrate products carry a risk of contracting Creutzfeldt-Jakob disease (CJD).
   c. there is a risk of contracting HIV from plasma-derived factor concentrate, but the risk of bleeding is more serious.
   d. viruses for hepatitis A and parvovirus are lipid-coated viruses that are found in plasma-derived factor concentrate.

8. A nurse in the perioperative area is caring for a child with hemophilia B. Recombinant factor concentrate is prescribed as a continuous infusion. The nurse should:
   a. administer the factor concentrate at a total dose of 40 to 50 units/kg.
   b. calculate the dose by multiplying the patient's weight by 60% to 80% and dividing the dose by 2.
   c. ensure that the medication is available.
   d. flush the catheter with heparin once a shift.

9. Calculations are available to predict patient response to infusion of factor concentrates. For each unit/kg of recombinant factor IX (BeneFix) administered, the patient's normal factor IX should increase:
   a. 1%.
   b. 2%.
   c. 5%.
   d. 10%.

10. The most important factor when the prescriber is determining the proper dose of factor concentrate is:
    a. age.
    b. clinical response.
    c. target percentage of normal factor levels.
    d. weight.

▶ 11. Desmopressin nasal spray 150 mcg is prescribed preoperatively for a 4-year-old boy with mild hemophilia A. The pharmacy only carries the spray that delivers 10 mcg/spray. The nurse should:
    a. administer 15 sprays of the medication.
    b. administer 150 mcg intravenously.
    c. consult with the prescriber as to whether the nurse should attempt to administer the nasal dose in this concentration or should the order be discontinued and an intravenous dose ordered?
    d. consult with the prescriber as to whether the nurse should attempt to administer the nasal dose in this concentration or should the order be discontinued and an oral dose ordered?

▶ 12. The nurse should teach the parents to assess for allergy symptoms when administering factor concentrate. What should the parents do if the child experiences swelling around the face?
    a. Administer aminocaproic acid (Amicar).
    b. Administer diphenhydramine (Benadryl).
    c. Seek immediate emergency medical care.
    d. Slow the infusion.

13. Aminocaproic acid (Amicar) syrup may be prescribed to control bleeding from minor injuries to the nose and mouth for patient's with:
    a. hemophilia A and B.
    b. hemophilia A only.
    c. hemophilia B only.
    d. severe hemophilia A and B only.

14. The nurse knows that inhibitor antibodies to factor concentrate is most likely to occur in hemophiliacs of which of the following descent? (Select all that apply.)
    a. African American
    b. Asian
    c. Latino
    d. Middle Eastern
    e. Native American
    f. Northern European
    g. Scandinavian

15. When a patient is receiving factor VIIa (NovoSeven) he should be carefully assessed for:
    a. allergy to pork.
    b. anorexia and nausea.
    c. chest pain and shortness of breath.
    d. muscle weakness and fatigue.

## CASE STUDIES AND PATIENT TEACHING

*(Use a separate piece of paper for your responses.)*

### Case Study 1

*A 17-month-old boy has been newly diagnosed with hemophilia A. Review of his chart indicates he has not been immunized for hepatitis A.*

1. What teaching needs to be provided relating to hepatitis immunization and, what information relating to immunizations does the nurse need to obtain regarding caregivers?

2. The mother asks why aspirin should not be given to her son. Describe what the nurse should explain.

3. The nurse provides a comprehensive list of over-the-counter drugs that contain salicylate. Which of these drugs would the nurse include on this list? (Select all that apply.)
   a. Alka Seltzer
   b. Anacin
   c. Aspergum
   d. Arthropan
   e. Ascriptin
   f. Disalcid
   g. Doan's original
   h. Dolobid
   i. Empirin
   j. Keygesic
   k. Momentum
   l. Pepto Bismol
   m. St Joseph's baby aspirin
   n. Trilisate

4. The home health nurse goes to the boy's home to teach the mother how to administer recombinant factor VIII concentrate via a central venous catheter. What are nursing diagnoses that the nurse should consider when developing the plan of care for this family?

5. Administering factor concentrate carries a risk of complications. What should the nurse teach the caregiver to prepare for possible complications?

# 54 Drugs for Deficiency Anemias

## OBJECTIVES

See page 26 for the Objectives.

## CRITICAL THINKING AND STUDY QUESTIONS

1. Matching

| |  | |  |
|---|---|---|---|
| _____ | a. Erythroblast | 1. | Developing RBC in marrow after incorporates hemoglobin |
| _____ | b. Ferritinbone | 2. | Developing RBC in bone marrow before incorporates hemoglobin |
| _____ | c. Hematocrit | 3. | Immature nonnucleated RBCs |
| _____ | d. Hemoglobin | 4. | Iron-containing protein in muscle cells that stores oxygen |
| _____ | e. Hemosiderin | 5. | Measures color of RBCs |
| _____ | f. IBC (TIBC) | 6. | Measures size of RBCs |
| _____ | g. MCHC | 7. | Oxygen-carrying protein of RBCs |
| _____ | h. MCV | 8. | Percentage of RBCs in a volume of blood |
| _____ | i. Myoglobin | 9. | Saturation capacity of transferrin with iron |
| _____ | j. Proerythroblast | 10. | Storage form of iron |
| _____ | k. RDW | 11. | Storage form of iron in bone marrow |
| _____ | l. Reticulocyte | 12. | Transports absorbed iron to bone marrow |
| _____ | m. Transferrin | 13. | Variation in size of RBC |

▸ 2. The nurse is caring for an anemic cancer patient who is receiving chemotherapy that prevents the reproduction of rapidly dividing cells, including the cancer cells, hair, red blood cells, and epithelium of the GI tract. Which of the following laboratory results suggests that the anemia is getting worse?
   a. Hemoglobin 9 mg/dL
   b. Hematocrit 26%
   c. RBC $3.8 \times 10^{12}$/L
   d. Reticulocyte count 0.002%

▸ 3. The nurse should assess for symptoms of anemia in a patient who has a history of:
   a. chronic obstructive pulmonary disease.
   b. chronic renal failure.
   c. diabetes insipidus.
   d. hypertension.

4. Normally the body prevents excessive buildup of iron in the body by:
   a. decreasing intestinal absorption of iron.
   b. increasing metabolism of RBCs.
   c. increasing excretion of RBCs in bile.
   d. increasing excretion of RBCs in urine.

5. Which of the following foods should the nurse include in her dietary teaching for pregnant women regarding prevention of iron deficiency anemia? (Select all that apply.)
   a. Carrots
   b. Cheese
   c. Chicken
   d. Citrus fruit
   e. Egg white
   f. Egg yolk
   g. Fish
   h. Legumes
   i. Milk
   j. Red meat
   k. Squash
   l. Yogurt

6. Matching

| | | |
|---|---|---|
| _____ | a. Hyperchromic | 1. Excessive color |
| _____ | b. Hypochromic | 2. Large erythroblast |
| _____ | c. Macrocyte | 3. Large erythrocyte |
| _____ | d. Megaloblast | 4. Pale |
| _____ | e. Microcytic | 5. Small size cell |

7. In iron deficiency anemia, the nurse would expect which of the following tests to be elevated from normal levels?
   a. Hematocrit (Hct)
   b. Hemoglobin (Hgb or Hb)
   c. (Total) Iron-binding capacity (IBC or TIBC)
   d. Mean corpuscular volume (MCV)

8. When administering ferrous sulfate, the nurse should assess for the common symptoms including:
   a. discoloration of teeth.
   b. dyspepsia.
   c. hypotension.
   d. weak, rapid pulse.

9. A patient complains of intolerable nausea and heartburn from taking an oral iron preparation. The nurse should instruct the patient to:
   a. consult with prescriber for possible dose reduction.
   b. take a calcium carbonate antacid with the iron.
   c. take the iron with milk.
   d. take the iron with orange juice.

▸ 10. The nurse is providing care to a patient who is receiving an oral iron preparation. The patients stool is greenish black. Initially the nurse should:
   a. administer a dose of the iron preparation.
   b. consult the prescriber.
   c. determine if this stool is usual or a change for this patient.
   d. hold the iron preparation.

11. A 56-year-old man is admitted with unexplained severe shortness of breath with minimal activity. Lung sounds are clear. Pulse is rapid. Abnormal lab results include low hemoglobin and hematocrit, elevated MCV, very high levels of ALT. The nurse reviews the patient's history, which reveals alcohol abuse. The patient's wife states that she does not know how he could be anemic. He takes iron and eats red meat every day. The basis of the nurse's response is alcohol abuse:
   a. impairs the absorption of iron.
   b. increases urinary excretion of iron.
   c. is associated with thiamin deficiency anemia.
   d. prevents the absorption of vitamin $B_{12}$ (cyanocobalamin).

12. The nurse teaches a patient to take iron with food for the first few weeks of therapy because:
    a. early in therapy, toxicity is more likely.
    b. ferrous sulfate leaves a bad aftertaste, which disappears with continued therapy.
    c. food increases the absorption of iron.
    d. GI adverse effects are most intense during the first weeks of therapy.

▸ 13. A patient with peptic ulcer disease has developed severe anemia. Iron dextran (DexFerrum) has just been prescribed. The nurse has administered a test dose. It is most critical to observe the patient for:
    a. angioedema.
    b. hives.
    c. phlebitis at the site of injection.
    d. tissue damage from extravasation.

14. When iron must be administered by injection, how should it be administered?
    a. Intradermal
    b. Intrathecal
    c. Subcutaneous
    d. Z-track intramuscular

▸ 15. The dialysis nurse has administered iron sucrose (Venofer) and erythropoietin. A priority nursing concern relating to adverse effects is:
    a. gastrointestinal cramping.
    b. infusion site discomfort.
    c. maintaining adequate tissue perfusion.
    d. nausea and vomiting.

16. The nurse should teach the patient with pernicious anemia to report:
    a. fatigue.
    b. joint pain.
    c. paresthesias.
    d. temperature >100.4° F (38° C).

▸ 17. A patient with pernicious anemia complains of numbness and tingling of the hands and feet. What data relating to possible neurologic damage should the nurse collect before notifying the physician of the patient's complaint?
    a. Blood pressure
    b. DTR
    c. Capillary glucose
    d. Skin color

▸ 18. To prevent damage to the developing neural tube of a fetus, it is important for women of child-bearing age to have adequate daily intake of folate, which can be found in: (Select all that apply.)
    a. asparagus.
    b. egg yolks.
    c. lentils.
    d. liver.
    e. meat.
    f. milk.
    g. oranges.
    h. spinach.
    i. whole wheat.
    j. Yogurt.

## CASE STUDIES AND PATIENT TEACHING

*(Use a separate piece of paper for your responses.)*

### Case Study 1

*An 11-month-old, who drinks 8-ounce bottles of whole milk 5 to 6 times a day, is diagnosed with iron deficiency anemia.*

1. What can the nurse teach the parents about factors that could be contributing to the anemia and measures to change the factors that can be altered?

2. The pediatrician prescribes ferrous sulfate drops 25 mg twice a day. The child weighs 22 lbs, and the recommended dose is 5 mg/kg/day. Is the dose safe and effective?

3. Ferrous sulfate drops are available as 75 mg in 0.6 mL. How much should the parents administer with each dose?

4. What should the nurse teach the parents about ferrous sulfate therapy?

### Case Study 2

*A 28-year-old female has gastric bypass surgery. She has lost 25 lbs in the past 2 months. She comes to her primary care provider (PCP) with complaints of fatigue and glossitis (smooth, beefy, red tongue).*

1. Because of a history of this surgery, the patient is at risk for what type of anemia? Why?

2. The patient is prescribed parenteral injections of vitamin $B_{12}$ (30 mcg) and folic acid 200 mcg daily for 1 week. She then will receive oral cyanocobalamin 10,000 mcg/day and folic acid 400 mcg/day. The patient tells the nurse that she had learned that oral administration of cyanocobalamin is ineffective. How should the nurse respond?

3. The nurse teaches the patient to report which symptoms that suggest the uncommon, but significant, adverse effect of hypokalemia when taking cyanocobalamin (Vitamin $B_{12}$)?

4. Because this woman is of child-bearing age, the nurse teaches this patient that adequate daily consumption is important because:

5. The patient states that she will take extra folic acid from the health food store because she wants to get pregnant. How should the nurse respond?

# 55 Hematopoietic Growth Factors

## OBJECTIVES

See page 26 for the Objectives.

## CRITICAL THINKING AND STUDY QUESTIONS

▸ 1. A patient with a history of diabetes mellitus type 2 (DM2) and chronic renal failure (CRF) is receiving epoetin alpha (Procrit) because her failing kidneys do not produce adequate amounts of erythropoietin, and she has become anemic. Considering the vascular complications of diabetes mellitus, an appropriate outcome for this drug therapy would be hemoglobin:
   a. 8 gm/dL.
   b. 11 gm/dL.
   c. 14 gm/dL.
   d. 17 gm/dL.

2. Epoetin alpha (Procrit) is scheduled to be administered at 0800. The patient is scheduled for hemodialysis at 1000. The nurse should:
   a. administer the drug as ordered.
   b. administer the drug during hemodialysis.
   c. do not administer the drug on a dialysis day.
   d. hold the drug until after dialysis.

▸ 3. Which of these findings would be most significant if a patient was receiving darbepoetin alpha (Aranesp)?
   a. Blood pressure 170/120 mm Hg
   b. Pulse 104 beats/min
   c. Respirations 26
   d. Temperature 100.4° F (38° C)

4. A chemotherapy patient has received three injections in the past week of epoetin alpha (Procrit). The patient's hemoglobin has not increased. The nurse should:
   a. hold the next dose.
   b. administer the medication as ordered.
   c. consult the prescriber regarding assessing for renal failure.
   d. consult the prescriber regarding assessing for neutralizing antibodies.

▶ 5. Epoetin alpha (Procrit) 4000 units subcutaneous is ordered at 0900 pending endogenous erythropoietin levels for an anemic HIV-infected patient receiving zidovudine (AZT). Lab results arrived at 0830 including endogenous erythropoietin level of 578 milliunits/mL. The nurse should:
   a. administer the epoetin alpha (Procrit) STAT.
   b. administer the epoetin alpha (Procrit) with the 0900 medications.
   c. hold the medication and consult the prescriber.
   d. hold the medication.

▶ 6. Nursing considerations regarding epoetin alfa (Procrit) include: (Select all that apply.)
   a. administer depot preparation intramuscularly for extended action.
   b. assess for allergy to albumin.
   c. check for dose adjustments.
   d. dilute in 5 mL of bacteriostatic water for injection.
   e. discard if preparation is discolored.
   f. freeze for up to 1 month.
   g. monitor hemoglobin results.
   h. refrigerate until ready for use.
   i. shake well to ensure that all particles have dissolved.

7. Generally leukopoietic growth factor, filgrastim (Neupogen), is contraindicated in myelogenous cancers. Why is it prescribed for patients with acute myelogenous leukemia?

8. When administering filgrastim (Neupogen), how often should the nurse expect to review the WBC count?
   a. Once a week
   b. Twice a week
   c. Once a month
   d. Twice a month

▶ 9. Elevation of uric acid is an adverse effect of filgrastim (Neupogen) therapy. The most important assessment for the nurse to evaluate relating to possible elevations of uric acid is:
   a. fever.
   b. joint pain.
   c. kidney functioning.
   d. presence of tophi.

▶ 10. The nurse is teaching administration of filgrastim (Neupogen) to the mother of a child with congenital neutropenia who weighs 88 lb. The prescribed dose is 240 mcg (6 mcg/kg). The medication is available in a concentration of 300 mcg/mL in 1.6-mL vials. The nurse should teach the mother to administer:
   a. 0.6 mL, discarding the vial after the first dose.
   b. 0.6 mL, obtaining 2 doses from each vial.
   c. 0.8 mL, discarding the vial after the first dose.
   d. 0.8 mL, obtaining 2 doses from each vial.

11. Administration directives for filgrastim (Neupogen) for a patient receiving chemotherapy include:
   a. administer after each dose of chemotherapy.
   b. consult prescriber once absolute neutrophil count has reached 10,000/mm$^3$.
   c. must be kept refrigerated at all times.
   d. wipe rubber stopper with alcohol when re-entering vial.

12. Advantages of using pegfilgrastim (Neulasta) instead of filgrastim (Neupogen) include that:
   a. it can be administered immediately before or after chemotherapy.
   b. the course of therapy is one injection lasting 2 weeks.
   c. it does not cause bone pain.
   d. there is less elevation of LDH, alkaline phosphatase, and uric acid.

13. Hematopoietic growth factors cannot be taken orally because:

14. Which of the following would be a contraindication to administration of sargramostim (Leukine)?
   a. Allergy to chocolate
   b. Allergy to eggs
   c. Allergy to milk
   d. Allergy to yeast

▸ 15. Which of the following would be a symptom of a severe adverse reaction to sargramostim (Leukine)?
   a. Crackles (rales)
   b. Gurgles (rhonchi)
   c. Pleural friction rub
   d. Wheezes

16. If the final concentration of sargramostim (Leukine) is to be less than 10 mcg/mL, the drug should be diluted in 0.9%:
   a. sodium chloride.
   b. sodium chloride with 20 mEq KCl.
   c. sodium chloride with albumin.
   d. sodium chloride with 5% dextrose in water.

17. Oprelvekin (Neumega): (Select all that apply.)
   a. peaks in action in 24 hours.
   b. decreases count of abnormal platelets.
   c. increases production and maturity of megakaryocytes.
   d. is eliminated more rapidly in children than adults.
   e. is excreted in active form in the urine.
   f. is identical in structure to human interleukin-11.

▸ 18. What assessments for adverse effects should be performed before the nurse administers oprelvekin (Neumega)? (Select all that apply.)
   a. Blurred vision
   b. Bone pain
   c. Dehydration
   d. Edema
   e. Palpitations
   f. Pulse for tachycardia and dysrhythmias
   g. Rash
   h. Red eyes
   i. Shortness of breath

## CASE STUDIES AND PATIENT TEACHING

*(Use a separate piece of paper for your responses.)*

### Case Study 1

*A 65-year-old patient has had diabetes mellitus for 40 years and chronic renal failure for 20 years. He has been maintained at home leading a relatively normal life. Recently, he has become more anemic, and the diagnosis is a lack of erythrocyte production. He is prescribed epoetin alfa (Procrit) to help maintain his erythrocyte count. The prescriber has ordered baseline laboratory tests including BUN, creatinine, phosphorus, potassium, RBC indices, hemoglobin, transferring saturation, and ferritin. The patient is tired of "being jabbed" and asks the nurse why these tests have to be done.*

1. Describe the rationale for each test in a way the patient can understand.
   a. BUN/creatinine
   b. Phosphorus
   c. Potassium
   d. RBC indices
   e. Hemoglobin
   f. Ferrintin

2. What adverse effects should the nurse assess in this patient?

3. The physician has ordered 75 units/kg for maintenance therapy 3 times a week. The patient weighs 80 kg. How many units should the nurse administer in 1 dose?

4. The nurse is reviewing laboratory results for this patient. Hemoglobin is 13.5 gm/dL. What should the nurse do?

### Case Study 2

*Bobby Carter, a 5-year-old with acute lymphoblastic leukemia, has had a bone marrow transplant. Sargramostim (Leukine) 250 mcg/m² is ordered.*

1. What is the rationale for this therapy?

2. What should the nurse do or not do if the child experiences these adverse effects?
   a. Diarrhea
   b. Weakness
   c. Rash
   d. Bone pain

# 56 Drugs for Diabetes Mellitus

## OBJECTIVES

See page 26 for the Objectives.

## CRITICAL THINKING AND STUDY QUESTIONS

1. The nurse is caring for several patients who receive insulin therapy for diabetes. Which of the following symptoms, if exhibited by one of these patients, would be of most concern to the nurse?
   a. Fatigue and blurred vision
   b. Perineal itching and copious urine
   c. Profuse sweating and difficult to arouse
   d. Thirst and constant hunger

2. Which of these outcomes would be appropriate for a patient who is taking insulin glargine once a day?
   a. Premeal glucose level of 70 mg/dL
   b. Premeal glucose level of 130 mg/dL
   c. Premeal glucose level of 180 mg/dL
   d. Premeal glucose level less than 200 mg/dL

3. The nurse assesses for which of these symptoms of the electrolyte imbalance that is most likely when a patient is receiving large doses of insulin?
   a. Muscle weakness
   b. Restlessness
   c. Spasm of the wrist and fingers when circulation of the upper arm is constricted for several minutes
   d. Twitching of the facial nerve when the face is tapped over the nerve

4. The nurse is developing a teaching plan for a 15-year-old female newly diagnosed as a type 1 diabetic. This teaching plan should include: (Select all that apply.)
   a. blood sugar control will best be achieved if the patient follows a plan created by the healthcare providers.
   b. clear insulin is always short acting.
   c. insulin therapy with one long-acting agent that mimics the body's basal insulin secretion and another short-acting agent to cover eating is best.
   d. once the patient's blood sugar is stabilized, she should be able to maintain control with oral drugs.
   e. saturated fats should be limited to less than 10% of the total calories.
   f. taking insulin and not eating can cause serious effects from the blood sugar going too low.
   g. tight glucose control decreases the incidence of kidney failure.
   h. treatment can be monitored by blood or urine.
   i. weight loss is needed to decrease the patient's insulin requirements.

5. Whenever a patient's self-monitoring of blood glucose (SMBG) is within normal limits and the glycated hemoglobin (Hemoglobin $A_{1C}$) is above goal, the first nursing intervention should be to:
   a. assess the patient's technique of performing SMBG.
   b. check the expiration date on the insulin bottle.
   c. explain that the glycated hemoglobin indicates that the blood sugar has been high.
   d. teach the patient to count carbohydrates and calculate insulin needs.

▶ 6. The nurse is caring for a 62-year-old who has been a type 2 diabetic for 15 years. She is prescribed Humulin N 25 units in the AM. Recently the patient has experienced several hypoglycemic episodes despite maintaining her usual medication, diet, and exercise regimen. The patient's lab studies include C-peptide 1 ng/mL (normal 5 to 12 ng/mL). It would be most important for the nurse to assess this patient's:
a. calibration of her glucose meter.
b. intake of carbohydrates.
c. level of daily exercise.
d. sight for administering the proper amount of insulin.

7. When teaching about the onset, peak, and duration of different insulins, the nurse explains that which of the following insulin is most like the "natural" insulin produced by the body?
a. Aspart (NovoLog)
b. Lispro (Humalog)
c. Regular (Humulin R)
d. Neutral protamine Hagedorn (NPH) (Humulin N)

▶ 8. When obtaining a new vial of NPH insulin from refrigeration, the nurse notes that the suspension is partially frozen. The nurse should:
a. discard the vial and obtain a new one from the pharmacy.
b. shake the vial vigorously to produce heat.
c. warm the suspension in warm water.
d. withdraw the unfrozen portion then discard the rest.

▶ 9. A patient is admitted in a state of diabetic ketoacidosis. Orders include insulin lispro 0.1 mg/kg/hr to be administered by intravenous drip. The nurse should:
a. calculate the insulin dose and mix it with 100 mL of normal saline.
b. calculate the insulin dose and mix it with 100 mL of $D_5W$.
c. calculate the insulin dose and infuse the solution prepared by the pharmacy.
d. consult the prescriber STAT.

▶ 10. The nurse has done an initial assessment on assigned patients and is preparing to administer prescribed insulin. All patients are alert and oriented. It is 8:00 AM, and breakfast trays are scheduled to arrive at 8:20 AM. To which of the following patients should the nurse administer the insulin first?
a. 7:00 AM SMBG 60 mg/dL; prescribed NovoLog 3 units
b. 7:00 AM SMBG 90 mg/dL; prescribed 70% NPH/30% regular insulin (Humulin 70/30) 15 units
c. 7:00 AM SMBG 130 mg/dL; prescribed insulin aspart (NovoLog) 5 units
d. 7:00 AM SMBG 180 mg/dL; prescribed insulin glulisine (Apidra) 7 units

11. A patient has been prescribed 5 units of insulin aspart (NovoLog) and 25 units of insulin detemir (Levimir) to be administered at 0800. The nurse should:
a. draw up the two insulins in different syringes.
b. draw up 5 units of aspart first, then 25 units of detemir insulin in the same syringe.
c. draw up the clear insulin then the cloudy insulin in the same syringe.
d. inject the insulins in a different subcutaneous site (abdomen versus arm versus thigh) than the previous morning.

12. What special administration techniques must the nurse use when administering NPH insulin?
a. Never mix with another insulin.
b. Only administer this insulin at bedtime.
c. Roll the vial gently to mix particles in solution.
d. When mixing with another insulin, draw the NPH into the syringe first.

13. A patient with type 2 diabetes asks the nurse what is known about inhaled insulin. The best response by the nurse is inhaled insulin:
a. absorption is increased by smoking.
b. effects on the lung are not known.
c. is not effective in type 2 diabetes.
d. is only recommended for children.

14. A nursing student asks an emergency department (ED) nurse why premixed intravenous regular insulin solutions are not available in the ED as a stock drug. The best explanation is:
   a. insulin can be absorbed into the plastic altering the concentration.
   b. insulin is affected by light, and intravenous bags are clear.
   c. insulin rapidly biodegrades when mixed with a diluent.
   d. the appropriate insulin diluent cannot be refrigerated.

15. Research suggests that intensive insulin therapy (tight control) in type 1 and 2 diabetes is most effective in preventing:
   a. cerebral vascular accidents (CVAs).
   b. neuropathic pain.
   c. peripheral vascular disease requiring amputation.
   d. visual damage.

▶ 16. When performing the initial morning assessment on a diabetic patient, the nurse notes that a diabetic patient is very difficult to arouse. The nurse checks the SMBG, which is 37 mg/dL. Before administering orange juice, it is most important for the nurse to assess the patient's:
   a. blood pressure.
   b. deep tendon reflexes.
   c. swallowing reflex.
   d. temperature.

17. Which of the following statements, if made by a patient who has been prescribed tolbutamide (Orinase), would indicate the patient understood the teaching?
   a. "I can eat what I want as long as I take enough of the drug."
   b. "I need to notify my doctor if I have episodes of sweating and shakiness."
   c. "I should not experience low blood sugar with this drug because it does not stimulate the release of insulin."
   d. "This drug is less potent than the newer drugs."

18. The nurse teaches the diabetic patient who is prescribed tolbutamide (Orinase) and metoprolol that the metoprolol: (Select all that apply.)
   a. can prevent the patient from feeling the symptoms of hypoglycemia.
   b. is prescribed to prevent reflex tachycardia.
   c. prevents cardiac toxicity caused by tolbutamide.
   d. should be administered 1 hour after insulin administration.

▶ 19. Which of the following would warrant the nurse not administering nateglinide (Starlix) and consulting the prescriber?
   a. Fasting blood glucose 75 mg/dL
   b. Glycated hemoglobin ($HbA_{1C}$) 5.5%
   c. Patient is NPO for a colonoscopy
   d. Patient is scheduled to have hemodialysis

▶ 20. The nurse is reviewing the laboratory results of a patient who is prescribed metformin (Glucophage). Results include ALT 112 International Units/L, BUN 38 mg/dL, creatinine 2.6 mg/dL, hemoglobin 11 gm/dL, and hematocrit 33%. The nurse assesses the patient. Which of the following would be of most concern to the nurse?
   a. Dorsalis pedis pulse difficult to palpate
   b. Respirations 32 per minute and deep
   c. Pulse 100 beats/min
   d. Severe frontal headache

▶ 21. The nurse is preparing to perform the first assessment of the 3- to 11-shift at 3:30 PM (1530). Several assigned patients are diabetics. The patient receiving which of the following drugs should be assessed for hypoglycemia first?
   a. Acarbose (Precose) 50 mg 3 times a day with meals
   b. Glargine (Lispro) insulin units every evening plus insulin aspart according to dietary intake and SMBG
   c. Metformin (Glucophage) 500 mg before breakfast and supper.
   d. Neutral protamine Hagedorn (NPH) (Humulin N) 35 units every morning

▶ 22. The nurse is assessing a diabetic patient who is prescribed rosiglitazone (Avandia) and Novolin 70/30. The nurse notes the patient has become increasingly restless and short of breath with exertion. Which of the following is most important for the nurse to assess and report them to the physician?
   a. Heart sounds
   b. Peripheral edema
   c. SMBG
   d. Temperature

23. Which of these nursing outcomes would be most appropriate for a patient who is prescribed acarbose (Precose)?
    a. Bedtime SMBG 160 mg/dL
    b. Fasting blood glucose less than 90 mg/dL
    c. Glycated hemoglobin ($HbA_{1C}$) 7%
    d. Two-hour postprandial blood sugar less than 180 mg/dL

▶ 24. A blind, diabetic hospitalized patient is receiving acarbose (Precose) 50 mg 3 times a day with meals. The nurse plans interventions that include the fact that the patient is at risk for:
    a. activity intolerance.
    b. ineffective coping.
    c. injury.
    d. powerlessness.

▶ 25. A diabetic patient who receives glipizide and miglitol (Glyset) is diaphoretic, tachycardic, and anxious. The SMBG is 43 mg/dL. Which of the following would be most effective to quickly raise the patient's blood sugar?
    a. Glucose tablet
    b. Honey
    c. Orange juice
    d. Sugar cube

26. The nurse is teaching a type 1 diabetic patient who has been prescribed pramlintide (Symlin). Which of the following information should be included? (Select all that apply.)
    a. A common adverse effect of pramlintide is nausea.
    b. Patients need to estimate calorie and carbohydrate content of meals to determine if pramlintide should be administered.
    c. Pramlintide can interfere with the absorption of oral drugs.
    d. Pramlintide decreases the need for insulin.
    e. Pramlintide increases the release of glucagon.
    f. Pramlintide is more effective if prescribed along with acarbose (Precose).
    g. Pramlintide is used in place of insulin.
    h. Pramlintide should be administered with the daily long-acting insulin dose.
    i. Pramlintide speeds gastric emptying.
    j. Risk for hypoglycemia is greatest within 3 hours of administration.

27. The nurse knows that the best drug to treat type 2 diabetes during pregnancy and lactation is:
    a. acarbose.
    b. insulin.
    c. metformin.
    d. pioglitazone.

28. After administration of glucagon for severe hypoglycemia, the nurse anticipates treatment to:
    a. correct acidosis.
    b. correct cachexia.
    c. restore stores of glycogen in the liver.
    d. treat the adverse effect of diarrhea.

29. Matching possible drug interactions with insulin.

| | | |
|---|---|---|
| ______ | a. Need less insulin | 1. Alcohol binge |
| ______ | b. Need more insulin | 2. Beta blockers |
| | | 3. Glucocorticoids |
| | | 4. Meglitinides |
| | | 5. Pramlintide |
| | | 6. Sulfonylureas |
| | | 7. Thiazide diuretics |

## CASE STUDIES AND PATIENT TEACHING

*(Use a separate piece of paper for your responses.)*

### CASE STUDY 1

*A 28-year-old man, who is 5 feet 8 inches and 132 lbs, is admitted to the hospital after experiencing nausea, vomiting, and increasing confusion. BP 90/50 mm/Hg, apical pulse 112 beats/min, respirations 29 and deep with fruity odor. His skin is hot, dry, and flushed. Urine is pale in color and smells like rotting apples. The patient responds to verbal and tactile stimuli, but has become increasingly lethargic. According to a family member, the patient has had diabetes for 6 years and takes Humulin N 35 units and Humulin R 15 units every morning and Humulin N 17 units at dinnertime. He had stopped exercising this week and has not taken his insulin for 2 days because of having a "stomach flu."*

*Lab results include serum glucose 545 mg/dL; BUN 20 mg/dL; serum osmolarity 400 mOsm/kg; creatinine 2.0 mg/dL: urine + acetone, + sugar; potassium 3.3 mEq/L; sodium 139 mEq/L; WBC 18.3 × 103/μL. The physician orders:*

- *Intravenous fluid infusion of 1000 mL of half-normal saline (0.45% NaCl) with 10 mEq of KCl*

*to be infused in 1 hour followed by 1000 mL of 0.45% sodium chloride at a rate of 300 mL/hr.*
- *Regular insulin bolus of 0.15 units/kg.*
- *Intravenous infusion of regular insulin at 0.1 units/kg/hr.*
- *Bedside blood glucose level determination every 30 minutes.*
- *I&O every hour.*
- *Repeat serum osmolality, BUN, and creatinine in 4 hours.*
- *Once serum glucose reaches 250 mg/dL, change intravenous infusion to 1000 mL of 5% dextrose in water ($D_5W$) at a rate of 125 mL/hr.*

1. Why is it important for the nurse to initiate the intravenous solution first?

2. Based on the physician's orders, how much insulin should the nurse administer by bolus injection?

3. The insulin comes mixed as a solution of 25 units in 100 mL of normal saline. The intravenous pump calibration is in milliliters per hour. What rate should the nurse program for the continuous intravenous insulin drip?

4. The patient's wife asks why regular insulin is being infused instead of the patient's usual NPH. How should the nurse respond?

5. The patient is stabilized and transferred to the medical-surgical unit. The patient's wife is frightened that the patient will experience another episode. What teaching can the nurse provide to help prevent another episode like this one?

6. The patient states that he has been rotating injection sites. What information should the nurse provide about current recommendations for rotating insulin injection sites?

7. While in the hospital, the patient is on a sliding scale insulin program before meals and at bedtime. The patient admits to being afraid of administering insulin at bedtime because he is not eating during the night. How should the nurse respond?

   The schedule is as follows:
   - SMBG <150, give no insulin.
   - SMBG 151 to 200, give 2 units regular insulin.
   - SMBG 201 to 250, give 4 units regular insulin.
   - SMBG 250 to 300, give 6 units regular insulin.
   - SMBG >300, call the physician.

8. His Accucheck reading is 202. How much regular insulin should the nurse administer?

9. The physician has discussed changing the patient's insulin regimen to insulin glargine for once-a-day basal insulin needs and insulin lispro based on eating patterns. After meeting with a diabetic educator the patient, asks the nurse to explain again why he needs to count "carbs."

10. The patient is scheduled to come back to see the diabetes nurse educator in 1 week. Why should he do this even though he has had diabetes for some time and has been given additional information while in the hospital?

## Case Study 2

*A 46-year-old married construction worker with a history of hypertension has been admitted for testing after experiencing transient acute visual disturbances that caused a fall from a scaffold. The patient is a smoker, 5 feet 9 inches and weighs 203 lbs and is often nonadherent with his antihypertensive medication. He has been generally healthy, except for noting that he has been urinating more frequently. Neurologic examination and laboratory results are within normal limits, except for glycated hemoglobin ($HbA_{1c}$) 6.8% and triglycerides 438 mg/dL. The physician has just reviewed the laboratory results with the patient and informed the patient that a 75-gm 2-hour oral glucose tolerance test (OGTT) has been scheduled for tomorrow. The nurse is instructed to explain the test procedure to the patient. After the physician leaves, the patient asks the nurse why he needs to have this test done if his fasting blood sugar is normal.*

1. How should the nurse respond?

2. The patient asks how blood sugar could be related to visual changes. How should the nurse respond?

3. What factors in the patient's history suggest that this patient is developing type 2 diabetes?

4. Besides safety related to visual changes, why is it important to identify and treat if this patient is a diabetic?

5. The patient's 3-hour glucose tolerance test results are:

| | Blood glucose | Urine glucose | Urine ketones |
|---|---|---|---|
| Fasting | 97 mg/dL | negative | negative |
| 30 min | 225 mg/dL | 45 mg | negative |
| 1 hr | 283 mg/dL | 111 mg | negative |
| 2 hr | 261 mg/dL | 387 mg | negative |

The physician explains the impairment of glucose tolerance to the patient. What teaching should the nurse provide to assist this patient with controlling his blood sugar and preventing complications?

## Case Study 3

*A 17-year-old high school sophomore is a type 1 diabetic. She has been attempting to maintain tight control of her serum glucose levels using intensive insulin therapy.*

1. Why is it important to monitor this patient's weight?
2. Recently the teen has been experiencing frequent occurrences of hypoglycemia. After establishing rapport with the patient, what questions should the nurse ask in a attempt to identify factors that could be causing these episodes?
3. The patient is concerned about being different from her friends and has verbalized resentment that she must alter her diet or excuse herself from activities to take needed insulin. Her pediatric endocrinologist has recommended an insulin pump. The physician asks the diabetes nurse to explain how the pump works. What information should the nurse provide?
4. The patient asks if the pump can be removed when she wears something special, such as a prom gown. How should the nurse respond?
5. The patient confides in the nurse that she will not wear the pump to the prom. What is a possible solution to this problem?

# 57 Drugs for Thyroid Disorders

## OBJECTIVES

See page 26 for the Objectives.

## CRITICAL THINKING AND STUDY QUESTIONS

1. A patient asks why thyroid hormone effects decline slowly. The basis of the nurse's response is that thyroid hormone:
   a. contains iodine.
   b. is excreted by the kidneys.
   c. interacts with many other drugs.
   d. is primarily protein bound.
2. The primary function of tetraiodothyronine ($T_4$) in the body is:
   a. catalyzing the oxidation of iodide to iodine.
   b. enzymatic conversion to thyroxine ($T_3$) in tissues.
   c. modulating gene transcription.
   d. producing proteins that promote thyroid hormone effects.

3. Which of the following best explains control of the release of thyroid hormone?
   a. High plasma levels of $T_3$ and $T_4$ signal the hypothalamus to decrease production of thyrotropin-releasing hormone (TRH).
   b. High plasma levels of $T_3$ and $T_4$ signal the hypothalamus to decrease production of thyrotropin (TSH).
   c. Low plasma levels of $T_3$ and $T_4$ signal the pituitary to increase production of thyrotropin-releasing hormone (TRH).
   d. Low plasma levels of $T_3$ and $T_4$ signal the hypothalamus to increase production of thyrotropin (TSH).

▶ 4. The nurse is preparing to administer synthetic levothyroxine (Synthroid). A significantly low level of which of the following laboratory values would be a reason for the nurse to withhold the medication and consult the prescriber?
   a. Free $T_3$
   b. Free $T_4$
   c. TSH
   d. $T_3$

5. Adequate maternal thyroid hormone replacement therapy during pregnancy is most important to the fetus during the:
   a. first week of pregnancy.
   b. first trimester of pregnancy.
   c. second trimester of pregnancy.
   d. third trimester of pregnancy.

6. Which of the following statements, if made by a patient receiving the antithyroid drug propylthiouracil (PTU), would indicate a need for further teaching?
   a. "After this drug gets to a therapeutic level, it should help my heart to stop feeling like it is racing."
   b. "I should gain weight while eating less when I am on this drug."
   c. "This drug should help decrease the bulging appearance of my eyes."
   d. "This drug should stop the feeling that I am always too hot."

▶ 7. Which of the following assessment findings would be most critical for the nurse to report to the prescriber immediately if noted in a patient with urosepsis who has a history of Graves' disease treated by an antithyroid drugs?
   a. Blood pressure 150/88 mm Hg
   b. Pulse 90 beats/min
   c. Respirations 24 per minute
   d. Temperature 104° F (40° C)

8. The nurse is caring for a patient who receives levothyroxine. Which of the following drugs, if also prescribed, should be separated by hours from the administration of levothyroxine?
   a. carbazamepine (Tegretol)
   b. ferrous sulfate (iron supplement)
   c. rifampin (Rifadin)
   d. sertraline (Zoloft)

▶ 9. Because of drug interactions, the nurse should monitor a patient who has been taking warfarin and has recently been prescribed levothyroxine for:
   a. bleeding.
   b. dysrhythmias.
   c. insomnia.
   d. tachycardia.

10. A patient tells the nurse that for her insurance company to pay for prescription drugs her insurance requires that she use a generic drug if one is available. Up to now, she has been taking brand name Synthroid. The nurse should advise the patient to:
    a. ask the pharmacist what is best.
    b. discuss this change with her prescriber.
    c. pay for the brand name.
    d. use the generic brand; there is no difference.

11. A patient has received instructions regarding administration of levothyroxine (Synthroid). Which of these statements made by the client would indicate that the patient understood the directions?
    a. "I should take the drug in the morning with breakfast."
    b. "Stomach upset occurs if the drug is taken with an antacid."
    c. "Taking the drug first on an empty stomach 30 minutes before breakfast increases drug absorption."
    d. "Taking the drug with orange juice increases drug absorption."

▶ 12. Because of the risk of agranulocytosis, the nurse should teach the patient who has been prescribed propylthiouracil (PTU) to report which of the following symptoms?
    a. Anorexia
    b. Bleeding gums
    c. Pale conjunctiva
    d. Sore throat

13. A 34-year-old female is prescribed Iodine$^{131}$ for toxic nodular goiter. Which statement, if made by this patient, would indicate a need for further teaching?
    a. "I can develop inadequate thyroid hormone secretion from this therapy."
    b. "I must stay at home during therapy to avoid exposing others to radiation."
    c. "I need to use two reliable methods of birth control."
    d. "This drug takes months before it is fully effective."

14. Which of these factors, if identified in a patient receiving Lugol's solution, would be a concern to the nurse?
    a. Decrease in free $T_3$
    b. Gain of 2 lbs in 2 weeks
    c. States beverages have a brassy taste
    d. Takes the drug with grapefruit juice

## CASE STUDIES AND PATIENT TEACHING

*(Use a separate piece of paper for your responses.)*

### Case Study 1

*A 30-year-old mother of two notices that she is gaining weight. She visits her family physician complaining that she has been experiencing unusual fatigue, lethargy, and intolerance to cold. At the visit her vital signs are BP 100/58 mm HG, P 62, R 16, and T 97.8°F.*

1. What thyroid disorder do these symptoms suggest?

2. What laboratory test results would the nurse expect to see on this patient if she is hypothyroid?

3. After appropriate history, physical examination, and laboratory studies, she is diagnosed with primary hypothyroidism and started on levothyroxine (Synthroid) 112 mcg once a day. What teaching should the nurse provide about expected timing for relief of symptoms?

4. What teaching should the nurse provide to this patient about administration of levothyroxine (Synthroid)?

5. The nurse should teach about possible adverse effects of levothyroxine. What adverse effects warrant notification of the prescriber?

6. The patient tells the nurse that her sister has asked for some of her thyroid pills to help her lose weight. She wants to know if this would be a problem. How should the nurse respond?

7. The patient returns for her 1-year checkup. She wonders if she still needs the medication because she sometimes forgets to take the drug and does not feel any different on those days. How should the nurse respond?

### Case Study 2

*Propranolol (Inderal) 10 mg and propylthiouracil (PTU) 100 mg 3 times a day are prescribed for a 25-year-old woman who was recently diagnosed with Graves' disease.*

1. What laboratory results would the nurse expect to see when reviewing this patient's chart?

2. The patient asks the nurse why two drugs have been prescribed. What information should the nurse provide regarding the need for both drugs?

3. The drug methimazole (Tapazole) only needs to be taken once a day, and propylthiouracil (PTU) needs to be taken 3 times a day. What would be a reason why the prescriber chose PTU for this patient?

4. What assessments should the nurse teach the patient to monitor, and what findings should be reported to the prescriber?

5. Six months later, the patient's heart rate, blood pressure, TSH, and free $T^3$ levels are within normal limits. The prescriber provides a plan for gradual decrease, then discontinuation of propranolol (Inderal). Why was this drug dose tapered rather than discontinued if vital signs are normal?

# 58 Drugs Related to Hypothalamic and Pituitary Function

## OBJECTIVES

See page 26 for the Objectives.

## CRITICAL THINKING AND STUDY QUESTIONS

1. Which of the following findings would the nurse expect to find in a child who has a deficiency in secretion of growth hormone?
   a. Cognitive deficiency
   b. Long trunk and short extremities
   c. Profuse sweating
   d. Thin arms and legs

2. Which of the following laboratory results would the nurse expect in an otherwise healthy child who is receiving growth hormone?
   a. Decrease in blood urea nitrogen
   b. Decrease in fasting blood sugar
   c. Increase in blood urea nitrogen
   d. Increase in fasting blood sugar

3. A patient who is receiving octreotide (Sandostatin) for acromegaly should be assessed for which of the following symptoms of the underlying condition?
   a. Bradycardia
   b. Hypertension
   c. Hyperthermia
   d. Hypoglycemia

▸ 4. Which of these assessment findings, if identified in a patient who is receiving pegvisomant (Somavert), suggests possible liver injury and should be reported to the prescriber?
   a. Headache
   b. Nasal congestion
   c. Malaise
   d. Tea-colored urine

▸ 5. A patient who was recently diagnosed with hypothalamic diabetes insipidus and prescribed vasopressin reports weight gain of 1 to 2 lbs per day for the past week. The nurse should recognize that this may indicate:
   a. failure to comply with directions for administration of the drug.
   b. failure to limit water intake.
   c. improper diagnosis.
   d. the drug dose is inadequate.

▸ 6. When administering vasopressin to a patient with diabetes insipidus, which of the following urine specific gravity results would indicate that therapy has achieved the desired effect?
   a. 1.0002
   b. 1.002
   c. 1.02
   d. 1.2

7. An adolescent girl with schizophrenia that is being treated with haloperidol (Haldol) is prescribed carbegoline Dostinex. The patient's mother asks why this drug is being prescribed. The nurse explains that the drug counteracts which adverse effect of the antipsychotic drug?
   a. Breast tenderness
   b. Constipation
   c. Dry mouth
   d. Orthostatic hypotension

## CASE STUDIES AND PATIENT TEACHING

*(Use a separate piece of paper for your responses.)*

### Case Study 1

*The nurse works in an endocrine clinic at a major pediatric center that sees children with short stature. When growth hormone therapy with somatropin (Humatrope) is prescribed, the nurse must teach the patient and parents self-administration of the drug.*

1. What should the nurse include in the teaching of the technique of subcutaneous injection of this drug?

2. What will the nurse include when explaining the importance of monitoring weight while on this drug?

3. A patient is prescribed somatropin (Humatrope) 0.18 mg/kg/wk to be divided into three doses administered on Monday, Wednesday, and Friday. The nurse teaches the parents of the child who weighs 28 kg to administer how much somatropin (Humatrope) at each dose?

4. Some parents want therapy with growth hormone for their child, but the physician decides that risks are greater than benefits. What information can the nurse provide to reinforce physician teaching about why therapy with growth hormone may not be advisable for children with the following conditions?
   a. Prader-Willi Syndrome
   b. Diabetes mellitus
   c. Uncontrolled asthma

### Case Study 2

*Intramuscular vasopressin 5 units now and 5 units every 4 hours as needed are prescribed for a patient with postoperative abdominal distention.*

1. What should the nurse assess before administering this drug?

2. What assessment findings would be a reason to withhold the drug and contact the prescriber?

# 59 Drugs for Disorders of the Adrenal Cortex

## OBJECTIVES

See page 26 for the Objectives.

## CRITICAL THINKING AND STUDY QUESTIONS

1. Intramuscular injection of glucocorticoids to a pregnant woman at risk for preterm birth is given to:
   a. accelerate maturation of the fetal lungs.
   b. lower maternal blood pressure.
   c. prevent uterine contractions.
   d. stimulate fetal weight gain.

2. To follow the normal circadian pattern of cortisol release, cortisol replacement therapy should be administered so that the drug peaks:
   a. early morning.
   b. just before awakening.
   c. midmorning.
   d. when the patient first falls asleep.

▸ 3. Which of these findings would be most significant if the nurse is caring for a patient with Cushing's syndrome?
   a. Fasting blood sugar 235 mg/dL
   b. pH 7.44, $HCO_3$ 28 mEq/L, $PCO_2$ 45 mm Hg
   c. Peaked T waves on ECG
   d. Sinus rhythm on ECG

4. Which of the following diuretic drugs are used to treat bilateral adrenal hyperplasia? (Select all that apply.)
   a. Amiloride
   b. Bumetanide
   c. Furosemide
   d. Eplerenone
   e. Hydrochlorothiazide
   f. Spironolactone

▶ 5. Recommended dose of hydrocortisone for a patient with adrenal insufficiency is 8 to 15 mg/m$^2$. A patient who is 5 feet 11 inches and weighs 176 lbs has been prescribed 10 mg/m$^2$. What is a safe and effective dose range for this patient?
   a. 8 to 15 mg
   b. 13 to 25 mg
   c. 16 to 30 mg
   d. 32 to 60 mg

▶ 6. Which of these findings would be most significant if a patient was receiving fludrocortisone?
   a. Blood pressure 150/90 mm Hg
   b. Flushed, dry skin
   c. Nausea and vomiting
   d. Weight gain of 2 lbs in 24 hours

7. The nurse is caring for a patient who is scheduled for an adrenalectomy for adrenal adenoma. During the night, the nurse should assess the patient for which of the following symptoms of the hyperaldosteronism?
   a. Cool, clammy skin, and hypoglycemia
   b. Kussmaul's breathing to compensate for metabolic acidosis
   c. Postural hypotension when getting up to the bathroom
   d. Vomiting, diarrhea, and subsequent electrolyte imbalances

▶ 8. Which of these laboratory results, if identified in a patient who is receiving 800 mg of ketoconazole to inhibit corticosteroid synthesis in a patient with Cushing's disease, should the nurse report to the prescriber immediately?
   a. ALT 150 International Units/L
   b. BUN 15 mg/dL
   c. Creatinine 1.5 mg/dL
   d. Glucose 150 mg/dL

▶ 9. The nurse discovers a maculopapular rash on the face and neck of a patient when assessing before administering aminoglutethimide (Cytadren). The nurse should:
   a. administer the medication and place the patient in an isolation room.
   b. administer the medication and notify the prescriber on rounds.
   c. hold the medication and place the patient in an isolation room.
   d. hold the medication and notify the prescriber.

## CASE STUDIES AND PATIENT TEACHING

*(Use a separate piece of paper for your responses.)*

### Case Study 1

*A 32-year-old male has been admitted with severe episodic right upper quadrant (RUQ) pain, anorexia, and nausea. Oral cholecystography reveals acute cholecystitis, and an open cholecystectomy is planned. When gathering data regarding past medical history (PMH), the patient reveals he has been experiencing extreme fatigue, dizziness when changing position, and muscle weakness. He has felt this way for a long time, but thought the symptoms were caused by his stressful job. He also states that he loves every kind of salty food and eats at least one bag of potato chips daily. He states that he has experienced impotence on occasion. The nurse notes that he has increased pigmentation around the face and hands and a decrease in body hair. Blood work includes fasting glucose 62 mg/dL, sodium 132 mEq/L, potassium 53 mEq/L, and blood urea nitrogen (BUN) 28 mg/dL. Synthetic ACTH is administered intravenously, and plasma cortisol levels were checked. Levels failed to rise from the ACTH stimulation. He is diagnosed with Addison's disease. He asks the nurse how this causes his symptoms.*

1. Describe how the nurse relates current and possible symptoms to decreased levels of adrenal cortex hormones.

2. The patient is prescribed hydrocortisone sodium succinate (Solu-Cortef) 50 mg IV every 8 hours. Text states that daily doses of hydrocortisone should mimic normal daily secretion (20 to 30 mg per day). Why is this patient receiving such a high dose?

3. Because the patient is ill with cholecystitis and adrenal insufficiency, what is the most critical concern of the nurse? What should be included in the nursing plan of care to address this concern?

4. The patient is prescribed hydrocortisone 20 mg/day. What administration regimen would be used for the hydrocortisone if the prescriber wanted to mimic the body's natural basal secretion of glucocorticoids?

5. What teaching should the nurse provide to a patient who has been prescribed oral glucocorticoids?

# 60 Estrogens and Progestins: Basic Pharmacology and Noncontraceptive Applications

## OBJECTIVES

See page 26 for the Objectives.

## CRITICAL THINKING AND STUDY QUESTIONS

▶ 1. A 45-year-old woman has not had a menstrual period for 2 months. The nurse is reviewing laboratory tests. Which of the following results suggest that the woman may be entering menopause (perimenopause)?
   a. Elevated estradiol
   b. Elevated human chorionic gonadotropin
   c. Elevated luteinizing hormone
   d. Elevated progesterone

2. Which of the following would not be an acceptable use of postmenopausal estrogen hormone replacement therapy?
   a. Discomfort during sexual intercourse
   b. Hot flashes after total abdominal hysterectomy and bilateral salpingo-oophorectomy
   c. Low bone mineral density
   d. Urinary incontinence

▶ 3. The nurse is caring for a 66-year-old female postoperative total knee replacement patient who has been taking estrogen to relieve menopausal symptoms and increase bone mineral density. Which of the following nursing assessment findings would be of most concern to the nurse?
   a. Dizziness with position changes
   b. Dyspnea while resting
   c. Nausea and vomiting
   d. Vaginal spotting of sanguineous discharge

4. Which of the following is not a function of progesterone during pregnancy?
   a. Formation of the cervical mucous plug
   b. Prevention of immune rejection of the fetus
   c. Proliferation of the endometrium
   d. Suppression of uterine contractions

5. The current recommendation for hormone therapy for menopausal symptoms is:

6. Current research suggests that hormone replacement does not provide which of the following benefits?
   a. Cardiovascular protection
   b. Increase in bone density
   c. Prevention of vaginal atrophy
   d. Protection from dementia
   e. Relief of insomnia and hot flushes (hot flashes)

7. Which of the following symptoms, if exhibited by a patient who is receiving estrogen therapy (ET), is most likely to be an effect of this therapy?
   a. Constipation
   b. Dyspepsia after medication administration
   c. Nausea
   d. Orthostatic hypotension

8. A patient with PMS has been prescribed fluoxetine (Prozac) for PMS. Which of the following statements, if made by the patient, would suggest that the patient understands the potential benefits of this drug therapy for PMS?
   a. "I must take this drug every day even though my symptoms are only present part of the month."
   b. "It takes 2 to 4 weeks of daily therapy before I should notice improvement in how I feel."
   c. "This drug will help reduce my breast tenderness, bloating, and headache."
   d. "This drug should improve my mood and interest in sex."

## CASE STUDIES AND PATIENT TEACHING

*(Use a separate piece of paper for your responses.)*

### Case Study 1

*A 46-year-old woman has just received the recommendation that she undergo a total hysterectomy and bilateral salpingo-oophorectomy for uterine fibroids.*

1. The patient should be informed that which symptoms should be expected postoperatively relating to the removal of both ovaries (surgical menopause)?

2. The physician orders laboratory tests, including a lipid panel, mammogram, and DEXA scan and tells the patient that results are needed before they can discuss options to prevent surgically induced menopausal symptoms. The patient asks the nurse why these tests have been ordered. What information can the nurse provide?

3. Lab results include bone mineral density 1.5 standard deviations below normal, LDL 150 mg/dL, HDL 55 mg/dL, and no evidence of lesions on mammogram. The patient is interested in postoperative hormone replacement. What additional information must be obtained before the physician considers prescribing hormone replacement?

4. There are no contraindications for estrogen replacement therapy. The woman states that her mother received relief of menopausal symptoms by taking estrogen-progesterone combination (Prempro). Why would this particular drug not be prescribed for this patient?

5. After discussing risks and benefits, the physician prescribes Climara, a transdermal estrogen patch, and asks the nurse to teach administration directives. What should the nurse include?

6. What teaching should the nurse provide that can help reduce the risk of cardiovascular events?

7. The patient asks if there are any alternative treatments for menopausal symptoms. What information can the nurse provide?

### Case Study 2

*A patient suspects that she is experiencing premenstrual syndrome (PMS) because she has been experiencing episodes of headaches, moodiness, irritability, bloating, and craving chocolate.*

1. What data would be helpful to collect before consulting with her CRNP?

2. After completing a diary of symptoms for 3 months, the patient consults with her CRNP who diagnoses PMS. What are the recommended initial approaches to relieve PMS symptoms?

3. The patient informs her CRNP that she was aware of these recommendations and has already tried these interventions for the past 6 months without relief. She has been successful with making these lifestyle changes except for not always getting adequate sleep because of working shifts. She has heard that progesterone is no longer recommended for PMS and asks the CRNP why. What is the basis of the CRNP's response?

4. The patient had previously been prescribed an SSRI antidepressant, but was unable to tolerate several preparations because of sexual dysfunction. She also has been experiencing a rise in her blood pressure. The CRNP prescribes spironolactone (Aldactone) 25 mg once a day, every day and calcium carbonate 400 mg 3 times a day. What symptoms should these drugs relieve?
   a. spironolactone (Aldactone)
   b. calcium carbonate

# 61 Birth Control

## OBJECTIVES

See page 26 for the Objectives.

## CRITICAL THINKING AND STUDY QUESTIONS

1. When developing a teaching plan regarding unplanned and unwanted pregnancies, the nurse should consider that:
   a. abortion is a common approach to deal with unplanned pregnancies.
   b. unplanned pregnancy rarely occurs after age 25 years.
   c. most unplanned pregnancies occur in adolescents and young adult women.
   d. only 5% of females aged 15 to 17 years are or have been pregnant.

2. Which of the following statements about birth control are true? (Select all that apply.)
   a. Cervical caps are more effective in women who have already had babies.
   b. Diaphragm with spermacide is more effective than male condoms with typical and optimal use.
   c. Failure rates during the first year of use are 50 times more common with typical use of combination oral contraceptives.
   d. Surgical sterilization is the most common form of birth control in the United States.
   e. The most effective pharmacologic forms of birth control have the most adverse effects.
   f. When used exactly as directed, combination oral contraceptives are more effective than vasectomy.

3. When assessing the history of a patient who is seeking an oral contraceptive prescription, it is important for the nurse to assess for use of the over-the-counter alternative therapy of:
   a. echinacea.
   b. garlic.
   c. ginkgo biloba.
   d. St John's wort.

▸ 4. The nurse is working in a women's health clinic. A 38-year-old woman who smokes two packs of cigarettes a day, has a history of diabetes and hypertension, and who has been pregnant nine times is given a prescription for oral contraceptives. What is the most logical reason why oral contraceptives (OCs) are being prescribed for this patient who has risk factors for serious adverse effects?

▶ 5. Which of the following patients would be at greatest risk for pregnancy when using the contraceptive patch (Ortho Evra) as a contraceptive?
a. A 19-year-old with multiple sexual partners
b. A 25-year-old who has a BMI of 32
c. A 37-year-old who is anemic
d. A 40-year-old who smokes 2 packs of cigarettes per day

▶ 6. A 19-year-old healthy patient who has been taking a combination OC for 2 years is involved in an automobile accident and undergoes surgical reduction and fixation of multiple fractures of both lower extremities. A critical assessment finding that should be reported to the physician because it could be related to adverse effects of the OC in this situation is:
a. capillary refill of 2 seconds.
b. diaphoresis.
c. severe headache.
d. temperature 100°F (37.8°C).

7. The Women's Health Initiative (WHI) study suggests OC use may decrease the incidence of: (Select all that apply.)
a. breast cancer.
b. cerebral vascular disease.
c. cervical cancer.
d. hyperlipidemia.
e. hypertension.
f. myocardial infarction.
g. peripheral vascular disease.
h. sexually transmitted disease.

8. Research suggests that OC use increases the risk of beast cancer in women who have:
a. BRCA1 gene mutation.
b. BRCA2 gene mutation.
c. a history of breast cancer in a first-degree relative.
d. a history of smoking more than 15 cigarettes per day.
e. a personal history of breast cancer.
f. used OC for more than 10 years.
g. used OC with high estrogen content.

▶ 9. A patient calls the gynecologist because she is concerned that she has not had a period since starting low-dose oral contraceptives 3 months ago. A priority nursing response is to explain:
a. that she needs to be seen by the gynecologist to determine if another OC should be used.
b. that some women do not have periods when taking oral contraceptives.
c. the need for biopsy for uterine malignancy.
d. the need for an immediate pregnancy test.

▶ 10. Because of the effect of oral contraceptives on glucose levels of diabetics, it is important for the nurse to assess for:
a. diaphoresis.
b. excessive thirst.
c. flushed skin.
d. tachycardia.

11. A nullipara patient, who plans to get pregnant after 1 year of using contraceptives, is discussing different pharmacologic agents for birth control with the nurse. Nursing teaching should include:
a. alternative forms of birth control should be used for 3 months after stopping oral contraceptives if the woman wants to minimize the risk of multiple births.
b. contraception usually continues for 2 to 3 months after subdermal implanted contraceptive capsules are removed.
c. fertility returns in 3 months after a depot intramuscular injection of medroxyprogesterone.
d. the Mirena IUD is ideal for this patient.

▶ 12. A patient on oral contraceptives complains of right upper quadrant discomfort. Because of the possibility of a highly vascular benign hepatic adenoma, which of the following assessment techniques should the nurse use for abdominal assessment after inspection?
a. Deep palpation
b. Light palpation
c. Percussion

13. Which of these laboratory tests would be most important for the nurse to assess when a patient is receiving an OC?
a. Calcium
b. Magnesium
c. Potassium
d. Sodium

14. Teaching regarding administration of OCs should include:
a. backup contraception should be used and is recommended during the first week of the first cycle.
b. successive cycles should start when menstrual flow has stopped.
c. the prescription should be started on the first day of the menstrual period.
d. triphasic OCs are sometimes prescribed continuously for several months.

15. Administration directives for progestin-only pills include:
    a. take for 21 days, then take inert pill for 7 days, then start a new cycle.
    b. if one dose is missed, take one pill as soon as the omission is noticed, discard the second pill, and take the next scheduled pill at the normal time.
    c. if two doses are missed, two doses should be taken together each day for the next two scheduled doses.
    d. if 3 doses are missed, the rest of that cycle should be discarded and a new cycle started 7 days after the last missed dose. An additional form of birth control should be used through the first 2 weeks of the new cycle.

16. A patient who is taking phenytoin for a seizure disorder has been prescribed a combination OC for contraception. The nurse should instruct the patient that if she should use alternative methods of birth control and notify her physician if she experiences:
    a. breast tenderness.
    b. nausea.
    c. spotting.
    d. weight gain.

17. The nurse instructs the patient who is prescribed the transdermal contraceptive patch, Ortho Evra, to apply the patch to: (Select all that apply.)
    a. breasts.
    b. buttocks.
    c. lower abdomen.
    d. upper torso.
    e. upper inner arm.
    f. wrist.

18. A patient who is using the vaginal contraceptive ring calls her gynecology practice because she found the ring when making the bed this morning. The nurse should instruct the patient to:

19. Advantages of subdermal contraceptive implants include:
    a. consistency of plasma levels of the hormones.
    b. easy to remove.
    c. highly effective contraception.
    d. low incidence of adverse effects.

▶ 20. Nutritional counseling by the nurse to counteract adverse effects for a patient who is using depot medroxyprogesterone (Depo-Provera) should include:
    a. decreasing intake of bananas and other foods high in potassium.
    b. decreasing intake of red meat.
    c. increasing intake of dairy products.
    d. increasing intake of green, leafy vegetables.

21. When a patient has an IUD in place, the nurse should assess for which symptom of a common adverse effect?
    a. Breast tenderness
    b. Dull pelvic pain
    c. Dysmenorrhea
    d. Edema

## CASE STUDIES AND PATIENT TEACHING

*(Use a separate piece of paper for your responses.)*

### Case Study 1

*A 17-year-old sexually active female has used condoms as a form of birth control and prevention of sexually transmitted diseases. She is monogomous at this time and has decided to start on an OC. The patient's history includes asthma that is controlled with Theo-Dur, dysmenorrhea, and irregular menses. Her last normal menstrual period was 2 months ago, but she says she is not concerned because this is a common occurrence for her. The patient is anxious and asks you about the medical exam and what procedures will be completed.*

1. Briefly describe what will be included in the preadministration assessment and how frequently she will need to have it repeated.

2. The patient asks the nurse, "How do oral contraceptives prevent pregnancy?"

3. When educating this patient in the use of OCs, it is important to stress the need to take them every day at the same time as prescribed. The patient is started on a triphasic OC and is concerned that she may forget to take the pills consistently. If she does forget, what procedures should she take to minimize the risk of pregnancy?

4. The patient asks about using an alternative form of contraception. What teaching should the nurse provide about the use of condoms and spermicides?

5. Knowing that the patient has asthma and is presently taking Theo-Dur (a form of theophylline), what assessments relating to interaction of OCs and theophylline need to be taken and why?

6. What possible adverse effects warrant discontinuation of the OC, and what symptoms of these conditions should the nurse teach the patient to report to her prescriber?

## Case Study 2

*A 19-year-old college student is being seen at the student health clinic requesting birth control. At this clinic the RN does the initial health history before the patient is seen by the CRNP.*

1. What data are important for the nurse to collect from this patient?

2. The patient states, "I thought contraceptives fool my body into thinking I'm pregnant. Why do I have to have a negative pregnancy test before getting a prescription to prevent pregnancy?" How should the nurse respond?

3. The patient becomes tearful and admits that she is pregnant. Her LMP was over 4 weeks ago, and she did a home pregnancy test. She was hoping to get a prescription for an OC because she has heard from other students that if you take a couple of birth control pills at the same time you will have a miscarriage. What should the nurse explain about emergency contraception?

4. The student asks about abortion. The health center does not provide these services. The student makes an appointment for discussion with a health counselor. She elects to have a medical abortion with mifepristone with misoprostol at an off-campus center and returns to the health center the day after the abortion complaining of cramping. The nurse should assess for which adverse effects and their symptoms relating to the medical abortion?

5. The patient requests a form of birth control that does not require daily "remembering." She is not in a monogamous relationship, and she does not plan to have sex. "It just happens." What is a priority teaching that the nurse needs to provide?

6. Based on the possibility of multiple partners, which of the following methods of birth control that do not require daily dosing is contraindicated for this patient?
   a. Contraceptive patch (Ortho Evra)
   b. Intramuscular medroxyprogesterone acetate (Depo-Provera)
   c. Levonorgestrel subdermal implant (Norplant)
   d. Progesterone T (Progestasert) IUD
   e. Vaginal contraceptive ring (NuvaRing)

# 62 Drug Therapy of Infertility

## OBJECTIVES

See page 26 for the Objectives.

## CRITICAL THINKING AND STUDY QUESTIONS

1. Matching: Follicular maturation agents

| | | |
|---|---|---|
| _____ | a. Act on ovaries to promote follicular maturation (Clomid) | 1. Clomiphene |
| _____ | b. Promote ovulation | 2. Follitropin beta (Follistim) |
| _____ | c. Stimulate release of FSH and LH | 3. HCG (Pregnyl) |
| | | 4. Menotropin (Pergonal) |

2. Patients who are prescribed clomiphene (Clomid) may experience increased viscosity of cervical mucus hindering sperm motility. Estrogen is a possible treatment to thin the cervical mucus. Estrogen therapy would be of particular concern if the patient also has chronic:
   a. asthma causing bronchoconstriction when exposed to mold.
   b. hypertension requiring diuretic therapy.
   c. diabetes mellitus type 2 with peripheral neuropathy.
   d. venous stasis resulting in thrombophlebitis.

▸ 3. For early detection of the serious adverse effect of ovarian hyperstimulation syndrome from therapy with menotropins (Pergonal, Repronex, and Menopur), the nurse would be most concerned if, after starting therapy, the patient reported:
   a. fever higher than 100.4° F.
   b. gain of 2 lbs in 24 hours.
   c. pulse higher than 80 beats/min.
   d. redness across cheeks and nose.

▸ 4. The nurse is caring for a patient who experienced ovarian hyperstimulation syndrome after infertility therapy with HCG. Which of the following assessment findings warrant immediate notification of the physician?
   a. Headache
   b. Irritability
   c. Restlessness
   d. Rigid abdomen

5. Matching: Administration

| | | |
|---|---|---|
| _____ | a. Intramuscular | 1. Cetrotide (cetrorelix) |
| _____ | b. Oral | 2. Clomid (Clomiphene) |
| _____ | c. Subcutaneous | 3. Follistrom (follitropin beta) |
| | | 4. Gonal-F (follitropin alfa) |
| | | 5. Menopur (menotropins) |
| | | 6. Ovidrel (choriogonadotropin) |
| | | 7. Pergonal (menotropins) |

6. The nurse is explaining drug therapy to a patient who is prescribed cetrorelix. Which statement, if made by the patient, indicates a need for further teaching?
   a. "I should have someone else perform the injection because it must go into a muscle."
   b. "I should inject the drug into the fat below my skin about 2 inches away from my belly button."
   c. "I must stop taking the drug when instructed or I will not ovulate."
   d. "This drug prevents immature eggs from being released."

## CASE STUDIES AND PATIENT TEACHING

*(Use a separate piece of paper for your responses.)*

### Case Study 1

*A couple, who are in their late 30s and are childless, have been trying to conceive for the past 2 years, but have not been successful. During a lengthy diagnostic work-up for infertility, the wife was found to have no increase in her basal body temperature throughout her menstrual cycles. Her husband is healthy with a normal sperm count. The physician diagnoses primary infertility and decides to induce ovulation. Clomiphene (Serophene) and HCG (Pregnyl) are prescribed to promote ovarian follicular maturation and ovulation.*

1. What organ functioning must be present for this drug to work?

2. Which of the following laboratory results would be most important to have before the patient starts taking clomiphene (Clomid)?
   a. ALT
   b. HCG
   c. LDL
   d. UA

3. The nurse is explaining possible adverse effects of clomiphene (Clomid). Which of the following adverse effects, if experienced by the patient, would be most important for the patient to report to the prescriber?
   a. Breast engorgement
   b. Hot flushes (hot flashes)
   c. Low abdominal pain
   d. Nausea

4. One year later, the couple still has not conceived. Menotropins, aka hMG, (Pergonal) 1 ampule intramuscularly for days 9 through 12 of the menstrual cycle followed by HCG 5000 units are prescribed. The nurse provides counseling relevant to the need for follow-up and early detection of ovarian hyperstimulation syndrome. What symptoms should the nurse teach the patient to report immediately?

5. What will the nurse teach the patient about the timing of administration of HCG?

6. The couple ask whether she is more likely to have a multiple pregnancy (i.e., more than one fetus) with this drug regimen. How should the nurse respond?

### Case Study 2

*The nurse is caring for a patient who has been admitted with a diagnosis of ovarian hyperstimulation syndrome.*

1. What are outcomes, assessments, and interventions that the nurse should employ for each of the following nursing diagnoses for this patient?
   a. Acute pain
   b. Activity intolerance
   c. Anxiety and/or powerlessness and/or spiritual distress
   d. Decreased cardiac output
   e. Fluid volume excess
   f. Ineffective breathing pattern
   g. Pain
   h. Risk for injury
   i. Risk for impaired skin integrity

# 63 Drugs That Affect Uterine Function

## OBJECTIVES

See page 26 for the Objectives.

## CRITICAL THINKING AND STUDY QUESTIONS

1. The nurse may be able to decrease the incidence of the most common cause of preterm labor by teaching health promotion that includes:
   a. avoiding the use of alcohol during pregnancy.
   b. behaviors that decrease the incidence of sexually transmitted diseases (STDs).
   c. nutrition and exercise for healthy weight gain during pregnancy.
   d. smoking cessation counseling.

2. When performing a nursing assessment on a patient receiving magnesium sulfate to suppress uterine contractions of preterm labor, which of the following observations would be a reason to hold the medication and contact the prescriber?
   a. Fetal heart rate 90 beats/min
   b. 3+ maternal deep tendon reflexes (DTR)
   c. Maternal heart rate 90 beats/min
   d. Uterine contractions occurring more often than every 10 minutes

3. Which of these laboratory test results, if identified in a woman in preterm labor receiving magnesium sulfate, would be of most concern to the nurse?
   a. ALT 50 International Units/L
   b. Calcium 11 mg/dL
   c. Creatinine 4 mg/dL
   d. Magnesium 1.2 mEq/L

4. Which of the following magnesium levels suggest that magnesium sulfate is being administered at a therapeutic dose to suppress preterm labor?
   a. 2 mEq/L
   b. 5 mEq/L
   c. 8 mEq/L
   d. 11 mEq/L

5. A nursing outcome that best indicates that intravenous Pitocin therapy has achieved the desired effect in the first hour after delivery of the placenta is:
   a. blood pressure 120/80 mm Hg.
   b. pulse 80 beats/min.
   c. saturation of a perineal pad takes longer than 20 minutes.
   d. skin warm and dry.

6. Contraindications for magnesium sulfate therapy include: (Select all that apply.)
   a. bacterial vaginosis.
   b. hypernatremia.
   c. hypokalemia.
   d. myasthenia gravis.
   e. preeclampsia.
   f. renal failure.

7. Which of the following assessment findings in a woman receiving magnesium sulfate would most likely constitute an emergency?
   a. Dizziness
   b. Feeling of warmth
   c. Pink-tinged frothy sputum
   d. Urine output of 180 mL in 4 hours

8. The nursery nurse is caring for a neonate who was exposed to magnesium sulfate and delivered at 36 weeks of gestation. The neonate has experienced episodes of apnea and bradycardia. If these symptoms are related to the magnesium sulfate, the nurse would expect improvement by day:
   a. 3.
   b. 5.
   c. 7.
   d. 9.

9. The nurse is administering terbutaline (beta$_2$-adrenergic agonist) to a woman experiencing preterm labor. A possible adverse effect that the nurse should assess for is:
   a. bradycardia.
   b. diaphoresis.
   c. nausea and vomiting.
   d. shortness of breath.

▸ 10. Which of the following findings, if identified by the nurse in a patient receiving nifedipine (CCB) to suppress labor, would cause the greatest concern?
   a. Headache
   b. Fetal heart rate 88 beats/min
   c. Maternal heart rate 110 beats/min
   d. Skin flushed

▸ 11. Which of the following assessments would be reason to not start or to stop the infusion of oxytocin (Pitocin)? (Select all that apply.)
   a. Contractions lasting longer than 1 minute
   b. Contractions occurring more frequently than every 4 to 5 minutes
   c. Late decelerations of fetal heart rate
   d. Intrauterine pressure exceeds 20 mm/Hg during contractions
   e. Painful perineal vesicles
   f. Umbilical cord palpable in cervix

12. The labor and delivery nurse is preparing to administer ergonovine to a woman who has just delivered the placenta. Before administering the medication, it is critical that the nurse assess the patient for:
   a. hypertension.
   b. lochia flow.
   c. respiratory depression.
   d. uterine firmness.

▸ 13. A patient who is receiving ergotamine after delivery of the placenta has a soft uterine fundus. The nurse should:
   a. assess for cramping sensation.
   b. document the findings and continue to assess the patient.
   c. increase the rate of ergotamine infusion.
   d. notify the obstetrician or midwife.

▸ 14. In the postpartum unit, a patient receives methylergonovine (Methergine) 0.2 mg by mouth every 6 hours for 3 days to promote involution of the uterus. What assessment would warrant not administering this drug?
   a. Bradypnea
   b. Fever
   c. Hypertension
   d. Tachycardia

15. Dinoprostone for cervical softening is contraindicated in patients with a history of: (Select all that apply.)
   a. acute pelvic inflammatory disease (PID).
   b. blood sugar greater than 200 mg/dL.
   c. history of asthma.
   d. hypertension.
   e. hypotension.
   f. previous cesarean section.
   g. wheezing.

16. Which type of drug would the nurse administer to prevent a common adverse effect of dinoprostone?
   a. Analgesic
   b. Antiemetic
   c. Anti-inflammatory
   d. Antipyretic

▸ 17. Dinoprostone (Cervidil) vaginal insert pouch has been inserted in a patient's posterior fornix. Monitoring indicates that moderate contractions lasting 15 seconds have begun. The nurse should:
   a. immediately begin infusion of oxytocin (Pitocin).
   b. instruct the patient that she must lie on her back for at least 2 hours.
   c. place the patient on a fetal monitor.
   d. remove the dinoprostone pouch.

## CASE STUDIES AND PATIENT TEACHING

*(Use a separate piece of paper for your responses.)*

### Case Study 1

*A 25-year-old multipara (gravida 2, para 1) is admitted to the labor and delivery unit for induction of labor. She is 41 weeks of gestation. Vital signs and fetal heart rate are stable. Dinoprostone gel (Prepidil) is ordered for cervical ripening.*

1. What will the nurse teach the patient about this therapy?

2. The cervix has softened and is 50% effaced. The fetal head was at 0 stations in a left occiput anterior position. The medication order reads: "oxytocin (Pitocin) 10 milliunits. May increase 1 to 2 milliunits per minute every 30 minutes until normal pattern of uterine contractions are established." What is a normal pattern of uterine contractions?

3. When is oxytocin augmentation of labor contraindicated?

4. An intravenous infusion of 1000 units of oxytocin in 100 cc of 5% dextrose and 0.45% normal saline is infusing via a secondary line into a primary infusion line. The oxytocin infusion was regulated by an infusion pump and was initiated at 1 mU/min. Why is the oxytocin infusion "piggybacked" into the primary infusion line rather than added to the primary infusion solution?

5. The patient has suddenly started having contractions lasting 90 seconds every 2 minutes. What should the nurse do?

6. When reporting the patient's response to oxytocin therapy to the obstetrician, the nurse should include?

7. The patient has delivered her 6 lb-4-ounce baby boy. She received one dose of carboprost tromethamine (Hemabate) 250 mg IM to control postpartum hemorrhage. The next day she spiked a temperature of 101.6° F. Acetaminophen (Tylenol) 650 mg every 4 hours as needed is included in the postpartum orders. Fever is a common adverse effect of carboprost. Why is it important to notify the obstetrician rather than just administer the antipyretic?

### Case Study 2

*A woman who is 34 weeks of gestation has been admitted for tocolytic therapy with magnesium sulfate. She is concerned that the benefits of preventing preterm labor only for a few days does not outweigh risks of drug therapy on the neonate.*

1. The basis of the nurse's response is that suppressing labor, even if only for a short time, allows for what actions that can improve fetal outcomes to occur?

2. The patient's husband has read that taking an NSAID is as effective as magnesium sulfate for suppressing labor. He thinks that because NSAIDs can be purchased over-the-counter they must be safer than an infused drug. How should the nurse respond?

3. What are adverse effects of magnesium sulfate therapy used for suppressing labor, and what are critical nursing assessments relating to preventing the adverse effects and their complications?

# 64 Androgens

## OBJECTIVES

See page 26 for the Objectives.

## CRITICAL THINKING AND STUDY QUESTIONS

1. The body regulates testosterone levels by:
   a. blocking the effect of testosterone on receptors.
   b. decreasing release of testosterone from the adrenal gland.
   c. decreasing the release of testosterone from the testes.
   d. suppressing the release of stimulating hormones from the anterior pituitary.

2. A female patient with renal failure and anemia has been prescribed an androgen. The patient asks how this drug will help improve her red blood cell (RBC) count. The basis of the nurse's response should be that the drug:
   a. delays the destruction of old red blood cells.
   b. increases absorption of iron from the GI tract.
   c. promotes the release of intrinsic factor.
   d. stimulates the production of blood cells.

3. The nurse should explain the importance of adhering to monitoring of liver function tests when a patient is prescribed:
   a. methyltestosterone.
   b. testolactone.
   c. testosterone cypionate.
   d. testosterone enanthate.

▶ 4. Which of these findings would be most significant if a patient was receiving an androgen?
   a. ALT 45 mg/dL
   b. Bilirubin 1 mg/dL
   c. HDL 22 mg/dL
   d. LDL 120 mg/dL

▶ 5. When a patient is prescribed an androgen, it is important for the nurse to assess for:
   a. gain of weight.
   b. gynecomastia.
   c. orthostatic hypotension.
   d. symptoms of hyperglycemia.

6. A patient has received instructions regarding administration of testosterone buccal tablets (Striant). Which of these statements made by the client would indicate the patient needs further teaching?
   a. "I should apply the tablet to my gum above an incisor."
   b. "I should alternate sides of my mouth with each dose."
   c. "I should hold the tablet in place by pressing over the tablet from the outside of my mouth for 30 seconds to ensure adhesion."
   d. "I should remove the tablet when drinking hot fluids."

7. The pediatrician's triage nurse receives a call at 2:00 PM (1400) from a 14-year-old patient who was recently prescribed testosterone buccal tablets. The patient applied the buccal tablet at 7:00 AM (0700), and it fell out while eating lunch. He asks what he should do. The nurse should direct the patient to:
   a. not replace the tablet until the next dose is due at 7:00 PM.
   b. replace the tablet with a new one and remove it as scheduled for the original tablet at 7:00 PM (1900).
   c. replace the tablet with a new one and remove it 12 hours later (0200).
   d. replace the tablet with a new one and remove it the following morning at 7:00 AM (0700).

▸ 8. The high school nurse is planning a teaching presentation on the use of anabolic steroids. Developmentally, discussion of which effects of anabolic steroid use would most likely discourage the use of anabolic steroids by male high school athletes?
   a. Atherosclerosis
   b. Hypertension
   c. Liver damage
   d. Testicular shrinkage

9. Subjects in a 1996 study who received an equivalent of 6 to 8 times the amount of testosterone as normally produced by the testes did not experience:
   a. acne.
   b. increased ability to bench press weights.
   c. manic episodes, aggressiveness, and depression ("roid rage").
   d. muscle mass increase greater than subjects who only exercised.

10. Deepening of the voice and changes in hair patterns in females from use of androgens is usually:
   a. irreversible.
   b. reversible.

▸ 11. Which of these assessment findings, if identified in a patient who is receiving oxandrolone for muscle wasting associated with advanced HIV disease, should the nurse report to the prescriber immediately?
   a. Acne
   b. Fatigue, jaundice, and nausea
   c. Loss of hair
   d. Weight gain of 1 lb/wk

## CASE STUDIES AND PATIENT TEACHING

*(Use a separate piece of paper for your responses.)*

### Case Study 1

*A 16-year-old male has come to the healthcare provider because of his small testes and penis. The nurse notes that he is very tall (6 feet 10 inches) and thin (160 lbs). His legs are unusually long for his trunk. He tells the nurse that he frequently has been in trouble in school, and he will finally be a freshman in high school this year. He is considering dropping out of school. Laboratory test results reveal the absence of sperm in the semen and the presence of two more X chromosomes than would be expected for a male. The diagnosis of Klinefelter's syndrome is made. The nurse knows that this is not extremely rare, occurring in 1 of every 500 live male births, but is often not discovered until the male comes in for an infertility work-up. Therapy will be directed toward administration of the male hormone testosterone. The patient is prescribed 1% testosterone transdermal gel (Androgel). He asks "Why can't I take a pill?"*

1. How should the nurse respond?

2. The patient's mother is 36 years old. What precautions does the nurse need to teach the mother and patient?

3. What teaching should the nurse provide to the patient about administration of the gel?

4. The patient asks if there are any alternative routes of administration of testosterone. How should the nurse respond?

5. What information does the patient need regarding the adverse effects of testosterone?

# 65 Drugs for Erectile Dysfunction and Benign Prostatic Hyperplasia

## OBJECTIVES

See page 26 for the Objectives.

## CRITICAL THINKING AND STUDY QUESTIONS

1. The mechanism of action of sildenafil (Viagra) is to:
   a. activate guanylyl cyclase, the enzyme that makes cyclic guanosine monophosphate (cGMP).
   b. inhibit removal of cyclic guanosine monophosphate (cGMP) by phosphodiesterase type 5 (PDE-5).
   c. stimulate the release of phosphodiesterase type 5 (PDE-5).
   d. stimulate sexual arousal, which activates the parasympathetic nervous system, causing the release of nitric oxide.

2. The nurse who works in a reproduction clinic counsels patients who are experiencing sexual dysfunction. Many patients ask if sildenafil (Viagra) will help. The nurse knows that this drug will not be effective if the basis of the male's problem is: (Select all that apply.)
   a. desire for a more intense experience in a normally functioning male.
   b. improving erection quality in patients with impaired blood flow.
   c. lack of desire for sexual activity.
   d. maintaining erection long enough to experience a satisfactory sexual experience.
   e. premature ejaculation.

▸ 3. Which of these findings would be a priority concern relating to use of sildenafil (Viagra)?
   a. Blood pressure 160/90 mm Hg
   b. Blue-tinged, blurred vision lasting 1 to 2 hours
   c. Diarrhea
   d. Erection not subsiding after ejaculation

▸ 4. It is most important to assess if a male patient uses sildenafil (Viagra) when the patient is newly prescribed:
   a. cimetidine (Tagamet).
   b. doxazosin (Cardura).
   c. finasteride (Proscar).
   d. isosorbide (Imdur).

▸ 5. The nurse should teach the patient who is receiving sildenafil (Viagra) to avoid which of these foods?
   a. Bananas
   b. Grapefruit juice
   c. Processed foods that are high in sodium
   d. Refined carbohydrates

▸ 6. Which of these history findings, if identified in a patient who uses sildenafil (Viagra), should the nurse report to the prescriber immediately?
   a. Anginal symptoms when engaging in any moderate physical activity
   b. Glaucoma
   c. Hypertension
   d. Urinary frequency or difficulty starting the stream of urine

▸ 7. A patient who takes vardenafil (Levitra) reports palpitations and dizziness. Assessment findings include heart rate 122 beats/min and BP 80/46 mm/Hg. The nurse should recognize that which serious adverse effect may be occurring?
   a. Cerebral vascular accident
   b. Long-QT syndrome
   c. Malignant hypertension
   d. Myocardial infarction

8. Injection of papaverine plus phentolamine differs in response from the oral drugs for erectile dysfunction (ED) in that:
   a. arterial inflow is increased.
   b. hypotension will not occur.
   c. outflow of venous blood is decreased.
   d. the drug causes an erection without sexual stimulation.

9. When administering finasteride (Proscar), which of the following outcomes would be appropriate?
   a. Erection lasts long enough to achieve sexual satisfaction.
   b. Prostate-specific antigen levels less than 4 ng/mL.
   c. Size of the prostate gland is reduced by 50%.
   d. Urinary symptoms are relieved.

10. Before the nurse administers terazosin (Hytrin) to a patient who has been diagnosed with BPH, which of these assessments is most critical to perform?
    a. Bladder distention
    b. Blood pressure
    c. Respirations
    d. Temperature

11. Protecting the skin from contact with the medication is important for women of childbearing age when administering:
    a. alfluzosin (Uroxatral).
    b. dutasteride (Avodart).
    c. finasteride (Proscar).
    d. tamsulosin (Flomax).

12. A patient has received instructions regarding administration of tamsulosin (Flomax). Which of these statements made by the client about timing of dosing would indicate the patient understood the directions?
    a. "I should take the medication 30 minutes after a meal."
    b. "I should take the medication 30 minutes before a meal."
    c. "I can take the medication any time of day, as long as it is the same time every day."
    d. "I should take the medication first thing in the morning before taking any other medication and stay sitting up for 30 minutes after taking the medication."

13. Teaching for a patient prescribed doxazosin (Cardura) for BPH should include:
    a. adverse effects include gynecomastia.
    b. orthostatic blood pressure precautions.
    c. the drug reduces the size of the prostate, which improves urine outflow.
    d. the drug reduces PSA levels by approximately 50%.

14. Benign prostatic hyperplasia (BPH): (Select all that apply.)
    a. can cause kidney damage.
    b. can involve restriction of urine outflow from the bladder without significant increase in the size of the gland.
    c. is less common than prostate cancer.
    d. is not associated with risk for prostate cancer.
    e. symptoms are directly related to the size of the gland.
    f. treatment is based on presence of subjective symptoms, not objective findings.
    g. treatment when the gland is large involves blocking of $alpha_1$ receptors in the bladder neck.

15. A disadvantage of the herbal preparation saw palmetto is:
    a. it causes significant adverse effects.
    b. it is often toxic.
    c. it is only available in specialized stores.
    d. regulators do not check if the product contains the amount of product that the label states it contains.

## CASE STUDIES AND PATIENT TEACHING

*(Use a separate piece of paper for your responses.)*

### Case Study 1

*The nurse is providing medication teaching for a 45-year-old male patient who was admitted with cellulitis of the left lower leg. The patient has a history of diabetes mellitus type 2 and hypertension. During the discussion, the patient's wife mentions that he has been experiencing "difficulties with sex" since he started taking medication for his high blood pressure.*

1. Why is it particularly important to address sensitive adverse effects, such as erectile dysfunction, especially when they occur as a result of antihypertensive medications?

2. The nurse notifies the physician of the patient's and wife's concerns. After discussing the problem with the patient, the physician prescribes sildenafil (Viagra) 50 mg as directed and asks the nurse to explain administration of the drug. What should be included in this explanation?

3. Why is it important for the patient to have information on his person stating that he takes sildenafil (Viagra) and to share this information with all prescribers?

# 66 Review of the Immune System

## OBJECTIVES

See page 26 for the Objectives.

## CRITICAL THINKING AND STUDY QUESTIONS

1. Natural immunity:
   a. intensifies with each exposure to an antigen.
   b. involves lymphocyte receptors that recognize individual antigens.
   c. is specific to a particular antigen.
   d. protection includes the skin.

2. Matching

| | | |
|---|---|---|
| _____ | a. B cells | 1. Antigen-presenting cells |
| _____ | b. Basophils | 2. Attack and kill target cells |
| _____ | c. CTL | 3. Attack antigens tagged with IgE |
| _____ | d. Dendritic cells | 4. Attack helminths |
| _____ | e. Eosinophils | 5. Involved in immediate hypersensitivity |
| _____ | f. Helper T cells | 6. Make antibodies |
| _____ | g. Macrophage | 7. Mediate inflammation |
| _____ | h. Mast cells | 8. Phagocytize target cells |
| _____ | i. Neutrophils | 9. Promote production and differentiation of B cells and CTL |
| | | 10. Promote production of CTL and CD4 cells |

3. The nurse assesses for declining immune status of people who are infected with HIV by monitoring for declining levels of:
   a. basophils.
   b. CD4 cells (helper T cells).
   c. CD8 cells (cytotoxic T lymphocytes).
   d. macrophages.

4. Antibodies are also known as: (Select all that apply.)
   a. B lymphocytes.
   b. dendritic cells.
   c. gamma globulins.
   d. immunoglobulins.
   e. macrophages.
   f. monophils.

5. Matching

| | | |
|---|---|---|
| _____ | a. IgA | 1. Elevated in allergic reactions with histamine release |
| _____ | b. IgD | 2. First antibody produced in response to an antigen |
| _____ | c. IgE | 3. First line of defense in GI tract and lungs |
| _____ | d. IgG | 4. Most abundant antibody |
| _____ | e. IgM | 5. Only found on the surface of B cells |

6. Salk developed an injected vaccine for polio. When Sabin developed an oral vaccine, people who already had received the Salk vaccine were revaccinated with the Sabin vaccine. Based on the fact that polio is transmitted via the oral-fecal route, the rationale for these mass revaccinations is the:
   a. Sabin vaccine did not involve the pain of an injection.
   b. Sabin vaccine sensitized the GI mucosa to prevent the polio microbe from entering the bloodstream.
   c. Salk vaccine only stimulated the production of IgM.
   d. Salk vaccine did not cause adequate production of IgM on the surface of mature B cells.

7. Breast-feeding:
   a. does not affect the infant's immunity.
   b. produces life-long immunity for the diseases for which the mother has immunity.
   c. transfers maternal IgA to the infant's GI tract.
   d. triggers the release of mediators from mast cells.

8. The ability of the immune system to identify different antigens is a result of:

9. Autoimmune diseases occur when:
   a. a new antigen is introduced to the body, and the immune system does not recognize the antigen.
   b. a person has an inflammatory reaction to an antigen.
   c. an antigen is introduced, and the immune response fades too quickly.
   d. there is a failure in major histocompatibility complex (MHC) molecules' ability to identify self.

10. A person who is allergic to penicillin would expect a more severe reaction with exposure to the penicillin in the future because:
    a. helper T cells attack the penicillin molecule.
    b. higher doses of penicillin would have to be used.
    c. memory cells that identified the penicillin as an antigen allow for a more rapid, intense, and prolonged response.
    d. the immune system cannot eliminate the penicillin.

11. An immunologic reason for the fact that red blood cells can be transfused from one person to another is:
    a. human red blood cells do not have class I MHC molecules.
    b. human blood is exactly the same in all individuals.
    c. human blood does not respond to class II MHC molecules.
    d. the above statement is not true.

12. The nurse is reviewing the laboratory tests for a patient who is jaundiced. Laboratory results include an elevated tumor necrosis factor (TNF). This suggests the patient has:
    a. cirrhosis or hepatitis.
    b. diabetes mellitus or insipidus.
    c. inflammation or a tumor.
    d. kidney cancer or renal failure.

13. Cells that provide signals to regulate cell proliferation and function during immune responses are called:
    a. antigen-presenting cells.
    b. cytokines.
    c. MHC molecules.
    d. opsonins.

14. Activation of the complement pathway occurs when the first component of the complement system (C1) encounters:
    a. a free antibody.
    b. a free antigen.
    c. an antibody-antigen complex.

15. Antibodies neutralize viruses by:

16. A 45-year-old patient has been infected with *Mycobacterium tuberculosis*. What kind of immunity response has been activated?
    a. Activation of cytolytic T cells by recognizing *Mycobacterium tuberculosis* bound to a class I MHC molecule
    b. DTH where macrophage activates CD4 helper cell, which activates macrophage allowing it to kill the bacteria residing within the macrophage

17. Macrophages increase production of lysosome and reactive oxygen to kill bacteria within the macrophage in response to:
    a. granulocyte-macrophage colony-stimulating factor.
    b. interferon gamma.
    c. interleukins.
    d. tumor necrosis factor.

18. The principle job of cytolytic T lymphocytes is to kill self cells that are infected with:
    a. bacteria.
    b. fungi.
    c. helminths.
    d. viruses.

## CASE STUDIES AND PATIENT TEACHING

*(Use a separate piece of paper for your responses.)*

### Case Study 1

*The nurse is preparing to perform intradermal injection of house dust, molds, foods, and other common allergens.*

1. Why are the extracts that are injected called antigens?

2. The allergic reaction causes degranulation of mast cells. What cells respond in the skin, what do they release, and what dermal symptoms will the patient have if allergic to the antigen?

3. The patient is required to remain in the office for 20 minutes after injection of any antigen because that is the usual time frame for an immediate hypersensitivity reaction. What symptom is most important for the nurse to tell the patient to report?
    a. Itching
    b. Redness
    c. Rhinorrhea
    d. Tingling around the mouth

4. Why is it important to teach this patient about possible anaphylaxis?

# 67 Childhood Immunization

## OBJECTIVES

See page 26 for the Objectives.

## CRITICAL THINKING AND STUDY QUESTIONS

▸ 1. The nurse has volunteered to work triaging people who have been trapped in their homes during a flood. To be protected from contracting disease from contaminated areas during this work, the nurse should obtain what type of immunization?
    a. Live attenuated vaccine
    b. Killed vaccine
    c. Pooled immunoglobulins
    d. Specific immunoglobulins

2. The pediatric office nurse is responsible for obtaining vaccine information sheets to be provided to parents before they consent to vaccinations for their children. The best source of this information is:
    a. www.cdc.gov.
    b. www.immunize.org.
    c. pubmedcentral.nih.gov.
    d. www.webmd.com.

3. If smallpox has been eradicated from the planet earth, why has the Centers for Disease Control and Prevention (CDC) of the U.S. government recommended that certain healthcare providers consider vaccination against smallpox?

4. The nurse must be prepared for anaphylactic reactions after administering immunizations. The highest incidence of this type of reaction occurs with:
   a. diphtheria, tetanus, acellular pertussis (DTaP).
   b. *haemophilus influenzae* type b vaccine (Hib).
   c. measles, mumps, and rubella (MMR).
   d. oral poliovirus vaccine (OPV).

▶ 5. A 17-month-old child is late for receiving DTaP, MMR, varicella, and pneumococcal conjugate immunizations. The parent has brought the child to the pediatrician because she has been fussy, lethargic, and not eating. The child has a temperature of 100.1° F and is diagnosed with streptococcal pharyngitis. Amoxicillin is prescribed. The nurse expects that the immunizations will:
   a. be administered.
   b. be administered at the next scheduled well-child visit.
   c. not be administered until the child is afebrile.
   d. not be administered until the child has finished the antibiotic.

6. Research suggests that the most common serious adverse reaction that has been associated with the DTaP immunization is:
   a. anaphylaxis.
   b. autism.
   c. encephalitis.
   d. Guillain-Barré syndrome.

7. Matching: Communicable diseases or microbes and major concerns

| | | |
|---|---|---|
| _____ | a. Diphtheria | 1. Cerebellar ataxia and Reye's syndrome |
| _____ | b. Hepatitis | 2. Congenital defects including deafness |
| _____ | c. Hib | 3. One hundred-day cough |
| _____ | d. Measles | 4. Encephalitis |
| _____ | e. Meningococcal meningitis | 5. Liver damage |
| _____ | f. Mumps | 6. Neurologic disability or death |
| _____ | g. Pertussis | 7. Obstructed airway |
| _____ | h. Pneumococcal | 8. Orchiditis and possible sterility |
| _____ | i. Poliomyelitis | 9. Otitis media |
| _____ | j. Rubella | 10. Pneumonia and meningitis |
| _____ | k. Tetanus | 11. Skeletal muscle paralysis |
| _____ | l. Varicella | 12. Skeletal muscle spasm |

▶ 8. The literature states that wild-type polio has been eliminated from the Western Hemisphere. What type of polio is still present in the Western Hemisphere, and how could a person contract this type of polio?

▶ 9. The nurse would consult with the prescriber if which of the following immunizations was prescribed for a child who is receiving chronic high doses of prednisolone? (Select all that apply.)
   a. DTaP
   b. HAV
   c. HBV
   d. Hib
   e. IPV
   f. MCV4
   g. MMR
   h. OPV
   i. Varicella vaccine

▶ 10. Foster parents bring a 14-month-old child in for the first visit at the pediatrician's office. The child protective agency has been unable to obtain any immunization records. The office nurse would expect to:
   a. administer the immunizations scheduled for 12 to 14 months.
   b. delay immunizations until records can be found.
   c. immunize the child with the immunizations scheduled for 2 months of age.
   d. review the child's known history that will be used by the pediatrician along with a complete physical examination to determine which immunizations can be safely administered.

▶ 11. The nurse knows that the MMR vaccine should not be administered to a child who:
   a. has a mother receiving chemotherapy for breast cancer.
   b. has been diagnosed with leukemia.
   c. has had a positive Monospot test (EBV infection).
   d. is asymptomatic, but HIV positive.

▶ 12. The nurse is preparing to immunize an 18-year-old college-bound female. The nurse tells the patient "You cannot get pregnant for 2 months if I give you this shot." Why is this not a good statement for the nurse to make to this adolescent?
   a. Pregnancy is not contraindicated after MMR vaccination.
   b. The statement assumes that the teen is sexually active.
   c. The statement is a communication blocker.
   d. The teen may interpret the statement as the injection prevents pregnancy.

13. Which of the following would be critical to include when the office nurse is discussing a scheduled MMR vaccination with the parents of a 12-month-old boy? (Select all that apply.)
   a. The child has allergies to gelatin, eggs, or neomycin.
   b. Any adverse effects that occur from this vaccine should occur within 48 hours of receiving the vaccination.
   c. Has your child received any blood or blood products in the past 6 months?
   d. Is your child taking an antibiotic?
   e. Contact the office if you notice the child having any unusual bleeding or bruising.
   f. The child should not have close contact with anyone who is pregnant for 3 weeks after receiving the vaccine.
   g. There is a small risk that your child can experience seizures relating to a high fever.
   h. Vomiting and diarrhea are common adverse effects of this vaccine.

14. When choosing a site for vaccinations, the nurse is aware that it is generally recommended that live vaccinations be administered:
   a. intradermally.
   b. intramuscularly.
   c. orally.
   d. subcutaneously.

▶ 15. The triage nurse receives a call from a mother who is concerned about her 2-month-old son who received the first DTaP vaccination yesterday. Which of the following, if reported by the mother, would be of most concern to the nurse?
   a. Crying almost constantly for the past 5 hours
   b. Only nursing for 10 minutes every 5 to 6 hours
   c. Redness and swelling at the injection site
   d. Temperature of 103° F

16. The CDC currently recommends the inactivated poliovirus vaccine (IPV or Salk) instead of the oral polio vaccine (OPV or Sabin) because:
   a. immune compromised people can contract polio from OPV.
   b. IPV causes less adverse effects than OPV.
   c. IPV is less expensive than OPV.
   d. OPV is less effective than IPV.

17. Which of the following, if elicited by the nurse from the parent of a 15-month-old who is scheduled to receive the varicella vaccine, would be a reason to withhold administering the vaccine and consulting the prescriber?
   a. The child had a severe reaction to the MMR vaccine.
   b. The child is allergic to eggs.
   c. The mother's sister and her newborn are temporarily staying with the family.
   d. The office has used all of the syringes with 1-inch needles.

18. The triage office nurse receives a call from the father of a 16-year-old who received a varicella vaccine 10 days ago. The teen experienced a fever after the injection, which was treated with aspirin. Yesterday the teen stayed home from school with stomach flu. He has not vomited today, but the father is having difficulty awakening him. The nurse should direct the father to:
   a. allow the teen to rest and call back tomorrow morning.
   b. make an appointment to be seen in the office.
   c. reassess the teen's temperature.
   d. seek medical care immediately.

19. The nurse would expect to administer a booster dose of varicella vaccine to a child who is (has):
   a. not gotten a fever from the first dose.
   b. older than 12 years at the time of the first dose.
   c. seven years old at the time of the first dose.
   d. younger than 18 months.

20. The nursery nurse would expect to administer which of the following vaccinations to the neonate if the mother of the neonate is HbsAg positive? (Select all that apply.)
   a. Hepatitis A immunoglobulin (HAIG)
   b. Havrix
   c. Influenza vaccine
   d. Pneumovax
   e. Recombivax HB
   f. Twinrix

21. The nurse would withhold the vaccination and contact the prescriber if a patient who has a history of Guillain-Barré syndrome is scheduled to receive which of the following vaccinations?
   a. DTaP
   b. HBV
   c. MCV4
   d. MMR

22. A patient who has had a splenectomy asks why he needs to get a meningitis vaccine. The basis of the nurse's response is that the spleen:
   a. destroys old red blood cells.
   b. forms blood cells.
   c. is a critical defense whenever a patient has a fever.
   d. removes encapsulated bacteria from the bloodstream.

## CASE STUDIES AND PATIENT TEACHING

*(Use a separate piece of paper for your responses.)*

### Case Study 1

*A mother brings her 7-month-old child to the clinic. She states that she was told by the emergency department (ED) physician of the local hospital to bring the child in for "baby shots." The mother is concerned, stating that she has heard children die from these "baby shots."*

1. What teaching can the nurse provide about the safety and benefits of the immunizations?

2. The mother has difficulty understanding complex concepts. How can the nurse explain reactions to immunizations?

3. How would the nurse explain laws requiring children to have immunizations before they can attend school and, in some cases, day care?

4. What information does the mother need to collect when a child is scheduled for an immunization?

### Case Study 2

*Parents of an elementary school child in western Pennsylvania have verbalized to the school nurse that their children have never been "contaminated" with immunizations. The parent cites that her unimmunized child has not contracted the measles, mumps, diphtheria, or other illness for which immunizations are routinely administered.*

1. How should the school nurse respond?

2. The parents state that they are particularly concerned about MMR because of its association with autism. What has research suggested about the association of MMR and autism?

3. The school nurse is aware that exposure to certain populations or situations put unvaccinated children at risk for contracting vaccine-preventable disease. What are possible populations and situations that would put children at risk in this school and geographic area?

### Case Study 3

*What pediatric office procedure could be used to expedite identifying patients who have received specific vaccines in case of future issues with specific manufacturers?*

# 68 Immunosuppressants

## OBJECTIVES

See page 26 for the Objectives.

## CRITICAL THINKING AND STUDY QUESTIONS

▶ 1. The nurse is doing postoperative teaching for a patient who has had carpal tunnel release surgery and who is receiving immunosuppressant therapy for rheumatoid arthritis. Based on the surgery and medication, the priority nursing concern would be preventing:
   a. airway constriction.
   b. infection.
   c. pain.
   d. impaired tissue perfusion.

2. The nurse teaches a patient who has been prescribed immunosuppressant drugs to report early signs of infection, such as:
   a. chills and rigor.
   b. cough.
   c. rash.
   d. sore throat.

▶ 3. The nurse is administering intravenous cyclosporine (Sandimmune). Within 15 minutes after beginning the infusion, the patient complains of feeling hot. Her skin is flushed. The nurse assesses vital signs. Her blood pressure is 80/55 mm Hg, pulse is 108 beats/min, and respirations are 25 per minute. The nurse should discontinue the infusion and administer prescribed:
   a. azithromycin (Zithromax).
   b. epinephrine (Adrenalin).
   c. furosemide (Lasix).
   d. lorazepam (Ativan).

4. The nurse teaches sexually active female patients who are on cyclosporine that it is important to use which type of birth control:
   a. barrier, such as a latex condom.
   b. contraceptive patch containing norelgestromin and estradiol.
   c. oral contraceptive containing estradiol.
   d. oral contraceptive containing mestranol.

▶ 5. When reviewing the laboratory results of patients receiving cyclosporine (Sandimmune) and tacrolimus (Prograf), which of the following results would be a reason to contact the prescriber? (Select all that apply.)

| | |
|---|---|
| a. ALT | 28 International Units |
| b. Bilirubin, direct | 2 mg/dL |
| c. BUN | 17 mg/dL |
| d. Creatinine | 3.2 mg/dL |
| e. Potassium | 5.4 mEq/L |
| f. WBC | 7000/$mm^3$ |

6. A patient asks why he is prescribed ketoconazole in addition to cyclosporine. The nurse explains that the main reason these two drugs are administered concurrently is to:
   a. decrease adverse effects of cyclosporine while maintaining therapeutic blood levels.
   b. decrease cyclosporine levels to prevent nephrotoxicity.
   c. increase cyclosporine levels to therapeutic levels.
   d. lower doses and costs of cyclosporine while maintaining therapeutic blood levels.

7. When should the nurse draw cyclosporine trough levels?
   a. Just after administering a dose
   b. Just before the next dose
   c. One-half hour after administering a dose
   d. One-half hour before administering a dose

8. A renal transplant patient's orders include discontinuation of intravenous tacrolimus (Prograf) and starting oral tacrolimus. The last intravenous dose was administered at 10:00 AM. The first oral dose should be administered no sooner than:
   a. 2:00 PM.
   b. 4:00 PM.
   c. 6:00 PM.
   d. 8:00 PM.

▶ 9. A liver transplant patient who takes tacrolimus reveals that he has been drinking grapefruit juice, but he has made sure it has been at least 4 hours between the juice and the medication. Which of the following suggests a drug-food interaction?
   a. Blood sugar 235 mg/dL
   b. Sore throat
   c. Temperature 102° F
   d. Urine output 100 mL/4 hr

10. A 16-month-old child receives a heart-lung transplant. What teaching should the nurse provide about immunizations relating to immunosuppressant therapy? (Select all that apply.)
   a. The child may need more than the usual recommended doses of inactivated vaccines.
   b. The child may need more than the usual recommended doses of live vaccines.
   c. The child should not receive any inactivated vaccines.
   d. The child should not receive any live vaccines.
   e. The child should not receive any vaccines.

11. Body image is developmentally important to many patients. It is important for the nurse to discuss body image when cyclosporine has been prescribed to a young woman because the drug can cause:
   a. acne.
   b. facial hair.
   c. rash.
   d. weight gain.

12. The main reason why tacrolimus therapy is discontinued is toxicity. Which of the following drugs, if taken with tacrolimus. is most likely to cause toxicity?
   a. Erythromycin
   b. Phenobarbital
   c. Phenytoin
   d. Rifamycin

▶ 13. Trough levels of tacrolimus are 10 ng/mL. The nurse should:
   a. administer the medication.
   b. hold the medication.

14. Matching: Drug and adverse effect (Answer may be used more than once.)

| | Drug | Adverse effect |
|---|---|---|
| ____ | a. Azathioprine | 1. Decreased bone density |
| ____ | b. Cyclosporine | 2. Hyperglycemia |
| ____ | c. Prednisone | 3. Hypercholesterolemia and hypertriglyceridemia |
| ____ | d. Sirolimus | 4. Neutropenia and thrombocytopenia |
| ____ | e. Tacrolimus | 5. Tremor |

15. Because sirolimus has a half-life of 2.5 days and it is categorized as pregnancy category C, the nurse teaches women of child-bearing years to continue using birth control after stopping the drug for what period of time?
   a. 1 week
   b. 4 weeks
   c. 8 weeks
   d. 12 weeks

16. The nurse should teach patients who take sirolimus to take the medication:
   a. consistently with or consistently without food.
   b. on an empty stomach.
   c. with food.
   d. with 8 ounces of water.

17. A patient receiving azathioprine develops gout and is prescribed allopurinol. Because of the drug interaction, the nurse should consult the prescriber about possible need to:
   a. decrease the dose of allopurinol.
   b. increase the dose of allopurinol.
   c. decrease the dose of azathioprine.
   d. increase the dose of azathioprine.

18. The nurse should include in discharge instructions for a patient who is prescribed mycophenolate mofetil (CellCept) that which of the following over-the-counter drugs can prevent mycophenolate mofetil from reaching therapeutic concentrations in the blood?
   a. Acetaminophen (Tylenol)
   b. Antacids
   c. Diphenhydramine (Benadryl)
   d. NSAIDs

19. Which of the following should be employed when administering antilymphocyte globulin (Atgam)? (Select all that apply.)
    a. Administer using an in-line filter.
    b. Assess for flushing, dyspnea, and generalized anxiety
    c. Do not take aluminum or magnesium antacids because they decrease absorption of the drug.
    d. Infuse slowly—over 4 hours or more.
    e. Premedicate with a glucocorticoid to prevent adverse effects.
    f. Should be administered via a central line.
    g. Teach not to drink grapefruit juice.

20. The nurse is preparing to administer $Rh_o$(D) immune globulin. This drug should not be administered to which individuals?

## CASE STUDIES AND PATIENT TEACHING

*(Use a separate piece of paper for your responses.)*

### Case Study 1

*A 4-year-old girl received an allogenic heart transplant at age 16 months for transposition of the great vessels and only one ventricle, which resulted in cardiac failure.*

1. What is an allogenic transplant?

2. The patient was discharged on cyclosporine, azathioprine (Imuran) and prednisone. She is brought back to the transplant site monthly for blood work to monitor rejection status and performance of her new heart. During the past year, she has shown no sign of rejection or limitation of her activities. Her growth has more closely followed normal growth charts and outwardly she appears to be a healthy 4-year-old. Recently, following a trip to a national park, she developed fatigue and appeared tired. Blood work indicated evidence of macrophages and monocytes beginning the rejection process. She was hospitalized and diagnosed with evidence of transplant rejection. What are nursing priorities for this patient?

3. Intravenous muromonab-CD3 is added to the patient's medication regimen to prevent rejection of the transplanted heart. What actions should the nurse take in the hospital to prevent the patient from contracting an infection?

4. What special steps must be taken when administering this drug intravenously?

5. Four hours after receiving the first dose of muromonab-CD3 the mother tells the nurse that the patient is shivering. Her temperature is 102.6° F. These symptoms could be indicative of further organ rejection or adverse effects to the drug. What should the nurse do?

### Case Study 2

*A 38-year-old female heart transplant recipient is prescribed immunosuppressant therapy with intravenous cyclosporine (Sandimmune), prednisone, and ketoconazole.*

1. What teaching should the nurse provide relating to the adverse effect of increased risk of neoplasms from taking cyclosporine?

2. The patient has a history of knee pain and a seizure disorder. What should be included in the plan of nursing care relating to immunosuppressant therapy that she is receiving and her medical history?

3. Intravenous cyclosporine is discontinued, and the patient is started on oral cyclosporine (Gengraf) 9 mg/kg/day divided into 2 doses 12 hours apart. The patient weighs 132 lbs, and the medication is available as a solution of 100 mg/mL. What is the prescribed dose in mg?

4. How much medication should the nurse administer?

5. How should the nurse teach the patient to administer this dose of medication?

6. The hospital pharmacy sends the Sandimmune formulation (100 mg/mL). What should the nurse do?

# 69 Antihistamines

## OBJECTIVES

See page 26 for the Objectives.

## CRITICAL THINKING AND STUDY QUESTIONS

1. A patient is scheduled to receive a plasma expander. The patient has never received this treatment or any of its components before. Allergic reactions:
   a. are common because patients often are unaware if they have had plasma expander therapy in the past.
   b. are very likely to occur.
   c. can occur even without prior exposure to plasma expanders.
   d. will not occur because allergic reactions require prior exposure to the substance.

2. $H_1$ blocking drugs for allergic reactions: (Select all that apply.)
   a. are the active ingredient in most over-the-counter drugs to induce sleep.
   b. can cause excitement, nervousness, and tremors.
   c. can cause urinary retention.
   d. cause the skin to become red and warm.
   e. decrease release of histamine present in high levels in the skin and lungs tract.
   f. decrease pruritus.
   g. elevate the pH of stomach secretions.
   h. have sedation as the most common adverse effect.
   i. prevent local edema.
   j. prevent the release of histamine from mast cells and basophils.
   k. relieve the symptoms of a cold.
   l. reverse bronchoconstriction of an asthma attack.
   m. treat the anaphylaxis.
   n. thicken respiratory secretions.

3. The term "antihistamine" is commonly used to refer to drugs that block:
   a. $H_1$ receptors.
   b. $H_2$ receptors.
   c. $H_1$ and $H_2$ receptors.

4. Second-generation $H_1$ blockers cause less sedation than first-generation $H_1$ blockers because they:
   a. are less potent.
   b. bind reversibly to histamine receptors.
   c. do not cross the blood-brain barrier.
   d. are rapidly metabolized.

▶ 5. Which of these assessment findings, if identified by the delivery room nurse in a full-term neonate whose mother has taken diphenhydramine (Benadryl) just before going into labor should be reported to the pediatrician immediately?
   a. Systolic BP 60 mm Hg
   b. Temperature 39.2° C
   c. Pulse 180 beats/min
   d. Respirations

6. The nurse is teaching a patient who has a history of benign prostatic hypertrophy (BPH) and allergic rhinitis about taking desloratadine (Clarinex). Teaching should include that: (Select all that apply.)
   a. avoidance of alcohol and other CNS depressants.
   b. avoidance of any activity that requires coordination or alertness.
   c. high doses are more likely to cause sedation.
   d. many patients find hard candy relieves the adverse effect of dry mouth.
   e. monitoring of ECG for long QT syndrome should be done after starting the drug.
   f. taking doses higher than recommended does not help the drug work better.
   g. the drug may aggravate urinary retention from the enlarged prostate.

▶ 7. The nurse is administering 6 AM medications, including chlorpheniramine (Chlor-Trimeton) 4 mg every 6 hours for urticaria. The patient complains of nausea associated with the medication. The nurse should:
   a. change the timing of the medication to 8 AM (0800), 12 noon (1200), 4 PM (1600), and 8 PM (2000) to correspond to meals and bedtime snack.
   b. decrease the dose of the medication.
   c. hold the medication and consult the prescriber.
   d. provide a snack with each dose of medication.

8. A patient with asthma that is triggered by exposure to environmental allergens has been taking diphenhydramine to treat his allergy symptoms. He asks the nurse why his asthma attacks have not abated. The nurse's response should include:

▶ 9. A 3-year-old child is brought into the emergency room after ingesting an unknown quantity of his grandmother's cetririzine (Zyrtec). The child is restless, incoherent, skin is flushed and hot, pulse is 70 beats/min, BP 70/42 m/hg, respirations 35/minute. The nurse should be prepared to:
   a. assess for abnormal movements.
   b. administer an antidote.
   c. monitor for hypertension.
   d. warm the patient.

## CASE STUDIES AND PATIENT TEACHING

*(Use a separate piece of paper for your responses.)*

### Case Study 1

*A 25-year-old truck driver has come to his healthcare provider to obtain information and help for his "hay fever." He says he doesn't know what to take because over-the-counter (OTC) drugs seem so confusing. His condition is diagnosed as allergic rhinitis and is seasonal with reactions lasting from May until the end of June each year. He also says that he is occasionally bothered by dust during the rest of the year. He complains of headache, congestion, sneezing, rhinorrhea (runny nose), and itchy, burning, and watery eyes.*

1. What is the physiology involved in this allergic response?

2. What are the disadvantages to antihistamines for those who drive or use heavy equipment at work?

3. The patient is concerned about cost. He asks if prescription antihistamines are more effective than OTC diphenhydramine (Benadryl). How should the nurse respond?

4. How do second-generation antihistamines work but not cause sedation?

5. The physician orders azelastine (Astelin) 2 sprays of 250 micrograms in each nostril twice a day. Why is this medication ordered specifically for this patient?

6. What suggestions can the nurse make if the patient chooses to use one of the antihistamines that cause sedation?

# 70 Cyclooxygenase Inhibitors: Nonsteroidal Anti-Inflammatory Drugs and Acetaminophen

## OBJECTIVES

See page 26 for the Objectives.

## CRITICAL THINKING AND STUDY QUESTIONS

1. The nurse is administering celecoxib (Celebrex) 100 mg to an 82-year-old patient with osteoarthritis (degenerative joint disease, DJD). Which of the following adverse effects, if present, would be of most concern to the nurse?
   a. Edema
   b. Flatulence
   c. Headache
   d. Nausea

▶ 2. The following information was included in the change of shift report on patients who are prescribed aspirin for its anticoagulant effects. Which of the following patient symptoms, if present, would be most important for the nurse to report to the attending physician?
   a. Abdominal bloating
   b. Coffee ground emesis
   c. Heartburn when recumbent
   d. Two liquid stool in the past 24 hours

▶ 3. Which of the following would not be an appropriate reason for the nurse to administer aspirin 650 mg by mouth that has been ordered every 4 hours as needed?
   a. Hand pain and stiffness when arising
   b. Knee pain with ambulation
   c. Right temporal headache associated with a tense neck
   d. Right upper quadrant pain that occurs with deep inspiration

4. A 13-year-old girl has been prescribed ibuprofen 600 mg, 1 tablet every 6 hours as needed for severe cramping menstrual pain. Her mother contacts the telephone advice nurse and asks if she can give her over-the-counter (OTC) ibuprofen instead because it is less expensive and she does not have prescription insurance coverage. What information is most accurate for the nurse to include in her response?
   a. Aspirin is just as effective as ibuprofen at relieving menstrual cramps.
   b. Aspirin is ineffective in relieving menstrual pain, even at high doses.
   c. Brand-name preparations of ibuprofen are more effective than generic products.
   d. Three 200-mg generic over-the-counter ibuprofen tablets are equivalent to 600 mg prescription strength ibuprofen.

5. A patient is scheduled for a total knee replacement. Preoperative teaching by the nurse should include that the patient should discontinue high-dose aspirin therapy prescribed for joint pain for what period of time before surgery?
   a. One hour
   b. One day
   c. One week
   d. One month

6. A 52-year-old nurse has just read the results of the Women's Health Initiative (WHI) study published in 2005. Based on this research, it would be appropriate for the nurse to discuss which of the following aspirin therapy regimens with her primary care practitioner (PCP)?
   a. 81 mg once a day
   b. 100 mg every other day
   c. 325 mg once a day
   d. 650 mg once every other day

7. Research suggests that long-term low-dose aspirin use has been shown to prevent:
   a. Alzheimer's disease progression.
   b. colon cancer.
   c. hemorrhagic stroke.
   d. myocardial infarction.

▶ 8. To prevent the most common adverse effect of long-term aspirin therapy, the nurse should:
   a. administer the drug with food.
   b. assess lung sounds for wheezing before administering the drug.
   c. monitor urine output.
   d. teach the patient to report tarry colored stool.

9. Which of the following statements, if made by a patient who is receiving aspirin therapy for rheumatoid arthritis, suggests that the patient needs further teaching?
   a. "Drinking a full glass of water with my aspirin can help prevent the pill particles from getting trapped in the inside folds of my stomach."
   b. "I will know if aspirin is causing ulcers because it will cause abdominal pain."
   c. "If I drink alcohol, it can irritate my stomach and make it easier for aspirin to cause it to bleed."
   d. "I should stop taking aspirin and consult with my physician if I experience sudden watery runny nose and chest tightness."

▶ 10. It would be extremely important for the nurse to communicate self-prescribed aspirin use to the primary care provider of which of the following patients? (Select all that apply.)
   a. Abuses cocaine
   b. Admitted with status asthmaticus
   c. Has genetic hypercoagulability disorder
   d. History of hemorrhagic cerebral vascular accident (CVA, stroke)
   e. History of hypertension and diabetes mellitus type 2
   f. Sexually active woman using aspirin for dysmenorrhea and not using any form of birth control
   g. Smokes two packs of cigarettes per day

11. How many regular strength aspirin (325 mg) tablets are equivalent to the lowest dose of aspirin that is known to be potentially fatal?
   a. 12
   b. 16
   c. 20
   d. 24

12. The nurse should instruct patients to dispose of aspirin tablets if they develop an odor that smells like:
   a. ammonia.
   b. alcohol.
   c. vanilla.
   d. vinegar.

▶ 13. A child is brought into the hospital after ingesting an unknown amount of aspirin. It is most important for the nurse to monitor the child for:
   a. bronchospasm.
   b. changes in respiratory rate and depth.
   c. profuse watery nasal discharge.
   d. urticaria (hives).

▶ 14. The nurse notes a respiratory rate of 41 breaths/minute when assessing an 18-month-old child with suspected salicylate poisoning. Which of the following laboratory results support this diagnosis?
   a. pH 7.32; $PaCO_2$ 40mm Hg; $HCO_3^-$ 24 mEq/L
   b. pH 7.35; $PaCO_2$ 37mm Hg; $HCO_3^-$ 22 mEq/L
   c. pH 7.41; $PaCO_2$ 35mm Hg; $HCO_3^-$ 20 mEq/L
   d. pH 7.46; $PaCO_2$ 31mm Hg; $HCO_3^-$ 18 mEq/L

15. A patient has been prescribed aspirin 81 mg once a day after angioplasty. It is important for the nurse to teach this patient to avoid using which of the following over-the-counter (OTC) medications?
   a. acetaminophen (Tylenol)
   b. calcium carbonate (TUMS)
   c. guaifenesin (Robitussin)
   d. ibuprofen (Motrin, Advil)

16. A post-MI patient with a history of diabetes mellitus and hypertension is advised by his primary care provider to take 325 mg aspirin each day for antiplatelet effects. He asks the nurse which preparation would provide the best results for him and not irritate his stomach. The best response is:
   a. buffered aspirin solution.
   b. enteric-coated aspirin.
   c. four chewable children's aspirin.
   d. timed-release aspirin.

17. The daughter of a cardiac patient asks why her father has been instructed to take 1 baby aspirin every day. The basis of the nurse's response should be that low-dose aspirin:
   a. dissolves blood clots.
   b. is less irritating to the stomach.
   c. prevents platelets from sticking together.
   d. relieves chest pain.

18. The nurse instructs a preoperative coronary bypass patient to not take any nonaspirin traditional NSAIDs for 14 days before surgery because these drugs:
    a. cause irreversible inhibition of cyclooxygenase so anticoagulant effects are long lasting.
    b. increase the risk of bleeding during surgery.
    c. increase the risk of developing a blood clot.
    d. increase the risk that the graft will not improve coronary blood flow.

▶ 19. When obtaining a history from a patient, the nurse questions the patient on use of over-the-counter (OTC), herbal, and natural medications. The patient reports regular use of sodium salicylate for joint pain. The nurse would be most concerned about use of this OTC product if the patient has a history of:
    a. chronic obstructive pulmonary disease.
    b. heart failure.
    c. diabetes mellitus.
    d. excessive bleeding with dental procedures.

▶ 20. The nurse is teaching a patient who has just been prescribed over-the-counter (OTC) ibuprofen (Advil, Motrin). Which of the following is a symptom of a minor adverse effect that would not need to be immediately reported to the prescriber?
    a. Black, sticky stool
    b. Chest pain
    c. Frontal headache
    d. Vesicular rash

21. A patient has been prescribed naproxen plus lansoprazole (Prevacid NapraPAC). Teaching regarding administration of this drug has been successful if the patient states:
    a. "I should take 1 naproxen and 1 lansoprazole before breakfast and 1 naproxen 12 hours later."
    b. "I should take 1 naproxen and 1 lansoprazole before breakfast and again 12 hours later."
    c. "I should take 1 lansoprazole before breakfast and 2 naproxen 12 hours later."
    d. "I should take 1 combination pill with naproxen and 1 lansoprazole with breakfast."

22. A hospitalized patient is prescribed diclofenac plus misoprostol (Arthrotec) for knee pain associated with osteoarthritis. He had been taking ibuprofen at home. He asks the nurse how this drug differs from ibuprofen. When describing the misoprostol component of Arthrotec, the nurse explains that this drug prevents GI distress associated with NSAIDS by:
    a. decreasing stomach acid production.
    b. decreasing stomach acid production and promoting gastric mucus production.
    c. preventing gastric reflux and promoting gastric mucus production.
    d. promoting gastric mucus and acid production.

23. The parents of a premature neonate ask the nurse to explain the medications that are prescribed for their baby. The most logical explanation for indomethacin (Indocin) being prescribed for this neonate is to promote closure of the duct between the:
    a. inner ear and cochlea.
    b. liver and the duodenum.
    c. pulmonary artery and the aorta.
    d. umbilical vein and the neonate's abdomen.

24. It is most important for the nurse to know how long a patient has been prescribed:
    a. ketorolac (Toradol).
    b. nabumetone (Relafen).
    c. piroxicam (Feldene).
    d. sulindac (Clinoril).

▶ 25. The nurse works in a large university teaching hospital. A medical resident has prescribed ketorolac (Toradol) 15 mg IM for a woman who is requesting pain relief during labor. The nurse should:
    a. assess the patient's stage of labor and question the order if the patient is in transition.
    b. question administering an intramuscular injection for a woman in labor.
    c. monitor the neonate's respirations for depression after delivery.
    d. withhold the drug and question the prescriber.

▶ 26. The physician prescribes celecoxib (Celebrex) 100 mg twice a day. The nurse would withhold this drug and consult the prescriber if a patient is allergic to:
    a. amoxicillin.
    b. bactrim.
    c. ceftin.
    d. zithromax.

▸ 27. The only pain relief order on admission for a new patient is the routine order of acetaminophen 650 mg every 4 hours as needed. The nurse should consult the prescriber regarding possible prescription of an NSAID if the nurse identified that the patient was experiencing:
a. muscle cramping.
b. stress headache.
c. swollen, painful joints.
d. temperature greater than 102° F.

▸ 28. A patient is prescribed oxycodone-acetaminophen (Percocet) for postoperative pain. Based on the drug containing acetaminophen, it would be most important for the nurse to consult the prescriber before administering the drug if the patient developed:
a. bleeding gums.
b. dyspepsia.
c. jaundice.
d. peripheral edema.

29. Based on the Women's Health Study, the nurse should teach women who take acetaminophen on a regular basis the importance of frequent assessment of their:
a. blood glucose.
b. blood pressure.
c. pulse.
d. serum lipids.

▸ 30. A patient with a known history of chronic obstructive pulmonary disease (COPD) is admitted to an extended-care facility for rehabilitation after an open reduction and internal fixation (ORIF) of a hip fracture. The patient requests acetaminophen 325 mg-oxycodone 5 mg (Percocet) 1 tablet, ordered every 4 hours as needed, before going to physical therapy. The patient states that her pain is 3 of 10 currently, but she experiences unbearable pain if she does not take the Percocet before therapy. The patient has not received a dose of this drug in the last 4 hours. The nurse should:
a. administer the drug.
b. encourage the patient to wait until after therapy to take the drug so that it is longer between doses.
c. withhold the drug and question the prescriber because a patient with liver disease should never take acetaminophen.
d. withhold the drug because the patient's pain does not warrant administration of a narcotic.

▸ 31. The mother of a child calls the pediatrician's office stating that her 15-month-old child just ate an unknown quantity of children's chewable Tylenol tablets while she was busy preparing breakfast. The nurse should:
a. assess for the presence of nausea, vomiting, abdominal pain, or diaphoresis.
b. direct the mother to seek medical care for the child immediately.
c. make an appointment for the child to be seen as soon as possible.
d. take the opportunity to teach the mother about child proofing her home.

▸ 32. Acetylcysteine (Acetadote) 2250 mg intravenous to be infused over 30 minutes is prescribed for a 33-lbs child who drank Tylenol extra strength liquid. The drug is diluted in 200 mL of 5% dextrose. The infusion pump is calibrated in mL/hr. What rate should the nurse enter as the infusion rate?
a. 100 mL
b. 200 mL
c. 300 mL
d. 400 mL

▸ 33. While infusing acetylcysteine (Acetadote) for acetaminophen overdose, the nurse notes that the patient is scratching her arms. The initial response of the nurse should be to:
a. assess respirations, breath sounds, and vital signs.
b. consult the prescriber regarding slowing of the infusion.
c. report the itching to the prescriber.
d. stop the infusion and contact the prescriber STAT.

▸ 34. The pediatric nurse practitioner asks the office nurse to give a parent of a 13-month-old, who has just received an MMR vaccine, a sample of acetaminophen drops (80 mg/0.8 mL) and to explain the age-appropriate dose. The nurse teaches the mother to use the dropper to administer how many mL of the acetaminophen per dose?
a. 0.8 mL
b. 1.2 mL
c. 1.6 mL
d. 2.4 mL

35. A 3-year-old child is brought to the emergency department. Nursing triage assessment reveals a lethargic child who does not resist examination. The child's mother states that he had a runny nose, cough, and fever over a week ago. He vomited several times last night. This morning he was so drowsy that she could not arouse him, so she brought him in to the hospital. It is important for the nurse to ask the mother if she administered which of the following products to her child during his illness?
   a. Robitussin cough syrup
   b. Sudafed decongestant
   c. St. Joseph's baby aspirin
   d. Tylenol elixir

## CASE STUDIES AND PATIENT TEACHING

*(Use a separate piece of paper for your responses.)*

### Case Study 1

*The nurse is assisting an obese 58-year-old science teacher who is postoperative total abdominal hysterectomy and bilateral salpingoophorectomy (TAH-BSO) with ambulating in the hallway when the patient complains of knee pain and stiffness. The patient has a history of hypertension, impaired glucose tolerance, and osteoarthritis (degenerative joint disease, DJD). The patient had been taking the cyclooxygenase-2 (COX-2) enzyme inhibitor rofecoxib (Vioxx) and is upset because the drug has been removed from the market. She tells the nurse that the drug really helped her knee pain and did not cause stomach distress like other nonsteroidal anti-inflammatory (NSAID) drugs. She asks the nurse what the difference is between rofecoxib (Vioxx) and other drugs used for mild-to-moderate pain.*

1. What could the nurse include in her explanation?

2. The patient asks why rofecoxib (Vioxx) was removed from the market. What information can the nurse share with this patient?

3. The patient asks the nurse if this means she should not take celecoxib (Celebrex). How should the nurse respond?

4. The patient says "I am glad there is still one drug that I can take for my arthritis that does not cause side effects." How should the nurse respond?

5. What nonpharmacologic teaching can the nurse provide this patient?

### Case Study 2

*A 21-year-old female comes to the family planning clinic to determine what she can do for relief of moderate dysmenorrhea. She states that the pain is not incapacitating, but creates discomfort during the first day of her menses. She says she does not want anything that makes her sleepy and that she has tried acetaminophen without relief. After further assessment, the nurse practitioner suggests that she try ibuprofen as a beginning drug to see how she responds. She is told to take 2 ibuprofen (200 mg tablets) every 4 hours for the first 2 to 3 days of her menstrual period, starting with the first symptom of menses or cramping.*

1. Why is this schedule appropriate in this situation?

2. What information should be provided to this patient about possible adverse effects of this drug therapy?

3. Based on the developmental stage of this patient, what teaching should the nurse provide about use of ibuprofen and other over-the-counter NSAID drugs?

# 71 Glucocorticoids in Nonendocrine Diseases

## OBJECTIVES

See page 26 for the Objectives.

## CRITICAL THINKING AND STUDY QUESTIONS

1. The most appropriate nursing outcome for a patient who is receiving a glucocorticoid to treat rheumatoid arthritis is the patient will:
   a. be able to participate in desired activities without experiencing fatigue.
   b. be able to participate in desired activities without experiencing inflammation.
   c. be able to participate in desired activities without experiencing unacceptable levels of pain.
   d. have full range of motion of arthritic joints when participating in desired activities.

2. A patient with adrenocortical insufficiency verbalizes concern that she will loose muscle mass, gain weight, get a buffalo hump, and moon face if she takes the prescribed glucocorticoid. The nurse's response should be based on the fact that:
   a. doses to treat adrenocortical insufficiency are similar to amounts produced normally by the body and should not cause these adverse effects.
   b. drug therapy is necessary to sustain life so the patient will have to deal with these adverse effects.
   c. these adverse effects are caused by mineralocorticoids, not glucocorticoids.
   d. these adverse effects can be minimized with proper diet and exercise.

3. A tennis player has received an intraarticular injection of betamethasone for bursitis. The nurse should teach the patient to (that):
   a. not overuse the joint until pain has eased.
   b. limit activity, even if pain has eased.
   c. pain relief will occur within 2 to 3 weeks.
   d. the injection will only provide limited relief. Other anti-inflammatory drugs will be necessary.

4. The nurse should be especially vigilant in assessing for adverse systemic effects of a topical glucocorticoid therapy when administering the preparation: (Select all that apply.)
   a. as a cream.
   b. as an ointment.
   c. to dry cracked skin.
   d. on inflamed skin.
   e. to intertriginous areas.
   f. to mucous membranes.
   g. to well-hydrated skin.
   h. to infants.
   i. under an occlusive barrier.

5. The nurse is working in a primary care practice. An important nursing assessment in this scenario to assess for common adverse effects for patients who are receiving chronic oral glucocorticoid therapy is:
   a. BMI.
   b. height.
   c. pedal pulses.
   d. skin turgor.

6. Which of the following recommended immunizations for a 5-year-old child should not be administered by the nurse if the child is receiving glucocorticoid therapy? (Select all that apply.)
   a. Hepatitis A (Hep A)
   b. Diphtheria, tetanus, and acellular pertussis (DTaP)
   c. Inhaled influenza
   d. Injected influenza
   e. Injected polio vaccine (IPV)
   f. Measles, mumps, and rubella (MMR)
   g. Pneumococcal
   h. Varicella

7. Patients on chronic glucocorticoid therapy may minimize complications by having adequate servings of which of the following in their diet?
   a. Broccoli and cauliflower
   b. Dairy products
   c. Legumes
   d. Whole grains

8. Which of the following are common symptoms of fluid and electrolyte disturbances caused by glucocorticoids with high mineralocorticoid activity?
   a. Anxiety and flushed skin
   b. Hypotension and cool, clammy skin
   c. Muscle weakness and abdominal distention
   d. Tingling around the mouth and fingers

9. Alternate day glucocorticoid therapy is most appropriate for a patient who is:
   a. 9 years old.
   b. 29 years old.
   c. 45 years old.
   d. 65 years old.

10. Matching. Glucocorticoid drug interactions

| | |
|---|---|
| ____ a. Biphosphonates | 1. May need higher dose |
| ____ b. Insulin | 2. Increases potassium loss from drug |
| ____ c. Loop diuretics | 3. Do not develop antibody response |
| ____ d. NSAIDs | 4. Increases risk of GI bleed |
| ____ e. Tetanus toxoid | 5. Prevent osteoporosis |

11. A patient who has been receiving glucocorticoid therapy for 2 months is being tapered off the glucocorticoids. Which of the following symptoms suggest a withdrawal syndrome?
   a. BP 84/47 mm/Hg
   b. Fasting glucose 255 mg/dL
   c. Potassium 3.5 mEq/L
   d. Pulse 55 beats/min

12. A patient is taking dexamethasone for chronic obstructive pulmonary disease (COPD) and digoxin for heart failure (HF). The nurse should assess for: (Select all that apply.)
   a. anorexia.
   b. + Chvostek's sign.
   c. diarrhea.
   d. fever.
   e. flushed skin.
   f. irregular pulse.
   g. muscle weakness.
   h. visual halos.

## CASE STUDIES AND PATIENT TEACHING

*(Use a separate piece of paper for your responses.)*

### Case Study 1

*A 35-year-old female was diagnosed with systemic lupus erythematosus (SLE) 2 years ago and has been in remission for more than 6 months. Lupus is a progressive, relapsing-remitting connective tissue disease. It appears to be an autoimmune process in which abnormal antibodies are produced and then react with the person's own tissue. She is seen today with complaints of joint pain, fever, generalized weakness, and fatigue. She is afraid that she is experiencing an exacerbation. Glucocorticoid therapy is prescribed. The patient is reluctant to take the medication because she has heard that glucocorticoids cause diabetes.*

1. How should the nurse respond?

2. What assessments need to be made when the patient returns to the office for her healthcare visits?

3. The patient has been tapered from glucocorticoid therapy. What should the nurse teach the patient relating to the need for supplemental doses of glucocorticoids during times of stress for a period after the drug is discontinued?

4. Why is it important for the nurse to teach the patient symptoms of the disease that are important to report to the physician?

5. A nursing intervention for patients diagnosed with SLE is to enhance drug therapy. What type of environmental conditions and activities can trigger exacerbations and what realistic interventions can the nurse suggest?

6. The patient states she is planning to get pregnant. What counseling might she require?

## Case Study 2

*A 43-year-old man with severe persistent asthma is admitted with an acute exacerbation. After the crisis is averted, the patient is prescribed dexamethasone sodium succinate 4 mg IV push. The pharmacy sends dexamethasone acetate 16 mg/mL.*

1. How much should the nurse administer?

2. The patient is switched to oral glucocorticoid therapy. Because of the severity of the patient's asthma, the prescriber explains that long-term oral glucocorticoids will probably be necessary in addition to an inhaled glucocorticoid and bronchodilators. What instructions should the nurse provide this patient regarding minimizing the following adverse effects of glucocorticoid therapy?
   a. Adrenal insufficiency
   b. Osteoporosis
   c. Infection: suppresses immune response and phagocytic activity of neutrophils and macrophages
   d. Glucose intolerance
   e. Myopathy
   f. Edema, hypernatremia, and hypokalemia
   g. Mood
   h. Cataracts and glaucoma
   i. Peptic ulcer disease

# 72 Drug Therapy of Rheumatoid Arthritis and Gout

## OBJECTIVES

See page 26 for the Objectives.

## CRITICAL THINKING AND STUDY QUESTIONS

1. When planning the care of a patient with rheumatoid arthritis the nurse considers that this is a:
   a. complication of a joint infection.
   b. disease that primarily affects weight-bearing joints.
   c. reaction of joints to deposit of urate crystals.
   d. systemic inflammatory disorder.

2. The nurse is teaching a patient who has been diagnosed with rheumatoid arthritis. The patient asks why her joints are so painful and stiff. The nurse could include in the explanation that:
   a. an overgrowth of cartilage releases chemicals that damage the bone.
   b. the pain and swelling are due to overuse of the joint.
   c. the swelling and warmth are due to an infection.
   d. your body is producing substances that damage the joint.

3. The nurse is discussing with the patient interventions to protect joints affected by rheumatoid arthritis. The nurse determines that the patient does not understand the effect of activity on rheumatoid arthritis-afflicted joints if the patient states:
   a. "I can use tools that make it easier for me to keep using the joint."
   b. "I need to quit my walking with my co-worker at lunchtime because activity will make my pain worse."
   b. "I should try to alternate activities that involve painful joints with those that rest the joint rather than do the same thing for a long period of time."
   c. "Warm tub baths in the morning will help me get moving with less pain."

4. A housewife who has been recently diagnosed with rheumatoid arthritis tells the nurse that she is concerned about her ability to perform household chores. Referral to which of the following specialist would be most appropriate for developing strategies to allow the patient continue in this role, but protect her joints?
   a. Physical therapist
   b. Occupational therapist

c. Social worker
d. Specialist in vocational rehabilitation

5. Which of the following use of drugs for rheumatoid arthritis (RA) follows current guidelines?
   a. Do not discontinue glucocorticoid therapy once started because this will cause "flares."
   b. If symptoms cannot be controlled by an NSAID, add a DMARD.
   c. Start with a DMARD within 3 months of diagnosis.
   d. Start with an NSAID.

6. A patient has been prescribed methotrexate (DMARD) immediately after being diagnosed with rheumatoid arthritis (RA). The patient has heard that these drugs can be dangerous and asks the nurse why the physician has not ordered a prescription-strength NSAID. The best response by the nurse should include:
   a. methotrexate delays joint degeneration.
   b. methotrexate has less adverse effects than prescription-strength NSAID.
   c. methotrexate works faster than NSAIDS.
   d. prescription-strength NSAIDs can cause peptic ulcers; methotrexate does not.

▶ 7. A patient who is unwilling to take other drugs for his RA has been prescribed aspirin 975 mg (3 tablets) every 6 hours. Which of the following symptoms, if experienced by this patient, suggests aspirin toxicity?
   a. Bruising
   b. Epigastric pain
   c. Jaundice
   d. Ringing in the ears

8. A patient with rheumatoid arthritis (RA) is being treated with oral prednisolone for a flare of RA. Which of the following, if stated by the patient, would suggest to the nurse that this patient needs more teaching?
   a. "If I stop taking this drug suddenly, my body may not be able to deal with infection, healing, and stress."
   b. "It is important to keep active if I need to take this drug because it can make my bones weak."
   c. "I should not stop taking this drug without guidance from my doctor."
   d. "Taking this drug with food will prevent me from having any bad effects."

▶ 9. A 16-year-old female takes methotrexate once a week for juvenile rheumatoid arthritis. Which of the following laboratory test results for this patient would be of most concern to the nurse?
   a. Blood urea nitrogen (BUN) 20 mg/dL
   b. Erythrocyte sedimentation rate (ESR) 30 mm/hr
   c. Urine HCG +
   d. White blood cell count 11,000/mm$^3$

10. When a woman is prescribed hydroxychloroquine for RA, it is important for the nurse to assess the patient's adherence with follow-up care with a/an:
   a. endocrinologist.
   b. gastroenterologist.
   c. gynecologist.
   d. ophthalmologist.

11. Which of these laboratory test results would be most important for the nurse to monitor when a patient is receiving sulfasalazine (Azulfidine) for RA?
   a. CBC
   b. Electrolytes
   c. SMBG
   d. Urine specific gravity

▶ 12. Which of these assessment findings, if identified in a patient who is receiving a DMARD II-biologic agent, should the nurse report to the prescriber immediately?
   a. Dizziness
   b. Fever
   c. Headache
   d. Injection-site erythema

▶ 13. The pediatric office nurse is preparing a referral to a rheumatologist for a child who has juvenile rheumatoid arthritis that has been unresponsive to methotrexate. It would be most important for the nurse to identify whether the child has received which of the following immunizations, if scheduled to be administered in the near future, before the child sees the specialist? (Select all that apply.)
   a. DTaP
   b. IPV
   c. Influenza
   d. Varicella

14. A patient has returned to his PCP office for reading of the PPD tuberculin test administered 50 hours ago before initiation of treatment for RA with adalimumab (Humira). The nurse would document the test results as positive if the skin reaction was greater than:
   a. 5 mm of erythema.
   b. 5 mm of induration.
   c. 5 cm of erythema.
   d. 5 cm of induration.

▶ 15. When performing a nursing assessment on a patient receiving leflunomide (Arava), which of the following observations would be a reason for the nurse to hold the medication and contact the prescriber?
   a. Abdominal pain and dark urine
   b. Alopecia and skin rash
   c. Nausea and diarrhea
   d. Rhinorrhea and sneezing

16. It is most important for the nurse to counsel a male patient who has been receiving which of the following DMARD about the need for a specific procedure to clear the body of the drug before attempting to impregnate his spouse?
   a. adalimumab (Humira)
   b. anakinra (Kineret)
   c. infliximab (Remicade)
   d. leflunomide (Arava)

▶ 17. Because of common adverse effects of gold therapy for RA, the nurse would assess for symptoms suggesting the need for which of the following nursing diagnosis?
   a. Activity intolerance
   b. Excess fluid volume
   c. Fatigue
   d. Impaired oral mucous membrane

18. A hypertensive patient is scheduled for a Prosorba column treatment in combination with plasmapheresis for RA. It would be most important for the nurse to contact the prescriber if the patient had just received which of the following antihypertensive drugs?
   a. doxazosin (Cardura)
   b. hydrochlorothiazide (HydroDIURIL)
   c. quinapril (Accupril)
   d. valsartan (Diovan)

19. A patient who experiences infrequent attacks of gout has been self-treating with over-the-counter (OTC) drugs. Which of the following would the nurse expect to provide the least relief of gout pain?
   a. acetaminophen (Tylenol)
   b. aspirin
   c. ibuprofen (Advil, Motrin)
   d. naproxen (Aleve)

▶ 20. A patient on the Atkins diet develops an acute gouty attack of the left first toe, impairing mobility. He is prescribed colchicine and is able to walk and return to work in 48 hours. The patient's wife calls the physician stating that her husband reported experiencing nausea, abdominal pain, and vomiting. She wants to know what he should do. The nurse should advise the patient to:
   a. stop taking the medication.
   b. take the medication in the evening before going to bed.
   c. take the medication with food.
   d. take the medication with milk.

▶ 21. A male patient has been prescribed allopurinol (Zyloprim) for chronic tophaceous gout. The nurse would be most concerned about which of the following laboratory test results for this patient?
   a. BUN 22 mg/dL
   b. Creatinine 3.8 mg/dL
   c. ESR 28 mm/hr
   d. Uric acid 9 mg/dL

22. The nurse should withhold allopurinol (Zyloprim) if the patient experiences:
   a. diarrhea.
   b. drowsiness.
   c. fever.
   d. headache.

23. An important nursing action to prevent complications when administering drugs, such as probenecid, for gouty arthritis is to:
   a. avoid taking BP or drawing blood from the affected extremity.
   b. increase fluid intake to 2500 to 3000 mL/day.
   c. elevate the affected extremity.
   d. measure intake and output.

24. It is important for the nurse to teach a patient who is prescribed probenecid to increase renal excretion of uric acid to avoid which of the following over-the-counter (OTC) medications?
    a. Aspirin
    b. Docusate
    c. Milk of Magnesia
    d. Naproxen (Aleve)

## CASE STUDIES AND PATIENT TEACHING

*(Use a separate piece of paper for your responses.)*

### Case Study 1

*A 34-year-old single mother who works as a grocery store clerk has been diagnosed with rheumatoid arthritis (RA) after seeking care for carpal tunnel syndrome. The patient asks how she got the disease from carpal tunnel syndrome.*

1. How should the nurse respond?

2. The patient's physician has recommended that she see a vocational rehabilitation counselor. The patient asks the nurse "What type of job should I be thinking about?" What guidance can the nurse provide?

3. When developing a long-range plan of care for this patient, what interventions might the nurse include to address the four goals of RA therapy?
    a. Relieving symptoms
    b. Maintaining joint function
    c. Minimizing systemic joint involvement
    d. Delaying disease progression

4. The rheumatologist has recommended that the patient start a drug regimen including NSAIDs and methotrexate (Rheumatrex). Based on the developmental stage of this patient, what teaching would be especially important for the nurse to provide to this patient?

5. What symptoms of methotrexate toxicity to these organs should the nurse teach the patient to report to her prescriber?
    a. Liver
    b. Kidney
    c. Bone marrow
    d. GI
    e. Lungs

# 73 Drugs Affecting Calcium Levels and Bone Mineralization

## OBJECTIVES

See page 26 for the Objectives.

## CRITICAL THINKING AND STUDY QUESTIONS

▶ 1. A 62-year-old woman is receiving chemotherapy for metastatic breast cancer. Which of the following laboratory results would likely increase the risk that this patient will experience hypercalcemia?
   a. CPK 75 units/mL
   b. Creatinine 3.2 mg/dL
   c. HDL 35 mg/dL
   d. SMBG 145 mg/dL

▶ 2. The plan of nursing care for a patient with bone cancer should include teaching to avoid which of the following foods in the diet?
   a. Bran
   b. Canned sardines
   c. Spinach
   d. Whole-grain cereal

▶ 3. When taking a history from the parents of a 7-year-old who has been diagnosed with rickets, which of the following questions would be most important for the nurse to ask?
   a. "Does the child have any difficulties in school?"
   b. "Has your child ever had a kidney infection?"
   c. "Have you noticed a change in your child's energy level?"
   d. "How many hours a day does the child watch television?"

▶ 4. A priority nursing outcome for an asymptomatic patient with a history of Paget's disease is:
   a. able to work full 8-hour shift without fatigue.
   b. consumes 32 ounces of milk each day.
   c. does not experience a fall.
   d. performs activities of daily living independently.

▶ 5. The nurse is assessing a postoperative thyroidectomy patient. Which of the following assessments suggest that the parathyroid glands may have been damaged or removed during the surgery? (Select all that apply.)
   a. Dorsiflexion of the first toe and fanning of the other toes when the sole of the foot is stroked with a blunt object from lateral heel to medial toes
   b. Inflation of BP cuff for 3 minutes produces involuntary spasms of the wrist
   c. Involuntary flexion of the hips when the neck is flexed
   d. Loss of balance when standing with the eyes closed, arms at sides, and legs together
   e. Resistance to extension of the knee when the hip is flexed
   f. Sharp calf pain with dorsiflexion of the foot
   g. Twitching of facial muscles when the facial nerve is tapped

6. A 58-year-old woman is at risk for osteoporosis caused by a history of hypothyroidism treated with levothyroxine (Synthroid) 0.1 mg every morning. She has been instructed to take supplemental calcium. She is considering taking calcium carbonate (TUMS) with 400 mg of elemental calcium. Which of the following statements, if made by the patient, would indicate a need for further teaching?
   a. "I can take TUMS with food, but it will not be as well absorbed if I take it with bran cereal."
   b. "I should take the TUMS with a large glass of water."
   c. "The calcium will be better absorbed if I take each tablet at separate times throughout the day."
   d. "TUMS are not as good of a source of calcium as oyster shell calcium, but they are less expensive."

7. The pediatric nurse is providing anticipatory guidance for parents of a toddler. During the discussion, the parents question why vitamins need to be kept out of the reach of children. The nurse's explanation includes effects from vitamin D toxicity, which include: (Select all that apply.)
   a. diarrhea.
   b. growth suppression.
   c. hyperactive DTRs.
   d. kidney stones.
   e. loss of calcium from bones.
   f. nausea.
   g. tetany.
   h. vomiting.

8. Calcitonin (Miacalcin):
   a. is usually administered once a week.
   b. is the safest effective drug for osteoporosis in men.
   c. nasal pumps need to be primed before each use.
   d. promotes bone formation.

▸ 9. Which of these outcomes would be most important for a patient who is taking a biphosphonate for Paget's disease?
   a. Decrease in alkaline phosphatase (ALP)
   b. Decrease in aspartate aminotransferase (AST)
   c. Decrease in blood urea nitrogen (BUN)
   d. Decrease in erythrocyte sedimentation rate (ESR)

10. A patient has received information regarding a new prescription for alendronate (Fosamax). Which of the following would suggest understanding of the teaching?
   a. "Fosamax helps my bones build up."
   b. "Fosamax prevents the breakdown of bone."
   c. "Fosamax only works for women."
   d. "I should take Fosamax with food to prevent heartburn."

▸ 11. Which of these assessment findings, if identified in a patient who is receiving a biphosphonate, such as alendronate (Fosamax), should the nurse report to the prescriber immediately?
   a. Dysphagia
   b. Dysphasia
   c. Headache
   d. Muscular pain

12. Monitoring of creatinine clearance, urine output, weight, and intake and output is especially important for the nurse to monitor when a patient is receiving the biphosphonate:
   a. alendronate (Fosamax).
   b. etidronate (Didronel).
   c. tiludronate (Skelid).
   d. zoledronic acid (Zometa).

13. Taking calcium supplements at the same time as a dose of a biphosphonate for osteoporosis:
   a. increases bone building.
   b. interferes with absorption of the biphosphonate.
   c. potentiates the action of the biphosphonate.
   d. prevents adverse effects.

▸ 14. A patient with skeletal metastasis of breast cancer who has been prescribed etidronate (Didronel) has researched the drug on the Internet. She asks the nurse why this drug has been prescribed if its effects are not long lasting and it can weaken bones and increase the risk of experiencing a fracture. The basis of the nurse's response should be:
   a. adverse effects can be minimized by taking the drug with milk.
   b. at the doses prescribed, adverse effects are unlikely.
   c. high levels of blood calcium are more life threatening than the adverse effects of the drug.
   d. the drug is needed to treat her breast cancer.

▸ 15. A patient with hypercalcemia of malignancy (HCM) receives zoledronate (Zometa). Which of the following symptoms, if present, suggest that the patient may be experiencing drug-induced hypomagnesemia?
   a. Anorexia
   b. Dry, sticky mucous membranes
   c. Muscle weakness
   d. Neuromuscular irritability

16. When a patient is prescribed a biphosphonate, which of the following nursing measures would be most effective to prevent the possible adverse effect of osteonecrosis?
   a. Emphasizing the importance of excellent oral hygiene
   b. Taking calcium supplementation with the drug
   c. Teaching the importance of weight-bearing exercise
   d. Teaching the importance of avoiding alcohol and tobacco

17. Raloxifene (Evista), a selective estrogen receptor modulator (SERM):
    a. may damage the eyes so the nurse should teach to report blurring of vision.
    b. may stimulate the occurrence of hot flushes (hot flashes).
    c. reduces the risk of hip, forearm, and vertebral fractures.
    d. should be avoided in women with a history of breast cancer.

▶ 18. Which of the following, elicited from a patient who is receiving raloxifene (Evista), would be most important for the nurse to communicate to the prescriber?
    a. Has an aunt who has been diagnosed with estrogen receptor positive breast cancer
    b. Has had a hysterectomy
    c. Is experiencing hot flashes
    d. Work requires frequent, long airplane trips

▶ 19. Which of the following laboratory test results, if found in a woman who has just been prescribed raloxifene to prevent recurrence of breast cancer, would be of most concern to the nurse at this time?
    a. Calcium 11.1 mg/dL
    b. Hemoglobin (Hb)11.6 g/dL
    c. Hemoglobin $A_{1C}$ ($HbA_{1C}$) 6.8%
    d. Human chorionic gonadotropin (HCG) positive

20. To increase bone mineral density, teriparatide (Forteo) should be administered:
    a. continually.
    b. intermittently.
    c. intravenously.
    d. orally.

21. Which of the following should the nurse perform when scheduled to administer teriparatide (Forteo) to a patient with osteoporosis?
    a. Administer in the deltoid or vastus lateralis muscle with a 1-inch needle.
    b. Administer subcutaneously in the upper arm, alternating arms daily.
    c. Date the injection pen for disposal 28 days after first use.
    d. Remove the pen from refrigeration 20 minutes before administration to allow the solution to warm.

22. Teriparatide (Forteo) administration has a risk of bone cancer. A patient receiving teriparatide complains to the nurse of bone pain. Which of the following could be symptoms of an electrolyte imbalance often seen in bone cancer and should be included in the nurse's assessment of this patient?
    a. Constipation and bloating
    b. Diaphoresis and thirst
    c. Diarrhea and abdominal cramps
    d. Weakness and fatigue

▶ 23. The nurse would withhold cinacalcet (Sensipar) and consult with the prescriber if which of the following were new findings on patient assessment?
    a. Anorexia
    b. Diarrhea
    c. Headache
    d. Numbness

24. Intravenous furosemide has been prescribed for a patient in a hypercalcemic emergency. The nurse knows that which of the following imbalance would be least likely to occur as a result of this therapy?
    a. Hypocalcemia
    b. Hypoglycemia
    c. Hypokalemia
    d. Hyponatremia

## CASE STUDIES AND PATIENT TEACHING

*(Use a separate piece of paper for your responses.)*

### Case Study 1

*A 50-year-old woman, who states that she is going through menopause, is undergoing a thyroidectomy today. The literature states that the nurse should be sure intravenous (IV) calcium is available postoperatively. She has just been admitted to the nursing unit from the postanesthesia care unit (PACU).*

1. Knowing the anatomy of the thyroid gland, why would the nurse anticipate a potential need for IV calcium?

2. What is the average normal value for total serum calcium?

3. The patient's calcium level drops to 6.8 mg/dL. Intravenous 10% calcium gluconate 5 mL via intravenous (push) infusion is prescribed. The nurse's drug book recommends that the drug be infused at a rate of 0.5 to 2 mL/min. If the nurse infuses the solution at 0.6 mL/min, how long will it take to infuse the entire amount?

4. The patient is sitting in a chair when the nurse prepares to administer the calcium gluconate? Why is it important for the nurse to assist the patient back to bed before the drug is administered?

5. What should be monitored while the nurse is administering the calcium gluconate?

6. The patient's husband states that he thought calcium is in the bone. He asks how surgery on the neck can cause an imbalance in the calcium in the body. What could the nurse include in the discussion of the functions of calcium and the mechanism for calcium regulation?

## Case Study 2

*A 58-year-old man has stage III prostate cancer that has metastasized to the bone.*

1. What could the nurse include in the plan of care to address these symptoms of hypercalcemia that this patient is experiencing?
   a. Nausea and vomiting
   b. Constipation
   c. Lethargy and fatigue

## Case Study 3

*The orthopedic office nurse is preparing a 56-year-old woman a visit to review BMD test results after an ulnar and radial fracture occurred when she tripped and fell. DEXA scan results showing BMD 2.5 SD (standard deviations) below the norm are reviewed with the patient. She is diagnosed with osteoporosis and prescribed ibandronate (Boniva) 150 mg once a month.*

1. What information is essential to teach this patient regarding taking ibandronate?

2. The patient asks how it is possible to take a drug once a month to help improve bone density. What should the nurse include in the response?

3. The patient asks about taking calcium supplements. What recommendations can the nurse share?

4. Besides taking calcium supplements for osteoporosis, what other measures to promote bone density should the nurse include in teaching?

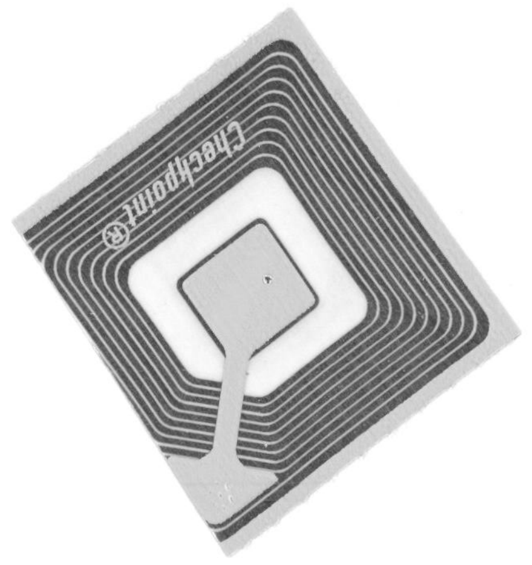

# 74 Drugs for Asthma

## OBJECTIVES

See page 26 for the Objectives.

## CRITICAL THINKING AND STUDY QUESTIONS

1. Which of these outcomes would be most important for a patient who has been diagnosed with asthma?
   a. Avoiding pollution
   b. Increasing exercise tolerance
   c. Preventing airway inflammation
   d. Stimulating release of eosinophils

2. Common triggers of asthmatic bronchospasm include: (Select all that apply.)
   a. airway inflammation.
   b. cold air.
   c. environmental allergens.
   d. exercise.
   e. mast cell degranulation.
   f. pain.
   g. tobacco smoke.
   h. upper respiratory infection.

3. When caring for a patient with asthma, the nurse should be prepared to administer which of the following drugs if an uncontrolled asthmatic episode occurs?
   a. Budesonide
   b. Epinephrine
   c. Terbutaline
   d. Theophylline

4. A patient has received instructions from the nurse regarding administration of 2 puffs of a $beta_2$-agonist drug via a metered-dose inhaler (MDI). Which of the following statements, if made by the patient, would indicate the need for further teaching?
   a. "I need to inhale more slowly if the spacer whistles."
   b. "I need to count the MDI doses that I use so that I know when it is empty."
   c. "I should inhale immediately after activating the inhaler."
   d. "It is best to wait 1 minute before I take the second puff."

▶ 5. A patient with a long history of asthma has developed peripheral muscle weakness after experiencing a cerebral vascular accident. It would be particularly important for the nurse to consult the prescriber of the patient's asthma drugs if the patient is receiving:
   a. flunisolide (AeroBid) MDI.
   b. fluticasone-salmeterol (Advair) DPI.
   c. nebulized levalbuterol (Xopenex).
   d. prednisolone oral tablets.

▶ 6. A hospitalized patient is scheduled to receive budesonide (Pulmicort Turbohaler) and salmeterol (Serevent) 2 puffs every 12 hours. She also has albuterol (Proventil) MDI 2 puffs prescribed every 4 hours as needed, which has not been administered in the last 24 hours. When preparing to administer the 0900 budesonide and salmeterol dose, the nurse notes audible wheezing, and the patient is anxious and short of breath. The patient states that she is having an asthma attack. The nurse should administer the:
   a. albuterol.
   b. albuterol, the salmeterol, and the budesonide.
   c. salmeterol and reassess in 15 minutes for the need for albuterol.
   d. budesonide and reassess in 15 minutes for the need for albuterol.

▶ 7. Which of these conditions, if identified in the history of a patient receiving an inhaled beta agonist for asthma, would be of most concern to the nurse?
   a. Heart failure (HF)
   b. Deep vein thrombosis (DVT)
   c. Gastroesophageal reflux (GERD)
   d. Rheumatoid arthritis (RA)

8. Which of the following statements, if made by an asthmatic patient who is prescribed inhaled beclomethasone (Qvar) would indicate a need for further teaching?
   a. "This inhaler decreases the secretion of mucus in my airways."
   b. "This inhaler helps to prevent bronchospasm."
   c. "This inhaler helps the hairs in my airways move the mucus upward."
   d. "This inhaler prevents swelling in my airway."

▸ 9. A 42-year-old female asthmatic patient who is prescribed budesonide (Pulmicort Turbohaler) and formoterol (Foradil Aerolizer) 2 puffs every 12 hours is admitted for a Roux-en-Y surgical procedure for morbid obesity. Which of the following information obtained in the patient's history is most critical for the nurse to share with the surgeon?
   a. This patient experiences an asthma attack whenever exposed to tobacco smoke.
   b. The patient has degenerative joint disease (osteoarthritis) of the knees.
   c. The patient is lactose intolerant.
   d. The patient was recently changed after long-term oral methylprednisolone to inhaled beclomethasone.

▸ 10. The nurse administers an "as needed" treatment of albuterol via nebulizer when an asthmatic patient experiences severe wheezing throughout the lung fields while attempting to eat lunch. After 1 minute of treatment, the patient is resting quietly with his eyes closed. The nurse should:
   a. allow the patient to rest.
   b. assess the patient's breathing.
   c. inform the dietary department that another lunch will be needed later.
   d. wake the patient and encourage him to try to finish his lunch.

▸ 11. Which of the following would be a reason for the nurse to withhold a prescribed beta$_2$-adrenergic agonist and contact the prescriber?
   a. BP 140/90 mm Hg
   b. SMBG 165 mg/dL
   c. Unexplained fainting
   d. Unexplained tremor

▸ 12. A patient has been prescribed intravenous methylprednisolone and inhaled fluticasone (Flovent) during a severe asthma attack. The prescriber discontinues the intravenous drug on the eighth day. The nurse should:
   a. administer the fluticasone as prescribed and continue nursing care.
   b. consult the prescriber regarding the need for an oral glucocorticoid drug.
   c. consult the prescriber regarding the need for an oral glucocorticoid drug that should have the dose tapered before the drug is discontinued.
   d. consult the prescriber regarding the need to taper the intravenous methylprednisolone before discontinuing the drug.

13. Which of the following drugs contains a component that has been associated with a risk of increased asthma severity and possibly death?
   a. Advair
   b. AeroBid
   c. Intal
   d. Pulmicort

▸ 14. If flunisolide (AeroBid) and pirbuterol (Maxair) are both ordered to be administered at 0900, how should they be administered?
   a. Flunisolide first, then pirbuterol 1 minute later, using a spacer for both drugs
   b. Flunisolide first, using a spacer, then pirbuterol 3 minutes later
   c. Pirbuterol first, then flunisolide 5 minutes later, using a spacer for both drugs
   d. Pirbuterol first, using a spacer, then flunisolide 10 minutes later

15. The nurse is explaining therapy with cromolyn (Intal) to an asthmatic patient. Which of the following would not need to be included in the teaching?
   a. Cromolyn must be taken on a regular basis to control inflammation.
   b. Rinse the mouth immediately after administration to remove the unpleasant taste.
   c. Timing of doses 15 minutes before activities involving exertion or exposure to known allergens may prevent bronchospasm.
   d. The drug is not effective to stop an episode once it has begun.

16. The nurse is caring for a patient who has a history of chronic stable asthma treated with long-acting oral theophylline. Which of the following serum levels of the drug would be considered safe and therapeutic?
   a. 2 mcg/mL
   b. 4 mcg/mL
   c. 7 mcg/mL
   d. 12 mcg/mL

▶ 17. Which of these assessment findings would be most significant if a patient who is receiving theophylline for asthma and is prescribed phenytoin for new onset seizures?
a. Diarrhea
b. Difficulty falling asleep
c. Restlessness
d. Wheezing

▶ 18. Which of these findings, if identified in a patient who has been prescribed ipratropium-albuterol (Combivent), should the nurse report to the prescriber immediately?
a. Allergy to peanuts
b. Complaint of sore throat
c. Consumes 4 to 6 cups of coffee per day
d. Smokes two packs of cigarettes per day

19. Which of the following adverse effects would the nurse expect a patient to experience when prescribed the anticholinergic bronchodilator drug tiotropium (Spiriva)?
a. Blurred vision
b. Constipation
c. Dry mouth
d. Urinary retention

20. The nurse should include in teaching about administration of tiotropium (Spiriva):
a. swallow whole with a full glass of water.
b. do not use as a rescue inhaler.
c. take 15 minutes before activities involving exertion or exposure to known allergens.
d. use of a spacer increases the amount of drug delivered to the lungs and decreases the amount deposited in the throat.

▶ 21. When a patient is receiving propranolol (Inderal), warfarin (Coumadin), and zileuton, (Zyflo), the nurse should assess for which possible symptoms of drug interactions among these drugs?
a. Deep vein thrombosis
b. Hypertension
c. Oliguria
d. Tachycardia

▶ 22. The nurse is caring for an asthmatic patient who is receiving zafirlukast (Accolate) and who complains of abdominal pain. Which of the following laboratory test results should the nurse review?
a. ALT
b. BUN
c. CBC
d. ESR

23. The nurse would be most concerned about drug interactions if an asthmatic patient was prescribed both zileuton (Zyflo) and:
a. albuterol.
b. prednisolone.
c. terbutaline.
d. theophylline.

▶ 24. Zafirlukast (Accolate) is scheduled to be administered at 7:00 AM (0700). Breakfast is served at 8:30 AM (0830). The nurse should:
a. administer the drug as ordered.
b. change the timing of the drug to 8:30 AM (0830).
c. change the timing of the drug to 10:00 AM (1000).
d. consult the prescriber.

25. A patient assesses his morning peak expiratory flow rate as 60% of his personal best. Current treatment recommendations state that he should:
a. continue regularly prescribed treatment.
b. use his rescue inhaler and continue his regularly prescribed treatment.
c. use his rescue inhaler and seek medical attention.
d. seek immediate emergency medical attention.

▶ 26. A child with moderate asthma is distressed because he has just learned that he is allergic to the family dog. Which of the following interventions would most effectively address the physical and psychosocial needs of the child?
a. Advise the family that there are no interventions that will help.
b. Advise the family to increase the dose of the child's asthma drugs when the dog is around.
c. Advise the family to take the dog to the local shelter.
d. Advise the family to train the dog to stay out of bedrooms and off of furniture.

## CASE STUDIES AND PATIENT TEACHING

*(Use a separate piece of paper for your responses.)*

### Case Study 1

*A 7-year-old boy, who was first diagnosed with asthma at 4 years of age, has been admitted to a medical unit from intensive care after experiencing status asthmaticus. Based on the frequency, characteristics, and severity of his symptoms, he is currently classified as having severe persistent asthma. The pediatrician has ordered oral prednisolone 10 mg every 8 hours, budesonide (Pulmicort respules) 0.2 mg and albuterol 1.25 mg via nebulizer every 6 hours as needed.*

1. What is the difference between administering budesonide and albuterol via nebulizer?

2. The budesonide is available as 250 mcg/2 mL. How much budesonide should be administered via nebulizer at each dose?

3. The boy's mother tells the nurse that she does not like steroids and is concerned about her son receiving them. What does the nurse need to teach regarding the importance of steroid therapy for this child?

4. The mother has heard that steroids prevent growth. What information can the nurse provide about the effects of steroids on growth?

5. What teaching does the nurse need to provide about the inhaled steroid therapy to prevent adverse effects?

6. The nebulizer is more time consuming to use than dry-powder inhalers (DPI) and metered-dose inhalers (MDI). What are possible reasons why this route was prescribed for this child?

7. Allergy work-up identified that this child was allergic to house dust mites. What teaching should be provided regarding exposure to allergens?

8. After 2 years of standard allergy treatment, the child is still experiencing asthma attacks 2 to 3 times a week, and he is missing many days of school. The allergist has prescribed omalizumab (Xolair) 200 mg to be administered subcutaneously every 4 weeks. What is the procedure for administering this drug?

### Case Study 2

*An 18-year-old college freshman has had asthma since she was 5 years old. During the past year, she has had occasional asthma attacks and used an albuterol (Ventolin) inhaler 2 to 4 times a week on an as needed (PRN) basis. As she tries to make the adjustment to college life and participate in all the various activities, her attacks begin to occur more frequently, and she has had to use her albuterol inhaler once or twice a day. She comes to the student health center for management of her asthma.*

1. What information would be helpful for the nurse to obtain before the student is seen by the CRNP?

2. The CRNP prescribes cromolyn (Intal) 3 puffs, 10 minutes apart, 3 times a day and montelukast (Singulair) 10 mg by mouth once a day. She is instructed that she may use her albuterol inhaler 2 puffs, every 4 hours as needed if asthma symptoms are present. The patient questions why cromolyn has been prescribed. What should the nurse include in the explanation?

3. The patient returns to the health center for follow-up care. She is still using her albuterol inhaler several times a day and is discouraged that her asthma is still "out of control." She provides a record of when she has been in the yellow zone and today was in the red zone. The CRNP discontinues the cromolyn and montelukast and prescribes fluticasone (Flovent HA) and formoterol (Foradil) 2 puffs each every 12 hours as her regular medication regimen in addition to the PRN albuterol. The student asks the college health nurse what the difference is between the formoterol and albuterol if they are both bronchodilators. How should the nurse respond?

4. What teaching should the nurse provide about administration of the prescribed drugs?

5. The nurse knows that many college students study before examinations for long periods at a time. Colas, coffee, and over-the-counter (OTC) drugs containing caffeine are commonly used to prevent drowsiness. How should the nurse use this knowledge?

### Case Study 3

*A patient has been prescribed high-dose oral prednisone every other day for severe persistent asthma. Every-other-day dosing increases the risk of medication errors.*

1. Why has this dosing schedule been prescribed?

2. What care should the nurse provide including prevention of adverse effects and when to notify the prescriber?

# 75 Drugs for Allergic Rhinitis, Cough, and Colds

## OBJECTIVES

See page 26 for the Objectives.

## CRITICAL THINKING AND STUDY QUESTIONS

1. A patient exhibits allergic rhinitis symptoms every winter when the house is closed and the forced-air furnace is running. This is classified as:
   a. perennial rhinitis.
   b. seasonal rhinitis.

2. Allergic rhinitis involves the release of: (Select all that apply.)
   a. epinephrine.
   b. glucocorticoids.
   c. immunoglobulins.
   d. histamine.
   e. leukocytes.
   f. leukotrienes.
   g. prostaglandins.

3. The nurse teaches a patient with allergic rhinitis that antihistamines are not effective in reducing the symptom of:
   a. nasal congestion.
   b. nasal itching.
   c. rhinorrhea.
   d. sneezing.

4. A patient has received instructions regarding administration of a second-generation oral antihistamine for seasonal allergic rhinitis. Which of these statements made by the client would indicate the patient needs further teaching?
   a. "I should only use the medication when I am experiencing symptoms."
   b. "I should take the medication as prescribed throughout the season when I have allergy symptoms."
   c. "This drug can still cause sedation, so I need to be careful when driving."
   d. "This drug is not any more effective than over-the-counter antihistamines."

5. The most effective drugs for prevention and treatment of symptoms of seasonal and perennial rhinitis are:
   a. first-generation oral antihistamines.
   b. intranasal corticosteroids.
   c. oral glucocorticoids.
   d. second-generation oral antihistamines.

▸ 6. The school office nurse notes that a child is receiving chronic therapy with intranasal glucocorticoids for seasonal rhinitis. It is important for this nurse to monitor the child's:
   a. blood sugar.
   b. hearing.
   c. height.
   d. weight.

▸ 7. Which of these assessment findings, if identified in a patient who is taking an oral decongestant should the nurse report to the prescriber immediately?
   a. Agitation
   b. Chest pain
   c. Epistaxis
   d. Sore throat

▸ 8. In which of the following situations would it be most beneficial for the nurse to administer an as needed dose of an antitussive medication?
   a. Barking cough of croup
   b. Cough that interferes with work because patient cannot carry tissues at work in which to expectorate the mucus
   c. Cough that is associated with upper respiratory infection and keeps the patient awake at night
   d. Severe episodes of coughing with sputum production that only occurs on arising

9. Research suggests that codeine, dextromethorphan, and diphenhydramine are not effective in suppressing coughs induced by:
   a. chemical irritation.
   b. common cold.
   c. mechanical irritation.
   d. smoking.

10. Matching

| | |
|---|---|
| ___ a. Acetylcysteine | 1. Acts in CNS but lacks potential for abuse |
| ___ b. Benzonatate | 2. Decreases sensitivity of cough-reflex pathway |
| ___ c. Dextromethorphan | 3. Potentiates action of opiate analgesics |
| ___ d. Diphenhydramine | 4. Smells like rotten eggs |
| ___ e. Guaifenesin | 5. Suppresses cough at doses that cause sedation |
| ___ f. Hydrocodone | 6. Toxicity can be reversed by naloxone |

11. A patient has received instructions regarding administration of benzonatate (Tessalon Pearls). Which of these statements made by the client would indicate the patient needs further teaching?
   a. "The drug should not be given to infants."
   b. "I can take the drug three times a day."
   c. "I need to be careful because the drug may make me drowsy."
   d. "I should crush the beads and mix them in a soft food such as applesauce."

12. Which statements are true about the common cold? (Select all that apply.)
   a. Antibiotics are not effective.
   b. Antihistamines do not help.
   c. It is best treated with multiple symptom medications.
   d. Fever usually means there is a bacterial infection.
   e. Zinc lozenges are not beneficial.

## CASE STUDIES AND PATIENT TEACHING

*(Use a separate piece of paper for your responses.)*

### Case Study 1

*A 19-year-old college student presents to the student health clinic during spring semester with complaints of runny and itchy nose, sneezing, and nasal congestion. He is diagnosed with allergic rhinitis. The student states that he has been using an over-the-counter nasal spray for 2 weeks. It really helps but the congestion comes back and seems to be getting worse.*

1. Explain what is happening and how he can discontinue use of this drug.

2. The nurse practitioner prescribes loratadine (Claritin) 10 mg daily and triamcinolone (Nasacort) 2 sprays twice a day. What teaching can the nurse provide?

3. If he develops a common cold, how should he change his medications?

# 76 Drugs for Peptic Ulcer Disease

## OBJECTIVES

See page 26 for the Objectives.

## CRITICAL THINKING AND STUDY QUESTIONS

1. Matching: Mechanism of action

| |  | |  |
|---|---|---|---|
| _____ | a. Aluminum hydroxide | | 1. Selectively blocks muscarinic receptors for gastric acid secretion |
| _____ | b. Bismuth (Pepto Bismol) | | 2. Neutralizes stomach acid |
| _____ | c. Clarithromycin (Biaxin) | | 3. Prostaglandin replacement |
| _____ | d. Cimetidine (Tagamet) | | 4. Creates a protective barrier against acid and pepsin |
| _____ | e. Misoprostol (Cytotec) | | 5. Topically disrupts and may prevent *H. pylori* from adhering to gastric wall |
| _____ | f. Omeprazole (Prilosec) | | 6. Suppresses acid secretion by inhibiting $H^+$ $K^+$-ATPase in parietal cells |
| _____ | g. Pirenzepine (Gastrozepine) | | 7. Antibiotic eradicates *H. pylori* |
| _____ | h. Sucralfate (Carafate) | | 8. Blocks histamine$_2$ receptors ($H_2RA$), decreasing amount and acidity of gastric secretions |

2. Hypersecretion of gastric acid is the etiology of:
   a. duodenal ulcers.
   b. gastric ulcers.
   c. peptic ulcers.
   d. Zollinger-Ellison syndrome ulcers.

3. Drug therapy that prevents recurrence of peptic ulcers associated with *H. pylori* must include:
   a. antacids.
   b. antibiotics.
   c. antisecretory agents.
   d. mucosal protectants.

4. Which of the following dietary alterations may promote ulcer healing?
   a. Avoiding caffeine intake
   b. Eating only bland foods
   c. Six small meals a day
   d. Frequent intake of milk

5. A patient with GERD who has difficulty following drug regimes with multiple doses has been prescribed cimetidine (Tagamet) 800 mg once a day at bedtime. The patient complains that the medication effects wear off before taking the next dose. To prolong the beneficial effects of the drug, the nurse instructs the patient to take the medication:
   a. twice a day.
   b. with food.
   c. on an empty stomach.
   d. with an antacid.

▶ 6. Cimetidine (Tagamet) inhibits the CYP2D6 and CYP3A4 hepatic enzymes. The nurse must be particularly cautious for toxic effects of which of the following drugs that are metabolized by these enzymes when administered with cimetidine because of their narrow margin of safety? (Select all that apply.)
   a. Chlorpheniramine (ChlorTrimeton)-antihistamine
   b. Finasteride (Proscar)-BPH
   c. Nateglinide (Starlix)-diabetes
   d. Phenytoin (Dilantin)-seizures
   e. Prednisone (Deltasone)-anti-inflammatory
   f. Theophylline-asthma
   g. Warfarin (Coumadin)-anticoagulant

7. The generic name of histamine$_2$ receptor antagonists ($H_2RA$) share the common suffix:
   a. (-azole). c. (-dine).
   b. (-lol). d. (-sartan).

8. A patient with Zollinger-Ellison syndrome asks why he was prescribed ranitidine (Zantac). His wife takes cimetidine (Tagamet) for GERD, and it would be easier if they both take the same drug. The nurse will base the response on the fact that: (Select all that apply.)
   a. ranitidine only needs to be taken as needed.
   b. Zollinger-Ellison syndrome requires a more potent acid reducer than cimetidine.
   c. long-term therapy with an acid reducer will be needed, and ranitidine has less adverse effects than cimetidine.
   d. ranitidine is less expensive than cimetidine.
   e. compliance wit drug therapy is important with Zollinger-Ellison syndrome, and ranitidine only needs to be taken once a day.

9. The generic name of proton pump inhibitors share the common suffix:
   a. (-azole). c. (-dine).
   b. (-lol). d. (-sartan).

▶ 10. A patient had been receiving omeprazole (Prilosec) for GERD. The patient recently had a PEG tube inserted, and the pharmacy substituted omeprazole (Zegerid) immediate release oral suspension because Prilosec capsules cannot be crushed. Because of differences between Prilosec and Zegerid, which of the following concurrent diagnoses would be a reason for consulting the prescriber? (Select all that apply.)
   a. COPD
   b. HF
   c. DM
   d. Grave's disease
   e. Hyperthyroidism
   f. Uncontrolled hypertension

▶ 11. It is important for the nurse to assess for what adverse effect related to the fact that all drugs that elevate the gastric pH provide an environment favorable bacterial colonization in a secondary site is:
   a. headache.
   b. neutropenia.
   c. pruritis.
   d. rales (crackles).

12. Matching: Administration of oral PPIs

| | |
|---|---|
| ___ a. Immediately before a meal | 1. esomeprazole (Nexium) |
| ___ b. With or without food | 2. lansoprazole (Prevacid) |
| ___ c. At least 1 hour before a meal | 3. rabeprazole (Aciphex) |
| | 4. pantoprazole (Protonix) |

13. The nurse is preparing to administer lansoprazole (Prevacid) IV. Administration directives include that it: (Select all that apply.)
   a. may be diluted in normal saline.
   b. may be diluted in lactated Ringer's solution.
   c. may be diluted in 5% dextrose in water.
   d. infuse over 15 minutes.
   e. must use an inline filter.

▶ 14. Which of the following laboratory results would be a reason for the nurse to consult the prescriber regarding administration of rabeprazole (Aciphex)? (Select all that apply.)

| | |
|---|---|
| a. ALT/SGPT | 350 U/L |
| b. Blood urea nitrogen (BUN) | 15 mg/dL |
| c. Creatinine | 1.0 mg/dL |
| d. Digoxin | 2.5 ng/mL |
| e. Lithium | 1.0 mEq/L |

15. A patient states she cannot swallow the esomeprazole (Nexium) capsule. An acceptable way to administer the medication to this patient is to:
   a. open the capsule and dissolve the contents in water.
   b. soak the capsule in water to dissolve the contents.
   c. open the capsule and crush the contents and mix them with applesauce.
   d. open the capsule and sprinkle on a tablespoon of applesauce and have the patient swallow the applesauce and medication beads immediately without chewing.

16. A patient who has recently been prescribed omeprazole (Prilosec) asks why he has been told to stop taking sucralfate (Carafate). The nurses response is based on:
    a. the two drugs are not necessary.
    b. the sucralfate prevents the absorption of the omeprazole.
    c. the adherent coating of sucralfate requires a gastric pH of less than 4.
    d. both drugs are metabolized by the CYP 450 cytochrome system.

▶ 17. A 48-year-old woman has been taking an NSAID for rheumatoid arthritis and an oral contraceptive. She was just prescribed misoprostol (Cytotec) because of GI distress relating to NSAID use. She informs the nurse that she has stopped taking her oral contraceptives because she has not had a period for 2 months and thinks she could be in menopause. The nurse should:
    a. administer all the medications as ordered.
    b. administer the NSAID and misoprostol (Cytotec), hold the oral contraceptive, and inform the prescriber.
    c. administer all the medications as ordered and inform the prescriber that the patient has not been taking the oral contraceptives.
    d. hold the medications and consult the prescriber regarding a pregnancy test.

18. Antacids for peptic ulcer disease should be administered:
    a. half an hour before meals and bedtime (four times a day).
    b. one hour before and 7 hours after meals and at bedtime (seven times a day).
    c. as soon as symptoms occur.
    d. as infrequently as possible.

19. Matching: Antacids (multiple answers)

___ a. Rapid acting
___ b. High acid neutralizing capacity
___ c. Adverse effect of diarrhea
___ d. Adverse effect of constipation
___ e. Adverse effect belching and flatus
___ f. May increase edema
___ g. May increase blood pH (alkalosis)
___ h. Associated with rebound of symptoms
___ i. Associated with milk alkali syndrome
___ j. Stop if undiagnosed abdominal pain occurs
___ k. Long duration
___ l. Caution in renal impairment
___ m. Binds phosphate, warfarin, and digoxin decreasing absorption

1. Aluminum hydroxide
2. Calcium carbonate
3. Magnesium hydroxide
4. Sodium bicarbonate

▶ 20. A patient with a history of chronic renal failure presents in the ED with a decreased level of consciousness. When taking the medication history from the family it is most important to assess for use of over-the-counter:
    a. Amphogel (aluminum hydroxide).
    b. baking soda (sodium bicarbonate).
    c. Mylanta (magnesium hydroxide).
    d. TUMS (calcium carbonate).

## CASE STUDIES AND PATIENT TEACHING

*(Use a separate piece of paper for your responses.)*

### Case Study 1

*A 47-year-old female with a history of obesity, type 2 DM, and hypertension is seen by her primary care practitioner (PCP) with the complaint of midepigastric pain, especially at night. The pain radiates to the back and is relieved by antacids, but returns within an hour. The pain is worse when bending forward and better after eating. The PCP wants to rule out peptic ulcer disease (PUD). A urea breath test and gastroesophogeal-duodenoscopy are ordered. The patient asks the nurse how breathing into a bag can test for the presence of bacteria in the stomach.*

1. Describe how the nurse explains this test.

2. Test results indicate a duodenal ulcer and the presence of *H. pylori*. What are the goals of drug therapy for PUD?

3. Initial therapy includes cimetidine intravenous infusion. The nurse is preparing to administer an IV bolus of 300 mg of cimetidine. What assessments, actions, and teaching should the nurse perform when administering this medication?

4. The cimetidine intravenous infusion is diluted in 100 mL of normal saline solution and is to be administered over 15 minutes. The intravenous tubing has a drip factor of 10 drops/mL. What is the drip rate per 15 seconds?

5. Assessment findings of the patient on the second day include severe pain and a rigid abdomen. What should the nurse do and why?

6. The patient is prescribed drug therapy, including bismuth subsalicylate, metronidazole, tetracycline, and famotidine for peptic ulcer disease (PUD) associated with *H. pylori*. The patient reveals to the nurse that she does not like taking medications. The nurse should explain that a priority reason for why it is important for the patient to take the therapy as prescribed is because if the drugs are used alone the:
   a. risk of developing resistance is increased.
   b. incidence of adverse effects is higher.
   c. dose of the individual drug must be increased.
   d. patient may experience nausea and diarrhea.

7. What teaching should the nurse provide relating to therapy with metronidazole?

8. The patient asks why she is not on a special diet. He has heard that ulcer patients should eat bland foods and drink a lot of milk. How should the nurse respond?

## Case Study 2

*A 47-year-old construction worker with a history of osteoarthritis has recently been experiencing GI distress attributed to use of NSAID for joint pain. Eating small frequent meals has helped, but not relieved, the GI distress. The patient asks how his arthritis medication can cause stomach distress.*

1. Describe the nurse's response.

2. Ranitidine (Zantac), a histamine$_2$ receptor antagonist ($H_2RA$), is prescribed. Based on the patient's need to take medications for his chronic conditions, his developmental level, describe why ranitidine is a better choice than cimetidine (Tagamet) for this patient.

3. Why is this patient at risk for accumulation of ranitidine and what laboratory tests should be monitored?

# 77 Laxatives

## OBJECTIVES

See page 26 for the Objectives.

## CRITICAL THINKING AND STUDY QUESTIONS

1. When clarifying a patient's complaint of constipation, it is most important for the nurse to obtain data regarding the:
   a. amount of stool.
   b. color of stool.
   c. consistency of stool.
   d. frequency of stool.

▶ 2. Which of the following conditions, if present, would warrant the nurse not administering a stimulant laxative and consulting with the prescriber?
   a. Aneurysm
   b. Anorectal lesions
   c. Appendicitis
   d. Cerebral vascular accident
   e. Diverticulitis
   f. Fecal impaction
   g. Myocardial infarction
   h. Parasitic infestation of the bowel
   i. Regional enteritis

3. Matching: Major types of laxative and mechanism of action.

| | |
|---|---|
| ___ a. Bulk forming | 1. Increase water and electrolyte secretion and decrease their reabsorption. |
| ___ b. Osmotic | 2. Facilitate penetration of feces by water. |
| ___ c. Stimulant | 3. Promote peristalsis by enlarging and softening fecal mass. |
| ___ d. Surfactant | 4. Retain water in amount that stimulates peristalsis. |

4. The nurse teaches a patient that the best source of fiber to promote proper colon functioning is:
   a. dietary bran.
   b. methylcellulose.
   c. psyllium.
   d. vegetable fiber.

5. A student nurse is sharing research on laxatives. Which of the following statements would indicate a need for further study?
   a. "Agents that produce a semiliquid stool are most commonly abused."
   b. "Bulk-forming agents can cause constipation if inadequate water is ingested."
   c. "Cathartics are useful as bowel preparations for colon procedures."
   d. "Laxatives that produce results in 6 to 12 hours are best for treating constipation."

▶ 6. The nurse is caring for a 45-year-old woman who is receiving antibiotic therapy. The patient regularly takes a fiber laxative twice a day. Which of the following assessment findings would be of the most concern?
   a. Bubbling sounds throughout the abdomen and dull sound with percussion of LLQ
   b. Gurgling bowel sounds throughout abdomen and one soft, liquid stool
   c. High pitched tinkling bowel sounds in RLQ and absent bowel sounds in other quadrants
   d. Soft bowel sounds throughout the abdomen occurring every 1 to 2 minutes in all quadrants on awakening

7. The most important teaching the nurse should provide regarding bulk-forming laxatives is:
   a. never take more than once a day.
   b. take with 8 ounces of water or juice.
   c. the fiber increases bulk, but has no effect on peristalsis.
   d. they are contraindicated if a patient is diagnosed with irritable bowel syndrome.

8. Directions for administration of bisacodyl tablets include:
   a. best response occurs if taken with a meal.
   b. chew the tablets for maximum effect.
   c. do not take antacids within 1 hour of this laxative.
   d. take with a full glass of milk.

▶ 9. It is important for the nurse to assess a patient who regularly uses milk of magnesia as a laxative for:
   a. hypertension and rapid, bounding pulse.
   b. paresthesias around mouth and fingers and toes.
   c. tremors, twitching, hyperactive DTR.
   d. weakness, diminished bowel sounds, bradycardia.

▶ 10. The nurse is administering lactulose 30 mL to a patient with hepatic encephalopathy. Which of these outcomes should receive priority as the nurse plans care with this patient?
   a. Ammonia 110 mcg/dL
   b. ALT 35 International Units/L
   c. One soft, formed stool within 24 hours
   d. Relief of constipation

11. A patient has been using mineral oil daily as a laxative. The nurse should assess for symptoms of deficiency of which vitamins? (Select all that apply.)
   a. A
   b. B
   c. C
   d. D
   e. E
   f. K

12. Polyethylene glycol-electrolyte solutions (GoLYTELY) can be safely used in patients with: (Select all that apply.)
   a. appendicitis.
   b. bowel obstruction.
   c. cardiovascular disease.
   d. dehydration.
   e. diabetes mellitus.
   f. fecal impaction.
   g. renal impairment.
   h. surgical abdomen.

▶ 13. A healthy pregnant patient complains of chronic constipation. Which of the following would be the best initial intervention?
   a. Bulk-forming laxative daily and increase fiber and fluid in diet
   b. Moderate exercise after meals and increase fiber and fluid in diet
   c. Stool softener and increase fiber and fluid in diet
   d. Stool softener and moderate exercise after meals

▶ 14. Which of the following laboratory results would be a reason to not administer milk of magnesia prescribed for constipation and to consult with the prescriber?
   a. Blood urea nitrogen (BUN) 10 mg/dL
   b. Creatinine 2.2 mg/dL
   c. Fasting glucose 135 mg/dL
   d. Sodium 146 mEq/L

## CASE STUDIES AND PATIENT TEACHING

*(Use a separate piece of paper for your responses.)*

### Case Study 1

*During a routine physical exam, the office nurse discovers that a 78-year-old widow who lives alone uses several over-the-counter (OTC) laxatives every day o have a daily bowel movement. She has a history of hypertension and heart failure.*

1. What additional information does the nurse need to know about this patient before she can address the problem of laxative overuse?

2. Further data collection reveals that this patient describes her daily bowel movement as light brown, mushy, and with some watery discharge. This patient is at risk for which fluid and electrolyte problems and symptoms?

3. What lifestyle changes are appropriate to help establish an acceptable bowel pattern for this patient?

4. What problems does this patient's medical history present when trying to address normalizing bowel patterns and laxative use for this patient?

5. Which of the following laxatives might be used to assist this patient with reestablishing normal bowel functioning when discontinuing her chronic laxative use?
   a. Castor oil
   b. Glycerin suppository
   c. Lactulose
   d. Mineral oil

6. What laxatives are contraindicated for this patient?

# 78 Other Gastrointestinal Drugs

## OBJECTIVES

See page 26 for the Objectives.

## CRITICAL THINKING AND STUDY QUESTIONS

▸ 1. The nurse has medicated a postoperative patient with ondansetron (Zofran) for vomiting. The drug has not relieved the patient's vomiting at 1 hour after administration. An important action for the nurse is to assess for:
   a. elevated temperature.
   b. hypertension.
   c. pain.
   d. purulent drainage.

▸ 2. Ondansetron (Zofran) 15 mg intravenous push is prescribed to be administered 15 minutes before, 4 hours after, and 8 hours after chemotherapy for a patient who weighs 143 lbs. The nurse should:
   a. administer the drug over 15 minutes.
   b. administer 7.5 mL of a 2mg/mL solution for injection.
   c. consult with the prescriber regarding the dose.
   d. premedicate the patient with acetaminophen to prevent headache.

3. A 38-year-old woman who is receiving chemotherapy for breast cancer has been using oral contraceptives (OC) for birth control. It would be particularly important for the nurse to discuss the need for alternative forms of birth control if the patient is receiving which of the following drugs to prevent chemotherapy-induced nausea and vomiting (CINV)?
   a. aprepitant (Emend)
   b. granisetron (Kytril)
   c. haloperidol (Haldol)
   d. metoclopramide (Reglan)

▸ 4. A patient with metastatic ovarian cancer has been receiving intravenous ondansetron (Zofran) 30 minutes before beginning infusion of cisplatin. The patient reports that she has been experiencing vomiting starting the day after chemotherapy that persists for 1 to 2 days. The nurse should:
   a. administer the ondansetron (Zofran) after chemotherapy.
   b. administer palonosetron (Aloxil) instead of ondansetron (Zofran) because of its prolonged action.
   c. consult the prescriber.
   d. recheck the dose calculation to ensure that the patient is receiving the correct dose per body weight.

5. The nurse needs to be especially vigilant in assessing for therapeutic effect and toxicity of drugs metabolized by the CYP3A4 and CYP2D6 hepatic enzymes when administering:
   a. aprepitant (Emend).
   b. granisetron (Kytril).
   c. haloperidol (Haldol).
   d. metoclopramide (Reglan).

▸ 6. The nurse is developing a plan of care to address adverse effects for a patient who receives aprepitant (Emend), ondresetron (Zofran), and dexamethasone to prevent CINV. Interventions should be planned to address:
   a. activity intolerance.
   b. constipation.
   c. ineffective management of therapeutic regime.
   d. sleep pattern disturbance.

▸ 7. A postoperative patient who is prescribed intravenous prochlorperazine (Compazine) as necessary for nausea and vomiting. After being transferred from the bed to a chair with the

assistance of three persons, the patient vomits and requests the medication. The nurse should: (Select all that apply.)
a. administer the medication while the patient is sitting in the chair.
b. assess vital signs before and after administration.
c. hold the medication if the patient is hypertensive.
d. incorporate safety precautions after medication administration.
e. transfer the patient back to the bed before administering the medication.

▶ 8. It is critical that the nurse instructs a patient who is receiving droperidol (Inapsine) or cisapride (Propulsid) to report:
a. headache.
b. dizziness when changing positions.
c. drowsiness.
d. sudden, unexplained fainting.

▶ 9. The triage nurse in the emergency department receives an 18-month-old child who is believed to have ingested an unknown quantity of diphenoxylate (Lomotil). An assessment finding that suggests an overdose has been taken is:
a. blood pressure 80/46 mm Hg.
b. pulse 120 beats/min.
c. respirations 16 per minute.
d. temperature 100° F (37.8° C).

10. A patient with severe pain during IBS episodes is prescribed amitriptyline (Elavil). She asks the nurse why she is prescribed this medication if she is not depressed. The nurse's response is based on the fact that:
a. action of this drug is not because of its antidepressant action
b. if the drug works, the patient is depressed but does not recognize this.
c. the drug reduces the patient's response to stress.
d. TCA also work as an antispasmodic.

11. A patient is prescribed alosetron (Lotronex) 1 mg once a day. How long after administration of the drug should the patient expect relief from her symptoms?
a. 1-4 hours
b. 1-4 days
c. 1-4 weeks
d. 1-4 months

▶ 12. It is important for the nurse to teach a patient who is taking alosetron (Lotronex) to stop taking the medication and immediately report:
a. abdominal pain and dyspepsia.
b. abdominal pain relieved by defecation.
c. fever and bloody diarrhea.
d. fever and headache.

▶ 13. A patient is prescribed mesalamine (Asacol) for moderate ulcerative colitis. The nurse would consult the prescriber if which of the following allergies was listed on the patient's chart? (Select all that apply.)
a. cefazolin (Ancef)
b. glipizide (Glucotrol)
c. meperidine (Morphine)
d. nafcillin (Unipen)
e. quinapril (Accupril)
f. trimethoprim/sulfamethazole (Bactrim)

▶ 14. Which of the following laboratory results for a 37-year-old female suggest possible adverse effects of sulfasalazine (Azulfidine)?
a. ANA positive
b. ESR 28 mm/hr
c. Potassium 5.2 mEq/L
d. WBC 2,500/$m^3$

▶ 15. A patient 43-year-old female with hypertension and ulcerative colitis who has been taking hydrochlorothiazide (HydroDiuril) and olsalazine (Dipentum) is admitted to the hospital. Nursing assessment findings include severe muscle weakness and paresthesias. It is critical for the nurse to review and communicate to the physician the results of which laboratory test?
a. Creatinine
b. Potassium
c. Sodium
d. WBC

16. A patient has received dexamethasone for an exacerbation of Crohn's disease with dramatic symptom relief. He is concerned because the prescriber is discontinuing this drug and prescribing budesonide (Entocort EC). How should the nurse respond?
a. Budesonide does not have the adverse effects of dexamethasone
b. Budesonide is released in the area of the colon where it needs to work
c. The drugs are the same, but budesonide is less expensive
d. Tolerance develops to long-term use of dexamethasone

17. The nurse teaches a patient with severe ulcerative colitis who is prescribed dexamethasone, methotrexate, and azathioprine that it is important to take both medications as prescribed because:
    a. onset of effect of azathioprine can take months to appear.
    b. the drugs prevent adverse effects from each other.
    c. the effect of one drug is dependent on the presence of other drugs.
    d. tolerance develops more rapidly if the drugs are not taken together.

▶ 18. Which of these outcomes would be appropriate for a patient who is taking palifermin (Kepivance)?
    a. Absence of nausea and vomiting after chemotherapy
    b. ALT/AST within normal limits
    c. Comfortably consume average of 70% of meals and snacks each day
    d. Weight gain of 1 lb/week

19. Which of the following is true about the administration of palifermin (Kepivance)?
    a. Administer 30 minutes before chemotherapy
    b. Administer by IV intermittent infusion over 1 to 2 hours
    c. Dose for a 70 kg woman is 4.2 mg
    d. Flush the line after administration with heparin

▶ 20. The school nurse cares for a student with cystic fibrosis. It is important that this child receive her pancrelipase:
    a. one half hour before lunch.
    b. one hour before lunch.
    c. two hours after breakfast and lunch.
    d. with lunch.

21. Drugs used to dissolve gallstones are most effective if the gall stones:
    a. consist of cholesterol.
    b. location is within the bile duct.
    c. location is within the gall bladder.
    d. show on x-ray.

22. Ursoidol is prescribed for a female patient with gallstones. The patient informs the nurse that she thinks she is pregnant. The nurse should:
    a. administer the medication.
    b. hold the medication and consult the prescriber.

## CASE STUDIES AND PATIENT TEACHING

*(Use a separate piece of paper for your responses.)*

### Case Study 1

*A patient who has a history of motion sickness receives a prescription for a scopolamine patch for use when she is flying cross country and embarking on a 7-day cruise. The patient has many questions, so the prescriber asks the office nurse to explain the use of this medication.*

1. How should the nurse describe the medication's action and administration?

2. Research the drug in a drug handbook and list precautions that the nurse should teach the patient to take.

3. What interventions can the nurse suggest to prevent adverse effects?

### Case Study 2

*A friend asks a nurse why her primary care practitioner is reluctant to prescribe antibiotics in case she and her family experience traveler's diarrhea on a vacation trip to Cancun.*

1. How should the nurse respond?

2. The friend states that she is packing a lot of diphenoxylate (Lomotil) "just in case." What precautions should be explained regarding the use of antidiarrheal medications for intestinal infections, especially in children?

## Case Study 3

*A freshman college student is diagnosed with diarrhea-dependent irritable bowel syndrome (IBS) at the college health center.*

1. What nonpharmacologic measures can the nurse teach to assist this patient with controlling her IBS?

2. Alosetron (Lotronex) is prescribed. The patient should stop taking the medication and return to the health center if she experiences what symptoms?

## Case Study 4

*A patient who has prescribed tegaserod (Zelnorm) for constipation-predominant IBS. The patient calls the office nurse 2 weeks later complaining of diarrhea.*

1. What data should the office nurse collect?

# 79 Vitamins

## OBJECTIVES

See page 26 for the Objectives.

## CRITICAL THINKING AND STUDY QUESTIONS

1. Vitamins are:
   a. essential for regulation of metabolic processes.
   b. inorganic compounds.
   c. required in megadoses for growth and maintenance of health.
   d. sources of energy.

2. Matching

| | | |
|---|---|---|
| ___ | a. Adequate intake (AI) | 1. Average daily intake of nutrient needs of most healthy adults |
| ___ | b. Dietary reference (DRIs) | 2. Estimate of average intake needed intakes |
| ___ | c. Estimated average requirement (EAR) | 3. Four values |
| ___ | d. Recommended dietary allowance (RDA) | 4. Highest amount that anyone can consume without significant adverse effects |
| ___ | e. Tolerable upper intake (UI) | 5. Meets nutrient needs of 50% of healthy individuals of any age level |

3. Published RDAs:
   a. include values for the elderly.
   b. may be excessive for a chronically ill person.
   c. need to been ingested every day.
   d. often are insufficient in pregnancy.

4. Routine vitamin supplementation is recommended with:
   a. alpha-tocopherol (E) to protect against heart disease and cancer.
   b. cyanocobalamin ($B_{12}$) to prevent anemia for people over age 50.
   c. vitamin C to prevent colds.
   d. vitamin D for growing children.

▶ 5. A patient with rough, scaling skin and sore tongue may be experiencing niacin deficiency. The nurse teaches that foods high in niacin include:
a. all enriched grain products, green leafy vegetables, and legumes.
b. chicken, peanuts, and cereal bran.
c. dairy and fortified cereal and bread.
d. pork and enriched breads and cereals.

▶ 6. The outpatient surgery nurse is completing the history of a 62-year-old female patient admitted for carpal tunnel surgery. Medication history includes hydrochlorothiazide 25 mg once a day, calcium 400 mg 4 times a day, senior multivitamin once a day, cholestyramine (Questran) 4 grams 4 times a day, and vitamin E 1000 mg twice a day. The patient has not consumed any food, fluids, or medication since midnight. The nurse should document the findings and notify the surgeon of the medication history because the patient is at risk for:
a. excessive bleeding during surgery.
b. hypotension during surgery.
c. poor wound healing.
d. vomiting during surgery.

7. Research suggests that vitamin E supplementation may be beneficial to:
a. prevent cancer.
b. prevent cardiovascular disease.
c. prevent age-related wrinkles.
d. slow progression of Alzheimer's disease.

▶ 8. The nurse would teach a patient who is a vegan the importance of supplementation with:
a. alpha-tocopherol.
b. ascorbic acid.
c. cyanocobalamin.
d. folic acid.

▶ 9. The nurse would be particularly concerned if which of the following patients was self-prescribing megadoses of vitamin A for healthy skin?
a. Adolescent female
b. Adolescent male
c. Elderly female
d. Elderly male

▶ 10. The nurse should be aware that which of the following disorders puts the patient at greatest risk for bleeding and bruising because of vitamin K deficiency?
a. Addison's disease
b. Celiac disease
c. Gastroesophageal reflux disease (GERD)
d. Peptic ulcer disease (PUD)

▶ 11. A neonate who was born in an automobile in a traffic jam is admitted to the hospital 3 hours after birth. Which of the following symptoms are of most concern to the neonatal nurse relating to delay of administration of vitamin K?
a. Bilateral edema over top of head
b. Deep blue color of skin over sacrum
c. Seizures 24 to 72 hours after birth
d. Yellow color of skin

12. The nurse includes in her health promotion teaching that vitamin C supplementation has been approved for:
a. decreased bronchoconstriction of asthma.
b. prevention of colds.
c. promotion of wound healing.
d. treatment of scurvy.

▶ 13. An oncology nurse is providing health teaching to a patient who is starting chemotherapy. The patient has heard that chemotherapy can cause painful "mouth ulcers." The patient would like to know if there is anything that she can do to help prevent these ulcers. The nurse's response would include trying to eat servings of which foods that are rich in the vitamin that protects mucous membrane integrity?
a. Citrus fruits, strawberries, red peppers
b. Deep yellow, orange, and green colored vegetables and fruits
c. Nuts and vegetable oils
d. Pork and enriched breads and cereals

14. The nurse is working with a patient with advanced esophageal cancer because of poor nutritional intake relating to nausea and epigastric discomfort. It is most important for the nurse to assess if the patient is self-medicating with which of the following vitamins that has been promoted as a treatment for cancer and can cause upper GI irritation?
a. Vitamin A
b. Vitamin B
c. Vitamin C
d. Vitamin E

15. Health promotion for aging adults should include the importance of adequate amounts of vitamin D because older adults often: (Select all that apply.)
    a. buy less fresh fruit because it is expensive.
    b. consume less dairy products.
    c. do not eat fresh vegetables because they cause gas.
    d. have difficulty chewing meat.

▶ 16. An 87-year-old male, who has become anxious, irritable, and is not sleeping, has been admitted with a diagnosis of change in mental status. One reason why it is important for the nurse not to assume this patient has Alzheimer's disease is because these symptoms can be caused by deficiency of which of the following foods in the diet?
    a. Chicken, peanuts, and cereal bran
    b. Dairy and fortified cereal and bread
    c. Meat, dairy, eggs
    d. Pork and enriched breads and cereals

▶ 17. A teacher sends a Hispanic migrant worker's child to the nurse's office because she is concerned that the child has a smooth, swollen tongue and cracks in the corners of her mouth and lips. The nurse knows that this may be a vitamin deficiency that can be caused by eating:
    a. guacamole.
    b. homemade corn bread.
    c. hot peppers.
    d. unpasteurized milk.

## CASE STUDIES AND PATIENT TEACHING

*(Use a separate piece of paper for your responses.)*

### Case Study 1

*A 46-year-old male has been admitted to a medical unit after 4 days in an alcohol detoxification center. He was admitted because of complaints of extreme weakness and an unsteady gait. His wife provided a history that his alcohol intake has steadily increased since he lost his job 3 years ago. During the past 6 months, he has been living on the street and drinking 1 to 2 quarts of wine daily. He is a poor historian and does not recall being admitted to the hospital. His response when asked about his diet is, "Whatever I can get." Physical assessment reveals ataxia, edema of the lower extremities, nystagmus, dry skin with cracks in the corners of his mouth, and multiple bruises. He states that the bruises are caused by any slight pressure. He is anorexic, taking sips of fluid and eating only a few bites of his lunch. He complains that his mouth is "too sore" to eat many foods. Endoscopy reveals severe gastritis with no obvious bleeding. The patient is diagnosed with vitamin deficiency and started on an IV drip with one ampule of vitamin C and B complex per liter.*

1. What symptoms led to a diagnosis of vitamin deficiency, and which vitamins are probably deficient?

2. Why is the patient less likely to be showing symptoms of fat-soluble vitamin deficiencies?

3. Blood studies include hemoglobin 8.4 grams, hematocrit 25%. Which vitamins are essential in red blood cell production?

4. The patient's wife has agreed that he may come home with her after his discharge from the hospital as long as he continues to stay in an outpatient rehabilitation program and does not drink. She asks the nurse to tell her some of the foods she should prepare to be certain that he gets the necessary vitamins. What foods or food groups would you suggest to her to ensure intake of the following vitamins?
    a. A
    b. C
    c. Niacin
    d. Pyridoxine
    e. Riboflavin
    f. Thiamine

5. The patient's wife asks the nurse whether it would be a good idea to go to the health-food store and buy him some high-dose vitamin pills with all vitamins included. What is the best response?

### Case Study 2

*The high school nurse has developed a relationship with a female student who has acne. The student states that she has been seeing a dermatologist without success. At the last appointment, the doctor stated that he would be considering isotretinoin (Accutane), a megadose form of vitamin A, as the next step in therapy.*

1. What precautions and instruction should the nurse provide?

# 80 Enteral and Parenteral Nutrition

## OBJECTIVES

See page 26 for the Objectives.

## CRITICAL THINKING AND STUDY QUESTIONS

1. Feeding a patient through a percutaneous endoscopic gastrostomy (PEG) tube is an example of:
   a. enteral nutrition.
   b. hyperalimentation.
   c. intravenous nutrition.
   d. parenteral nutrition.

2. The need for parenteral nutrition therapy is most critical for a patient who:
   a. is malnourished.
   b. has difficulty swallowing (dysphagia).
   c. cannot absorb nutrients via the GI tract.
   d. is unresponsive.

3. Matching

| | |
|---|---|
| ___ a. Bolus administration | 1. Infusion pump recommended |
| ___ b. Intermittent infusion | 2. Total feed delivered over several hours |
| ___ c. Cyclic infusion | 3. Often use a syringe |
| ___ d. Continuous infusion | 4. Three to six feedings lasting 30 to 60 minutes |

4. The nurse has been caring for a patient who has been experiencing diarrhea since she started to receive nutrition though a gastrostomy tube 5 days ago. The nurse should assess the patient history for:
   a. celiac disease.
   b. diabetes mellitus.
   c. hyperlipidemia.
   d. lactose intolerance.

▶ 5. The nurse is administering an every-4-hour bolus enteral feeding. Which of the following assessment would be a reason to hold the feeding? (Select all that apply.)
   a. Vomiting of 75 mL of milky liquid after last feeding
   b. Urine output of 300 mL during the past 8 hours
   c. Erythema of the skin around the feeding tube
   d. Residual of 50 mL of milky, yellow liquid
   e. Absence of a gag reflex
   f. Fasting blood sugar 230 mg/dL

▶ 6. A hospital nurse working on a medical-surgical unit is caring for a patient who is receiving a continuous parenteral nutrition infusion of an amino acid and dextrose solution. Recent lab tests include blood urea nitrogen (BUN) 17 mg/dL and creatinine 1.0 mg/dL. The nurse should:
   a. stop the infusion and notify the physician of the laboratory results.
   b. continue the infusion of the parenteral nutrition.
   c. decrease the rate of infusion of the parenteral nutrition.
   d. increase the rate of infusion of the parenteral nutrition.

7. Which of the following parenteral nutrition solutions must be administered through a central venous catheter? (Select all that apply.)
   a. 5% amino acid solution
   b. 10% amino acid solution
   c. 5% dextrose solution
   d. 10% dextrose solution
   e. Fat emulsion

▶ 8. Because insulin levels are elevated during parenteral nutrition therapy with dextrose solutions, the nurse should assess for symptoms of:
  a. Skeletal muscle weakness and absent bowel sounds (hypokalemia)
  b. Disorientation, psychosis, and seizures (hypomagnesemia)
  c. Muscle weakness, hypotension, and sedation (hypermagnesemia)
  d. Confusion, anxiety, heavy legs, and tall T waves on ECG (hyperkalemia)

▶ 9. A patient who was receiving amino acid-dextrose parenteral nutrition has the therapy discontinued. For 2 to 4 hours after discontinuing the therapy, it is important for the nurse to assess the patient for:
  a. hot, red skin and fruity breath.
  b. tachycardia and Kussmaul's breathing.
  c. shakiness and cool clammy skin.
  d. hypotension and sedation.

▶ 10. The nurse is administering a fat emulsion parenteral nutrition via a central line to a premature infant in neonatal intensive care. It is important for the nurse to assess for adverse effects specific to this population by assessing:
  a. urine output.
  b. lung sounds.
  c. liver enzymes.
  d. skin turgor.

▶ 11. A patient is receiving parenteral nutrition therapy via a triple lumen central venous catheter. The nurse is to draw blood for BUN, electrolytes, and glucose. The sample should be drawn from:
  a. the proximal port.
  b. the middle port.
  c. the distal port.
  d. a different vein than the one receiving the infusion.

## CASE STUDIES AND PATIENT TEACHING

*(Use a separate piece of paper for your responses.)*

### Case Study 1

*An 87-year-old patient who lives with his daughter's family is admitted with aspiration pneumonia. Medication history includes glyburide 5 mg for type 2 DM once a day. Nutritional consult reveals severe dysphagia. The patient is NPO, and the physician and family have agreed to initiate enteral tube feedings.*

1. What assessment is important for the nurse to communicate to the physician relating to choice of placement of the tip of the feeding tube in the stomach versus the duodenum or jejunum?

2. The patient receives a percutaneous endoscopic gastrostomy (PEG) tube. Twenty-four hours after the tube is inserted, half strength of a commercially prepared feeding is started at 50 mL/hr. The patient's daughter will be the primary caretaker when the patient is discharged. Describe teachings that the nurse should provide to the daughter to prevent aspiration of the enteral feedings.

3. The patient tolerates the initial feeding and amount, and concentration is increased to full strength at 100 mL/hr. This patient is at risk for what nursing problems (nursing diagnoses) relating to the enteral feeding tube, age, and the patient's past medical history?

### Case Study 2

*A 21-year-old college student who is admitted to the nursing unit for an exacerbation of Crohn's disease. She tells the nurse that her food and fluid intake have been limited for the last month because of cramping and diarrhea. She has lost 10 lbs (height 5 feet 6 inches and weight 98 lbs) and is extremely weak. Her physician inserts a central venous line and orders a dextrose-amino acid solution with a fat emulsion. Orders include daily weight, capillary blood sugar every 6 hours, intake and output, complete metabolic panel, and lipids. She is being evaluated for resection of the small intestine.*

1. Why is parenteral nutrition ordered rather than enteral feedings?

2. The parenteral nutrition tubing includes an in-line filter. Describe how the nurse will set up the infusion of the dextrose-amino acid solution and the fat emulsion.

3. Why has the physician ordered daily weights?

4. The nurse should monitor the patient for symptoms of which adverse effects to the parenteral nutrition?

# 81 Drugs for Obesity

## OBJECTIVES

See page 26 for the Objectives.

## CRITICAL THINKING AND STUDY QUESTIONS

▸ 1. What is the most important factor when the nurse is devising a weight reduction plan for a patient?
   a. Developing strategies to minimize stress
   b. Including aerobic exercise
   c. Limiting processed carbohydrates in diet
   d. Patient input in creating and revising the plan

2. Recommendations for drug therapy for obesity include to:
   a. expect at least 6 lbs of weight loss per week for the first 6 weeks.
   b. limit drug therapy to 6 months or less.
   c. only start drug treatment after a 6-month program of diet and exercise has failed to produce results.
   d. start regular exercise after the BMI is less than 40 to reduce the strain on the heart.

▸ 3. A patient who is prescribed fluoxetine (Prozac) for depression admits to taking her sister's prescription drug sibutramine (Meridia) to try to loose the weight she has gained while on the antidepressant. Which of the following assessment findings, if identified by the nurse, would be of most concern?
   a. Constipation and anorexia
   b. Diaphoresis and incoordination
   c. Difficulty falling asleep and nervousness
   d. Headache and dry mouth

4. Which of the following statements, if made by a patient receiving orlistat (Xenical), would indicate a need for further teaching?
   a. "I will eat less because my appetite should decrease."
   b. "Limiting the fat in my diet will decrease unpleasant adverse effects."
   c. "This drug may help reduce my bad fat and increase my good fat."
   d. "Unpleasant gas and oily bowel movements that are difficult to control may occur."

## CASE STUDIES AND PATIENT TEACHING

*(Use a separate piece of paper for your responses.)*

### Case Study 1

*A 48-year-old male with a history of sleep apnea, hypertension, and type 2 diabetes weighs 385 lbs and is 5 feet 8 inches tall. His waist circumference is 54 inches. His total cholesterol is 330 mg.*

1. What is this patient's BMI?

2. His physician has proposed a program of diet, exercise, and drug therapy. The patient's wife, who is 5 feet 5 inches and 165 lbs and has a pear shaped body, states that she has sought drug therapy for her weight, but her primary care provider (PCP) refused. She asks the nurse why drugs are being offered to her husband when drugs have adverse effects and he has a family history of heart disease. What could the nurse include in her explanation of guidelines for drug therapy for obesity?

3. The patient asks the nurse what is a realistic goal for weight loss, and how much does he need to cut back in eating. How should the nurse respond?

# 82 Basic Principles of Antimicrobial Therapy

## OBJECTIVES

See page 26 for the Objectives.

## CRITICAL THINKING AND STUDY QUESTIONS

1. Matching:

| | |
|---|---|
| ___ a. Antibiotic | 1. Using chemicals against invading organisms |
| ___ b. Antimicrobial | 2. Chemical produced by one microbe that can harm another microbe |
| ___ c. Bacteriocidal | 3. Drugs that slow microbe reproduction |
| ___ d. Bacteriostatic | 4. Any agent that can harm microbes |
| ___ e. Chemotherapy | 5. Drugs that kill microbes |

2. Which of the following are true about conjugation as a mechanism to change microbial DNA? (Select all that apply.)
   a. A single transfer of DNA can cause a formerly drug sensitive bacteria to become resistant to several antibiotics.
   b. Conjugation occurs primarily among gram-positive bacteria.
   c. Genetic material can only be transferred between members of the same species (staph to staph; strep to strep).
   d. Normal flora bacteria can transfer drug resistance to disease causing bacteria by conjugation.
   e. Results in resistance to only one drug.
   f. The resistance factor (R factor) of a donor microbe must include a DNA segment that codes for the mechanism of drug resistance and a sexual apparatus for DNA transfer.

3. Antibiotics promote drug resistance by: (Select all that apply.)
   a. altering the number of nonpathogenic microbes that produce toxins against pathogenic organisms.
   b. causing spontaneous mutation of microbes.
   c. creating a situation where there is less competition for nutrients.
   d. destroying drug-sensitive normal flora.
   e. encouraging DNA transfer between microbes.

▸ 4. A patient had a specimen sent for culture and sensitivity while in the emergency department. He was admitted to a medical unit and prescribed intravenous ampicillin/sulbactam (Unasyn) 1.5 gram every 6 hours. The nurse knows the priority reason for notifying the physician of culture results as soon as they become available is that this:
   a. antibiotic has many more adverse effects than many other antibiotics.
   b. is a broad spectrum antibiotic, and an effective narrow spectrum antibiotic may be effective.
   c. is an expensive antibiotic.
   d. is a narrow spectrum antibiotic and may not be effective for the cultured organism.

▸ 5. Which of the following patients would most likely have an infection that is resistant to antibiotic therapy?
   a. A child with asthma who develops pneumonia
   b. An adult construction worker who drinks from a work site water supply and develops giardiasis
   c. A adult who developed a wound infection while in the hospital after surgery
   d. An elderly adult who got an infected paper cut

6. Describe how microbial DNA can change to result in inheritable drug resistance with the different mechanisms of antibiotic action.
   a. Disrupt bacterial cell wall promoting cell lysis
      i. Increase production of enzymes that inactivate the antibiotic
   b. Inhibiting an enzyme needed for bacterial survival that is unique to the bacteria
      i. Make compounds that compensate for action of antibiotic
   c. Disrupt bacterial protein synthesis
      i. Change in the structure of microbial receptors to which the antibiotic binds that prevents the antibiotic from acting.
   d. Not dependent on mechanism of action of antibiotic
      i. Stop taking up the antibiotic into the cell

7. Which of the following would be classified as a suprainfection?
   a. Monial vaginal infection that developed during antibiotic therapy
   b. Peritonitis that developed after surgery for a ruptured appendix
   c. Pneumonia in a patient with emphysema
   d. Varicella outbreak after injection with varicella vaccine

▶ 8. The nurse has consulted the prescriber because a patient reports an allergy to the prescribed penicillin antibiotic. The prescriber is aware of the allergy, but the patient is experiencing a life-threatening infection and no other suitable antibiotic is available. The nurse should:
   a. administer the antibiotic.
   b. ask the patient if they are willing to take the antibiotic.
   c. obtain orders for treatment of a possible allergic reaction.
   d. refuse to administer the antibiotic.

▶ 9. The nurse is administering a sulfonamide antibiotic to a black male child who has not previously received this class of medication. The patient is a foster child and genetic history is unknown. Because of the possibility the child could have a glucose-6-phosphate dehydrogenase deficiency, the nurse should monitor:
   a. AST and ALT.
   b. BUN and creatinine.
   c. glucose and Hgb A1C.
   d. hemoglobin and hematocrit.

10. In most infections, the level of antibiotic at the site of infection needs to be:
   a. at the minimum inhibitory concentration (MIC).
   b. 2 to 3 times the minimum inhibitory concentration (MIC).
   c. 4 to 8 times the minimum inhibitory concentration (MIC).
   d. 10 to 20 times the minimum inhibitory concentration (MIC).

11. A valid reason for prescribing two different antibiotics is: (Select all that apply.)
   a. after receiving results of C & S and multiple drugs are effective.
   b. after receiving results of C & S and multiple organism sensitive to different drugs are present.
   c. severe infection in the immune compromised patient.
   d. suppressing the emergence of drug resistant enterococcus faecium.
   e. suppressing the emergence of drug resistant mycobacterium tuberculosis.
   f. when foreign material is present.
   g. when the microbe is sensitive to both penicillin and tetracycline.

12. It is important for the nurse to teach a patient who has had surgery for placement of a prosthetic heart valve to take prescribed antibiotic therapy:
   a. before dental procedures.
   b. before examination of the eyes where dilating drops are instilled.
   c. when experiencing yellowish or yellow-green nasal discharge.
   d. whenever they have a fever.

## CASE STUDIES AND PATIENT TEACHING

*(Use a separate piece of paper for your responses.)*

### Case Study 1

*A 78-year-old nursing home patient with a history of hypertension, type 2 DM, and COPD is brought into the emergency department with history of fever for 72 hours and moist cough. The extended care nursing report states that he was very irritable last night, then was difficult to awaken this morning. Assessment findings include temperature 103° F (39.4° C), pulse 112 beats/min,*

*BP 100/56 mm/Hg, respirations 26 and labored, fine late inspiratory crackles (rales) throughout the lung fields, Glasgow coma scale 12. Chest x-ray demonstrates lung consolidation. Intravenous fluids are infusing. Other orders include admit, sputum culture and sensitivity, and cefotetan (Cefotan) 1 gram every 12 hours.*

1. What are nursing responsibilities regarding these orders?

2. What type of antibiotic would the nurse expect to be ordered and why?

3. The intravenous antibiotic that was ordered is cefotetan (Cefotan) 1 gram every 12 hours. The unit nurse reviews the following culture and sensitivity results. What action should the nurse take?

| Organism: Moraxella catarrhalis | |
|---|---|
| **Antibiotic** | **Sensitivity (S = sensitive; R = resistant)** |
| Amikacin | R |
| Amoxicillin | R |
| Azithromycin | S |
| Cefepime | R |
| Cefotetan | R |
| Clarithromycin | R |
| Gatafloxicin | S |
| Levofloxacin | S |
| Pipericillin | R |
| Tobramycin | R |

4. The cultured organism is sensitive to more than one drug. In this case, what other factors are considered when choosing between the effective antibiotics?

5. What assessment should be monitored by the nurse to determine clinical response to the antibiotic?

## Case Study 2

*A neighbor asks a student nurse why her pediatrician does not prescribe antibiotics for her young son's "ear infections" like he used to for her older children, and her doctor will not phone in prescriptions when she has a "sinus infection" anymore.*

1. How can the nurse explain these changes in antibiotic prescription practices?

2. What type of chronic pediatric conditions would warrant earlier treatment of sinus and ear infections?

3. The neighbor states that she has antibiotics left over from the last infection. "I always save some in case I need it." She asks the nurse if it is okay to give this drug to her son since it was prescribed for him. How should the student nurse respond?

4. The neighbor asks what she can do to prevent resistance to antibiotics. What suggestions should the student nurse make?

5. Where can the student nurse direct people for more information on preventing antibiotic resistance?

## Case Study 3

*Student nurses are studying the immune system. During clinical conference, they are discussing why some patients are admitted when they have an infection and others are treated as outpatients.*

1. Discuss these questions.
   a. Why is a cancer chemotherapy patient admitted for two days of intravenous antibiotic therapy if the drug administered is available orally?
   b. Why do patients with an abscess have to have an incision and drainage (I & D) in order to effectively eradicate the infection?
   c. How can meningitis be treated if the effective antibiotics do not cross the blood-brain barrier?
   d. A severe infection warrants use of an ototoxic drug. The patient is breast-feeding. What teaching should the nurse provide?
   e. Why is it important to know the half-life of this drug?

# 83 Drugs That Weaken the Bacterial Cell Wall I: Penicillins

## OBJECTIVES

See page 26 for the Objectives.

## CRITICAL THINKING AND STUDY QUESTIONS

1. Penicillins: (Select all that apply.)
   a. are all broad spectrum antibiotics.
   b. cannot penetrate the gram-negative cell membrane.
   c. are generally bacteriocidal.
   d. are in the same antibiotic family as macrolides.
   e. are only active against bacteria that are undergoing growth and division.
   f. are more effective against gram-negative than gram-positive bacteria.
   g. must bind to PBPs to be effective.

▶ 2. Which of the following assessments is most critical for the nurse to complete before administering a penicillin antibiotic?
   a. Allergy history
   b. BUN and creatinine levels
   c. Temperature
   d. Wound drainage

3. A mother asks why her son has been prescribed amoxicillin and calcium clavulanate (Augmentin) if amoxicillin (Amoxil) has been ineffective in the past. The nurse's response is based on the fact that the addition of calcium clavulanate:
   a. aids the penicillin with attaching to microbial penicillin-binding proteins.
   b. affects a wider spectrum of bacteria.
   c. prevents penicillinase from inactivating the amoxicillin.
   d. provides additional activity to disrupt the bacterial cell wall.

4. A child is prescribed amoxicillin. When asking the mother of a child if her son is allergic to penicillin, she states that she does not know if he has ever received any medication before except immunizations. The nurse knows that it is important to assess for an allergic response despite this history because:
   a. most people who experience a penicillin allergy experience the first incident in childhood.
   b. most people who are allergic to penicillin do not know of the allergy.
   c. parents often are poor historians.
   d. people can have an initial exposure to penicillin present in foods.

5. Which of the following organisms was previously susceptible to penicillin but has developed the greatest resistance to penicillin G?
   a. Gas gangrene caused by *Clostridium perfringes*
   b. Gonorrhea caused by *Neiserria gonrrheae*
   c. Meningitis caused by *Streptococcus pneumoniae*
   d. Syphilis caused by *Treponema pallidium*

▶ 6. A pediatric office triage nurse speaks with a mother who calls complaining that her child gets diarrhea every time he is prescribed an oral antibiotic for an ear infection. An intervention that the nurse can suggest to restore normal flora is to teach the mother to offer her son which of the following foods 30 minutes after each dose of antibiotic?
   a. Cheese
   b. Ice cream
   c. Milk
   d. Yogurt

▶ 7. The nurse is preparing to administer 8 AM (0800) medications to a patient who is to receive nafcillin (Unipen) 2 grams via secondary intravenous infusion. The drug is dissolved in 100 mL of normal saline solution. The drug handbook states the drug should be infused over 30 to 90 minutes. Just before the nurse hangs the nafcillin, the nurse is informed the patient is to be placed on a cart to go off the unit for a critical test in 30 to 45 minutes. The patient is expected to be off the floor for 30 minutes. The nurse should:
   a. hold the drug infusion until the patient returns from the test.
   b. infuse the drug in 30 minutes before placing the patient on the cart.
   c. infuse the drug in 45 minutes while loading the patient on the cart.
   d. set the infusion to run over 90 minutes.

8. When the nurse is assisting with skin testing for penicillin allergy with the minor determinant mixture (MDM):
   a. the nurse instructs the patient how to assess for a local reaction during the following week.
   b. the nurse knows that test carries little risk of a systemic reaction.
   c. respiratory support and epinephrine should be available.
   d. the test involves injection of a small amount of penicillin under the skin.

9. The nurse would be concerned about the increased possibility of an allergic reaction when administering which of the following antibiotics if the patient's allergy record includes penicillin allergy? (Select all that apply.)
   a. ampicillin/sulbactam (Unasyn)
   b. azithromycin (Zithromax)
   c. carbenicillin (Geocillin)
   d. cefadroxil (Duricef)
   e. clindamycin (Cleocin)
   f. erythromycin (EES)
   g. gatafloxicin (Tequin)
   h. imipenem and cilastin (Primaxin)
   i. piperacillin/tazobactam (Zosyn)
   j. tobramycin (Nebcin)
   k. vancomycin (Vancocin)

10. A patient is prescribed intravenous ticarcillin (Ticar) every 4 hours and Amikacin (Amikin) every 8 hours. In order for the patient to receive maximum benefit from both of these antibiotics, the nurse should administer the drugs:
   a. with Amikin followed by Unasyn.
   b. at the same time.
   c. in the same solution.
   d. separated by at least 1 hour.

11. Ampicillin 1 g/sulbactam 0.5 g (Unasyn) is supplied in 50 mL of solution to be infused over 15 minutes. The nurse should program the intravenous pump to deliver how many milliliters per hour?

12. The drug of choice for methicillin resistant staphylococcus aureus (MRSA) is:
   a. dicloxacillin.
   b. nafcillin.
   c. oxacillin.
   d. vancomycin.

▶ 13. Which of these findings, if identified in a patient who is receiving ticarcillin (Ticar), should the nurse report to the prescriber immediately?
   a. Capillary refill 2 seconds
   b. Respirations 16 per minute
   c. Temperature 101° F
   d. Weight gain of 2 lbs in 24 hours

▶ 14. A patient has just been prescribed carbenicillin (Geocillin) 500 mg 4 times a day. Which of the following timing of administration would be most therapeutic?
   a. 2 AM – 8 AM – 2 PM – 8 PM
   b. 4 AM – 10 AM – 4 PM – 10 PM
   c. 9 AM – 1 PM – 5 PM – 9 PM
   d. 12 Midnight – 6 AM – 12 Noon – 6 AM

▶ 15. The nurse would be concerned about toxicity if a patient receiving penicillin had which of the following laboratory results?
   a. ALT 52 International Units/L
   b. BUN 20 mg/dL
   c. Creatinine 2.2 mg/dL
   d. Potassium 3.3 mEq/L

## CASE STUDIES AND PATIENT TEACHING

*(Use a separate piece of paper for your responses.)*

### Case Study 1

*An 8-year-old is diagnosed with streptococcal pharyngitis. She is prescribed amoxicillin 250 mg 3 times a day for 10 days.*

1. What important information should the nurse obtain before the penicillin is administered?

2. What information about the possible side effects and adverse reactions of penicillin does the nurse need to provide to the patient's mother?

3. Describe the types of allergic reactions that might develop with the administration of penicillin and the interventions that should be included in nursing care to prevent complications from an allergic reaction.

4. The patient's mother asks how and when amoxicillin should be given. How should the nurse respond?

5. Why is it critical that the nurse teach the patient's mother to not stop the medication even if the child's throat stops hurting in 4 to 5 days?

6. What outcomes would indicate that the antimicrobial effects were successful?

### Case Study 2

*The nurse is working in a public health clinic. A 15-year-old with no known allergies is diagnosed with syphilis and prescribed 1 dose of 2 million units of procaine penicillin G 2 intramuscularly.*

1. Developmentally, why is this drug a good choice for this patient?

2. The patient asks why she cannot get this medication in a pill. How should the nurse respond?

3. Describe the technique the nurse should use to administer this intramuscular injection, including precautions to prevent administration complications.

# 84 Drugs That Weaken the Bacterial Cell Wall II: Cephalosporins, Carbapenems, Vancomycin, Astreonam, Teicoplanin, and Fosfomycin

## OBJECTIVES

See page 26 for the Objectives.

## CRITICAL THINKING AND STUDY QUESTIONS

1. Characteristics of cephalosporins are most like:
   a. aminoglycosides.
   b. macrolides.
   c. penicillins.
   d. sulfonamides.
   e. tetracyclines.

2. Which of the following cephalosporins are most susceptible to cephalosporinases?
   a. Cefaclor (Ceclor)
   b. Cefadroxil (Duricef)
   c. Cefdinir (Omnicef)
   d. Cefepime (Maxipime)

3. What best describes the mechanism of staphylococci resistance to methicillin?
   a. Changing the structure of receptors, which decreases binding of the methicillin to the receptor
   b. Increasing production of enzymes that inactivate methicillin
   c. Making compounds that compensate for action of methicillin
   d. Stopping the uptake of methicillin into the cell

4. Nursing interventions when administering cephalosporins include:
   a. always administering on an empty stomach.
   b. assessment for severe allergy to carbapenems due to cross-allergy.
   c. oral suspensions to be kept at room temperature.
   d. warning patient that intramuscular injection is painful.

5. Which of the following cephalosporins would be best for meningitis caused by a gram-negative anaerobe?
   a. cefepime (Maxipime)
   b. cefotaxime (Claforan)
   c. cefoxitin (Mefoxin)
   d. cephalexin (Keftab)

▶ 6. A patient who is receiving ceftazidime (Fortaz) has three loose brown bowel movements in 24 hours. The nurse should:
   a. administer the drug and continue nursing care.
   b. continue to administer the drug and notify the prescriber of the change in bowel movements.
   c. discontinue administering the drug and notify the prescriber.
   d. page the prescriber stat.

▶ 7. A patient with hospital acquired pneumonia has just been prescribed cefotaxime (Claforan) and probenecid (Benemid). The patient has no history or evidence of gout. The nurse should:
   a. administer both medications as ordered.
   b. administer the cefotaxime as ordered and ask the patient if they were taking probenecid at home.
   c. administer the cefotaxime, but contact the prescriber before administering the probenecid.
   d. contact the prescriber before administering either of the medications.

▶ 8. An alert and oriented patient with a history of penicillin allergy is prescribed cephalexin (Keftab). The initial action by the nurse should be to:
   a. administer the cephalexin.
   b. administer the cephalexin and carefully assess for allergic reaction.
   c. assess the type of reaction that the patient had to the penicillin.
   d. notify the prescriber of the allergy and ask for a different antibiotic order.

▶ 9. The nurse is reviewing new laboratory results, including creatinine clearance results of 82 mL/min for a 74-year-old male patient receiving cefotetan (Cefotan) 2 grams every 12 hours. The nurse should:
   a. administer the medication.
   b. withhold the medication and notify the prescriber of the laboratory results.

10. Cefoperazone (Cefobid) has been prescribed at discharge for a patient with pelvic inflammatory disease. Due to the possibility of a disulfiram-like reaction, during discharge teaching it is important for the nurse to teach the patient to avoid:
   a. alcohol.
   b. antacids.
   c. aspirin.
   d. ibuprofen.

▶ 11. Which of the following laboratory results, if present, would be a reason to withhold administering cefotetan (Cefotan) to an adult male and notifying the prescriber?
   a. ALT 154 International Units/L
   b. BUN 34 mg/dL
   c. Creatinine 3.5 mg/dL
   d. FBS 380 mg/dL

12. Cefditoren (Spectracef) is prescribed on discharge for a patient diagnosed with chronic bronchitis caused by *Moraxella catarrhalis*, type 2 DM, GERD, and end stage renal failure. Why is this antibiotic a good choice for this patient?
   a. Absorption not affected by antacids
   b. Effective for beta-lactamase producing *M. catarrhalis*
   c. Low expense
   d. Once a day dosing

▶ 13. Ceftriaxone (Rocephin) 1 g intramuscular is ordered for a 130-lb woman. The drug is reconstituted to a solution of 250 mg/mL. The nurse should administer:
   a. 1 mL each in the right and left vastus lateralis and deltoid muscles.
   b. 2 mL each in the right and left ventrogluteal muscles.
   c. 2 mL each in the right and left deltoid muscle.
   d. 4 mL in the right or left gluteus maximus muscle.

14. The carbapenem antibiotic imipenem (Primaxin) is a combination of the antibiotic and cilastatin. The purpose of the additive cilastatin is to:
   a. decrease adverse effects of nausea and vomiting.
   b. improve absorption in the GI tract.
   c. prevent destruction of the antibiotic by beta-lactamases.
   d. prevent inactivation by a kidney enzyme.

▶ 15. The doctor has prescribed 250 mg every 8 hours for a 14-lb child who has been diagnosed with bacterial meningitis. The recommended safe pediatric dose of meropenem (Merrem) for meningitis is 40 mg/kg every 8 hours. Is this a safe dose?

16. The nurse is preparing to administer an intermittent infusion of ertapenem (Invanz). This drug cannot be administered concurrently with which of the following intravenous solutions? (Select all that apply.)
   a. 5% dextrose in water
   b. 0.9% sodium chloride (Normal saline)
   c. 0.45% sodium chloride
   d. 0.45% sodium chloride/5% dextrose solution
   e. 0.225% sodium chloride/5% dextrose solution
   f. Lactated Ringer's solution

▶ 17. Vancomycin is being administered by mouth for pseudomembranous colitis caused by *Clostridium difficile*. The nurse receives laboratory results on the patient that include creatinine 2.2 mg/dL. The nurse should:
   a. administer the medication.
   b. hold the medication and notify the prescriber.

## CASE STUDIES AND PATIENT TEACHING

*(Use a separate piece of paper for your responses.)*

### Case Study 1

*A 45-year-old, gravida 4, para 4, obese female admitted to the nursing unit with the diagnosis of cholelithiasis and cholecystitis. She complains of abdominal pain. She has a fever of 101°F and a white count of 12,000. A nasogastric tube is placed, an IV is started, and 1 g of cefazolin (Ancef) is ordered every 6 hours. Pain management is provided by IV meperidine (Demerol). Her cholecystectomy will be scheduled when her temperature returns to normal, probably in 2 to 3 days.*

1. The nurse should assess the patient for which possible adverse reactions to the antibiotic?

2. What are the steps the nurse must take when administering a slow bolus intravenous infusion (IV push) of the antibiotic?

3. How can the possibility of thrombophlebitis be minimized?

4. Why would a broader-spectrum antibiotic not be prescribed for this patient?

5. What should the nurse do if the nurse discovers the patient has had an anaphylactic reaction to penicillin?

## Case Study 2

*The nurse is caring for a patient who is prescribed intravenous cefoperazone (Cefobid) 2 grams every 12 hours and Amikacin (Amikin) 300 mg 3 times a day after surgery for a ruptured appendix.*

1. What assessments and laboratory results should be monitored while this patient is on this drug therapy?

2. What precautions does the nurse need to take when administering these two antibiotics through the same intravenous site?

3. The nurse notes that the patient's INR is 3.5. What should the nurse do?

4. Three days postoperatively, the patient has progressed to a soft diet and develops severe watery diarrhea. What are possible causes of the diarrhea?

5. What are possible electrolyte imbalances that could occur and what are their symptoms?

## Case Studies 3

*A patient is prescribed vancomycin (Vancocin) 1 g every 12 hours scheduled at 0900 (9 AM) and 2100 (9 PM). The pharmacy provides a solution of 1 g in 200 mL.*

1. Why is it critical to use an intravenous pump when administering this drug rather than hanging this drug by gravity?

2. If the drug is administered at 0900, at what time should blood be drawn to assess peak levels of the drug?

3. The drug will reach its therapeutic level after how many doses of the drug?

4. Describe red man syndrome and the nursing measures that can be taken to prevent this reaction?

5. Does experiencing red man syndrome create a contraindication for further administration of vancomycin?

6. Describe how the nurse will assess for the possible adverse effects of:
   a. Ototoxicity.
   b. Stevens-Johnson syndrome.

# 85 Bacteriostatic Inhibitors of Protein Synthesis: Tetracyclines, Macrolides, and Others

## OBJECTIVES

See page 26 for the Objectives.

## CRITICAL THINKING AND STUDY QUESTIONS

1. Tetracycline: (Select all that apply.)
   a. absorption of long-acting agents is decreased by food.
   b. easily crosses mammalian cell membranes.
   c. is active against the bacilli that cause anthrax.
   d. is a narrow spectrum antibiotic.
   e. kill bacteria.
   f. low doses prevent destruction of gingival connective tissue.
   g. reduces symptoms of rheumatoid arthritis.
   h. resistance is increasing.

2. The nurse teaches a patient who has been prescribed oral tetracycline (Sumycin) that the medication should not be taken with which of the following over-the-counter medications? (Select all that apply.)
   a. Ascorbic acid
   b. Centrum silver
   c. Ferrous sulfate
   d. Folic acid
   e. TUMs

▸ 3. A patient who was admitted with severe abdominal pain has been diagnosed with *H. pylori* associated peptic ulcer. Tetracycline 500 mg, metronidazole 250 mg, and bismuth subsalicylate 525 mg have been prescribed 4 times a day. The nurse notes that the patient's 24-hour fluid intake has been approximately 2500 mL and urine output has been 600 to 800 mL for each of the past 2 days. The nurse should:
   a. administer the medications and continue nursing care.
   b. administer the medications and report the changes.
   c. withhold the medication and continue nursing care.
   d. withhold the medication and notify the prescriber of the changes.

▸ 4. Tetracycline can cause esophageal ulceration. What can the nurse teach to minimize the risk of this adverse effect?
   a. Stay upright for 30 minutes after taking the medication
   b. Take the medication at bedtime
   c. Take the medication with an antacid
   d. Take the medication with milk

5. A patient is prescribed a tetracycline antibiotic. Which of the following are reasons that the medication should be withheld and the prescriber consulted?
   a. Allergic to penicillin
   b. 12-year-old child
   c. Pregnancy status unknown
   d. Theophylline for asthma is also prescribed

6. The nurse should assess for adverse effects of lightheadedness and dizziness when a patient is receiving:
   a. demeclocycline.
   b. doxycycline.
   c. minocycline.
   d. oxytetracycline.

7. An Amish baby has been diagnosed with diphtheria. The community health nurse has been assigned to attempt to obtain cooperation within the Amish community with identifying and treating carriers. When carriers are identified it is important for the nurse to note an allergy to:
   a. azithromycin.
   b. clarithromycin.
   c. dirithromycin.
   d. erythromycin.

8. A patient with a penicillin allergy is prescribed erythromycin ethylsuccinate 250 mg every 6 hours for pneumonia caused by haemophilus influenzae. The MAR has the medication scheduled at 0600, 1200, 1800, and 2400. On the second day of therapy, the patient complains that he does not like taking the drug because it causes heartburn. An appropriate intervention by the nurse would be to:
   a. administer the drug with food.
   b. change the timing of the drug to 0830, 1330, 1730, and 2400 so that most doses are administered with meals.
   c. explain that administering the drug with food or antacids will prevent absorption of the drug.
   d. withhold the drug and notify the prescriber.

▶ 9. Which of these findings would be most significant for the nurse if a patient was receiving erythromycin estolate?
   a. Abdominal pain and dark urine
   b. Cheesy vaginal discharge and vaginal itching
   c. Dyspepsia and flatulence
   d. Headache and insomnia

10. Enteric coated erythromycin base should be administered: (Select all that apply.)
   a. on an empty stomach.
   b. whole, not chewed.
   c. with a full glass of water.
   d. with food.

11. Erythromycin oral suspension 200 mg 4 times a day has been prescribed for a child. The pharmacy provided erythromycin 250 mg/5mL. How much erythromycin should the nurse teach the parent to administer per dose?

12. The nurse teaches that to be well absorbed, which of the following form of clarithromycin (Biaxin) must be administered with food?
   a. Standard tablets
   b. Extended release tablets
   c. Granules

13. What teaching can the nurse provide regarding administration of antibiotics that helps decrease the development of resistance?
   a. Only take antibiotics as prescribed
   b. Do not pressure prescribers for antibiotics
   c. When prescribed, take the full course as directed even if symptoms abate

▶ 14. It is important for the nurse to monitor which of the following laboratory tests when a patient is prescribed erythromycin and warfarin?
   a. BUN
   b. CK-MM
   c. INR
   d. RBC

15. A diabetic patient is receiving clindamycin (Cleocin) for gas gangrene. Which of the following is most suggestive of the development of antibiotic-associated membranous colitis (AAPMC) caused by *Clostridium difficile*?
   a. Dyspepsia and flatulence
   b. Five watery stools a day
   c. Hypoactive bowel sounds
   d. Nausea and vomiting

16. The nurse would consult the prescriber regarding administration of linezolid (Zyvox) if the nurse discovered the patient has a history of:
   a. asthma.
   b. celiac disease.
   c. gout.
   d. phenylketonuria.

17. A patient with a history of hypertension controlled by an angiotensin-conveting enzyme inhibitor is prescribed linezolid (Zyvox) for a vancomycin resistant enterococcal (VRE) infection. The patient should be instructed to avoid eating which of the following foods while on this antibiotic?
   a. Aged cheese
   b. Milk
   c. Red meat
   d. Seafood

18. It is important for the nurse to notify the prescriber if a patient is prescribed which of the following cholesterol lowering drugs and telithromycin (Ketek)? (Select all that apply.)
    a. atorvastatin (Lipitor)
    b. fluvastatin (Lescol)
    c. lovastatin (Mevacor)
    d. pravastatin (Pravachol)
    e. simvastatin (Zocor)

▸ 19. Which of these laboratory tests, if identified in a patient who is receiving dalfopristin/quinupristin (Synercid), should the nurse report to the prescriber immediately?
    a. ALT 250 International Units/L
    b. BUN 20 mg/dL
    c. CK-MM 50 units/mL
    d. FBS 250 mg/dL

▸ 20. The nurse is caring for a patient whose peak chloramphenicol level is 28 mcg/mL. It is a priority for the nurse to review the most recent results of which of the following ordered laboratory tests?
    a. ALT and AST
    b. BUN and creatinine
    c. CBC and differential
    d. Electrolytes

## CASE STUDIES AND PATIENT TEACHING

*(Use a separate piece of paper for your responses.)*

### Case Study 1

*A 30-year-old office worker reports to the healthcare facility with a fever of 101°F and a nonproductive cough that has lasted 10 days. Her medical history reveals that she is an asthmatic, takes theophylline (Theo-Dur), and is allergic to penicillin. On physical exam, her respiratory rate is 24 and nonlabored, and bilateral basilar crackles (rales) are heard. The patient is given a prescription for erythromycin 250 mg 4 times a day for 10 days to treat what is suspected to be mycoplasma pneumonia. She is advised to take Tylenol 325 mg q4hr for fever, to increase her fluids to 6 to 8 glasses of water per day, and to stay home from work for 2 to 3 days.*

1. What serious adverse effect is this patient at risk for based on drug interactions, and what symptoms would suggest this syndrome?

2. What should the nurse do regarding the possibility of this syndrome?

### Case Study 2

*A 15-year-old male patient is readmitted after being discharged post appendectomy with shaking chills, fever of 103° F, and purulent drainage from the incision site. Culture and sensitivity results of the wound drainage reveal entrococcus faecium that is resistant to vancomycin. Dalfopristin/quinupristin (Synercid) 500 mg intravenous every 12 hours.*

1. What laboratory tests and symptoms should the nurse monitor to assess for hepatotoxicity?

2. What nursing assessments and interventions should the nurse include in the plan of care relating to the significant risk of infusion-related thrombophlebitis?

3. Dalfopristin/quinupristin (Synercid) inhibits CYP3A4 hepatic drug-metabolizing enzyme. What are the ramifications for nursing care?

# 86 Aminoglycosides: Bacterial Inhibitors of Protein Synthesis

## OBJECTIVES

See page 26 for the Objectives.

## CRITICAL THINKING AND STUDY QUESTIONS

1. Aminoglycosides: (Select all that apply.)
   a. are administered intravenously to treat meningitis caused by *Escherichia coli* in infants.
   b. are all equally susceptible to inactivation by enzymes.
   c. are narrow spectrum antibiotics.
   d. are never administered orally.
   e. are primarily used to treat serious infections with aerobic gram-negative bacilli.
   f. can be toxic to the kidneys and nervous system.
   g. cannot kill bacteria when serum levels drop below the minimal bactericidal concentration.
   h. effectiveness correlates to serum concentration levels.

2. Facultative bacteria survive in the:
   a. absence of oxygen.
   b. both absence and presence of oxygen.
   c. presence of oxygen.

▸ 3. Neomycin topical drops have been prescribed for a patient with external otitis. Which of the following assessment findings would be a reason for the nurse to consult with the prescriber?
   a. Foul odor
   b. Pain when straightening the pinna to instill the drops
   c. Tasting the drops after they are instilled
   d. Temperature 100.4° F (38° C)

▸ 4. A patient, who is prescribed tobramycin (Nebcin), complains of a headache. The nurse should:
   a. assess the onset, characteristics, and associated symptoms of the headache.
   b. medicate with acetaminophen and reassess in 1 hour.
   c. withhold the Tobramycin and notify the prescriber when making rounds.
   d. withhold the Tobramycin and notify the prescriber stat.

▸ 5. The nurse is assessing a patient who is scheduled to receive a dose of gentamicin (Garamycin). In the last 12 hours, fluid intake has been 900 mL, urine output has been 300 mL, and the patient's bladder is not distended. The nurse should:
   a. administer the drug.
   b. administer the drug and notify the prescriber of the output.
   c. instruct the patient that he needs to drink a full glass of water each time the medication is administered.
   d. withhold the drug and notify the prescriber of the output.

▸ 6. The nurse is taking a history from the wife of a patient who was admitted in a septic state and prescribed an aminoglycoside antibiotic. Which of the following questions is most important to ask the wife about her husband's history?
   a. "Has he ever had any surgery performed?"
   b. "Has he been told to follow any specific diet?"
   c. "Has he received a flu vaccine this year?"
   d. "What medications is he currently taking?"

▶ 7. The nurse is assessing for adverse effects of intravenous Tobramycin. Which of the following changes would be most significant?
   a. Dilute urine
   b. Headache
   c. Limp, weak muscles
   d. Ringing in the ears

8. Matching: Interaction of drugs with aminoglycosides

| | |
|---|---|
| ___ a. Amphotericin B | 1. Aid aminoglycoside getting into cell |
| ___ b. Aspirin | 2. Inactivate aminoglycosides when in the same solution |
| ___ c. Cephalosporin | 3. Directly increase risk of damage to the inner ear |
| ___ d. Cyclosporine | 4. Indirectly increase risk of damage to the inner ear |
| ___ e. Ethacrynic acid | 5. Increase risk of kidney damage |
| ___ f. NSAID | 6. Risk of respiratory arrest |
| ___ g. Penicillin | |
| ___ h. Pancuronium | |
| ___ i. Polymyxin | |
| ___ j. Tubocurarine | |
| ___ k. Vancomycin | |

9. The nurse would be most concerned about the possibility of toxicity when a patient is prescribed the same daily dose of an aminoglycoside divided into which of the following regimes?
   a. Once a day
   b. Every 8 hours
   c. Every 12 hours

▶ 10. When aminoglycosides are prescribed intravenously as a once daily dose, it is critical to monitor the:
   a. peak levels 1 hour after completing the infusion.
   b. peak levels 30 minutes after completing the infusion and trough levels 1 hour before the next dose.
   c. peak levels 1 hour after completing the infusion and trough levels 30 minutes before the next dose.
   d. trough levels 1 hour before the next dose.

11. The most important reason why amikacin (Amikar) should only be used in cases where other aminoglycosides are known to be resistant is:
   a. it must be dosed more frequently.
   b. sensitivity to aminoglycoside-inactivating enzymes.
   c. to delay emergence of organisms resistance to amikacin.
   d. toxicity.

▶ 12. Which of these laboratory tests would be most important for the nurse to assess when a patient is receiving an aminoglycoside?
   a. Creatinine
   b. Fasting glucose
   c. Hemoglobin and hematocrit
   d. INR

▶ 13. A patient received a neuromuscular blocking agent during surgery. In the recovery room, the physician orders gentamicin 40 mg IV stat. What is the most appropriate nursing action?
   a. Administer the drug as quickly as possible
   b. Assess the patient's vital signs
   c. Clarify the order
   d. Refuse to administer the drug

## CASE STUDIES AND PATIENT TEACHING

*(Use a separate piece of paper for your responses.)*

### Case Study 1

*A 72-year-old man with a history of DM treated with metformin and rheumatoid arthritis treated for many years by non-steroid anti-inflammatory drugs is a 14 days postoperative prostatectomy patient. He is readmitted to a medical-surgical unit for a surgical site infection. Assessment findings include BP 100/70 mm/Hg, pulse 98 beats/min, respirations 24/minute, temperature 104° F (40° C). He is difficult to arouse and his skin is hot and dry. Escherichia coli cultured from the wound drainage is sensitive to amikacin (Amikar). The nursing drug handbook lists the recommended intravenous dose as a loading dose of 7.5 mg/kg followed by 15 mg/kg/day in 2 to 3 divided doses every 8 to 12 hours for 7 to 10 days. This patient weighs 65 kg and has been prescribed a loading dose of 250 mg of amikacin followed by 175 mg every 8 hours.*

1. Calculate the recommended dose of Amikacin for this patient.
2. What are possible reasons for the prescribed dose not being equivalent to the recommended dose?
3. The drug is to be administered at 0600 (6 AM), 1400 (2 PM), and 2200 (10 PM). Peak and trough levels of the Amikacin are ordered. When will the nurse schedule the collection of the blood sample for this testing?
4. Why are serum trough levels more significant than serum peak levels?
5. The trough level of the amikacin (Amikar) is 15 mcg/mL. What should the nurse do?

### Case Study 2

*A 40-year-old male patient is recovering in the trauma unit from a major accident. He is on a ventilator and has a central line for IVs and antibiotics, a Swan-Ganz catheter to measure cardiac status, an arterial line to measure continuous blood pressures, a small-bore feeding tube, 2 chest tubes, and a Foley catheter. After 3 days, he develops gram-negative septicemia and pneumonia and is started on gentamicin sulfate (Garamycin) and ampicillin (Unasyn) IV.*

1. Describe the assessments the nurse should perform to detect nephrotoxicity and neurotoxicity.
2. How does nephrotoxicity increase the risk of developing ototoxicity?
3. Which toxicity is most likely to be permanent?
4. How can the nurse prevent drug interactions?
5. What type of urine collection bag should the nurse use with this patient?
6. What changes in the dosages of medications would be necessary if the patient were 80 years old instead of 40?

### Case Study 3

1. Describe the teaching the nurse would provide to a mother who needs to instill antibiotic ear drops in her child's ear.

# 87 Sulfonamides and Trimethoprim

## OBJECTIVES

See page 26 for the Objectives.

## CRITICAL THINKING AND STUDY QUESTIONS

1. Sulfonamides: (Select all that apply.)
   a. are chemically related to glipizide, glyburide, furosemide, and hydrochlorothiazide.
   b. are narrow spectrum antibiotics.
   c. are no longer active against many microbes for which they initially were effective.
   d. are usually administered intramuscularly or intravenously.
   e. are widely used because of low toxicity.
   f. can cause folic acid deficiency in the patient.
   g. cross the placenta.
   h. do not cause toxicity when applied topically.
   i. inhibit microbial synthesis of folic acid.
   j. were the first systemic antibiotics developed.

2. The primary reason why the nurse teaches a patient who is prescribed sulfamethoxazole to take this medication with a full glass of water is to:
   a. decrease the risk of esophageal irritation.
   b. minimize crystal formation.
   c. prevent nausea.
   d. stimulate frequent voiding.

3. A patient who has liver impairment has been prescribed a sulfamethoxazole. The nurse should assess for which of the following symptoms that would be a result of increased acetylation of the drug?
   a. Clay-colored stool
   b. Pallor
   c. Rash
   d. Urine output of less than 30 mL per hour

4. A patient who takes glyburide for type 2 DM is prescribed sulfamethoxazole-trimethoprim (Septra). Because of a possible drug interactions, the nurse should assess for:
   a. bleeding and bruising.
   b. diaphoresis and tachycardia.
   c. hot, dry skin, and thirst.
   d. paresthesias and abdominal cramps.

5. The patient has been receiving mafendine (Sulfamylon) application to a second-degree burn for over 2 weeks. Which of the following laboratory results would be a reason for withholding mafendine application and consulting the prescriber?
   a. pH 7.32, $HCO_3$ 18 mEq/L, $PCO_2$ 36 mm/Hg
   b. pH 7.35, $HCO_3$ 22 mEq/L, $PCO_2$ 37 mm/Hg
   c. pH 7.41, $HCO_3$ 24 mEq/L, $PCO_2$ 40 mm/Hg
   d. pH 7.45, $HCO_3$ 21 mEq/L, $PCO_2$ 47 mm/Hg

6. The nurse is preparing to apply topical mafendine (Sulfamylon) to a second-degree burns on the anterior of a 7-year-old patient's arms, upper legs, and trunk. To gain compliance with this therapy, it would be important for the nurse to:
   a. employ aseptic technique.
   b. explain the importance of therapy.
   c. prevent pain.
   d. shield so the patient cannot see the wounds.

7. The nurse should assess for which of the following symptoms of an adverse effect for which an alcoholic would be at greater risk than the average patient if prescribed trimethoprim?
   a. Nausea and vomiting
   b. Rash and malaise
   c. Pallor and sore throat
   d. Photosensitivity and drug fever

8. Trimethoprim (Proloprim) is classified as pregnancy category C. This means:
   a. animal studies have shown a risk for fetal problems, but human studies have not shown any problems.
   b. controlled studies have shown no risk to the developing fetus.
   c. do not use this drug in pregnancy.
   d. risks are possible, but potential benefits may justify the risk.
   e. there is definite evidence of risk to the developing fetus.

9. Benefits of trimethoprim-sulfamethoxazole (TMP-SMZ) over the components used alone include:
   a. lack of interactions with drugs that have a have a narrow therapeutic range.
   b. less adverse effects.
   c. less resistance has developed.
   d. lower incidence of toxicity.

10. A physician who is on call for another physician's practice gives a verbal order for sulfamethoxazole-trimethoprim (Septra) for a patient. The nurse would consult the prescriber about this order if the patient had a history of:
    a. chronic obstructive lung disease.
    b. heart failure.
    c. diabetes mellitus.
    d. hypertension.

11. The recommended dose of sulfamethoxazole-trimethoprim (Septra) for children is 150 mg/m$^2$ BSA of trimethoprim and 750 mg/m$^2$ BSA of sulfamethoxazole daily in three doses; not to exceed 320 mg of trimethoprim and 1600 mg of sulfamethoxazole per day. What is the recommended dose for a child who is 96 cm tall and weighs 18 kg?

## CASE STUDIES AND PATIENT TEACHING

*(Use a separate piece of paper for your responses.)*

### Case Study 1

*A 30-year-old IV drug addict who is HIV positive has been treated with AZT for more than 1 year. She presents to the clinic with a low-grade fever, nonproductive cough, and shortness of breath. A chest x-ray shows diffuse infiltrates. A diagnosis of pneumocystis carinii pneumonia (PCP) is made. The patient is started on trimethoprim-sulfamethoxazole (TMP-SMZ).*

1. Why is TMP-SMZ a good choice for this patient?

2. Why is it important to wait for the results of hCG levels before this patient starts taking TMP-SMZ?

3. What adverse effects should the nurse teach the patient to report, should they occur?

4. What can the nurse teach to decrease the incidence and severity of these possible adverse effects to TMP-SMZ?
   a. Photosensitivity
   b. Stevens-Johnson syndrome
   c. Renal damage

5. What forms of sulfonamide drugs have less risk of Stevens-Johnson syndrome?

### Case Study 2

*The nurse has volunteered to do a health mission trip to provide healthcare to Rwandan refugees in Uganda. A clinic has been set up and doctors and nurse practitioners are diagnosing cases and providing donated samples of medications. The RN is providing teaching via an interpreter. Sulfonamides are being provided to patients with urinary tract infections.*

1. What adverse effect would these patients be at greater risk for than the general population?

2. What type of sulfonamides would be more likely to cause hemolytic anemia?

3. The nurse should assess for what symptoms that suggest possible development of hemolytic anemia?

4. An HIV positive mother comes to the clinic with a 2-week-old infant who appears toxic. The only antibiotic the team has in a liquid form is a sulfonamide. Why is this dangerous to give to this infant?

# 88 Drug Therapy of Urinary Tract Infections

## OBJECTIVES

See page 26 for the Objectives.

## CRITICAL THINKING AND STUDY QUESTIONS

1. An example of a complicated urinary tract infection (UTI) is a UTI:
   a. acquired in the hospital.
   b. caused by an enlarged prostate.
   c. caused by multiple organisms.
   d. of the kidney pelvis.

2. A female patient has been prescribed ciprofloxacin (Cipro) 250 mg by mouth twice a day for 7 days. The patient asks why she has to take the antibiotic for so long. Her friend had a urinary tract infection and only had to take her antibiotic for 3 days. The nurse knows that a possible explanation for the need for the longer therapy includes:
   a. fewer adverse effects.
   b. less potential for antibiotic resistance.
   c. lower cost.
   d. upper urinary tract involvement.

▶ 3. A physician's orders for a new admission include urine culture and sensitivity and ciprofloxacin 400 mg intravenously every 12 hours. A priority nursing responsibility is to:
   a. calculate the drip rate for the intravenous infusion.
   b. flush the intravenous cap.
   c. mix the antibiotic in the correct intravenous solution.
   d. obtain the urine culture specimen before administering the antibiotic.

4. Nitrofurantoin, methenamine, nalidixic acid, and cinoxacin:
   a. are first line agents for prostatitis.
   b. are not absorbed from the GI tract.
   c. concentrate in the urine much greater than in the blood.
   d. have few adverse effects.

▶ 5. Which of these assessment findings, if identified in a patient who is receiving nitrofurantoin (Macrodantin), should the nurse report to the prescriber immediately?
   a. Paresthesia
   b. Nausea
   c. Headache
   d. Drowsiness

▶ 6. The nurse is reviewing the other over-the-counter products taken by a patient who has been prescribed methenamine (Mandelamine). Which of these home treatments can reduce the urinary antiseptic action of methenamine?
   a. Baking soda in water for frequent heartburn
   b. Drinking 10 glasses of water each day for general health
   c. Ibuprophen for joint pain
   d. Megadoses of vitamin C (ascorbic acid) to prevent colds

7. A patient has been prescribed nalidixic acid (NegGram) for recurrent urinary tract infections. The nurse should teach the patient to: (Select all that apply.)
   a. report musculoskeletal pain.
   b. stop taking the drug if you note changes in your vision.
   c. take the medication with milk.
   d. use sunscreen.

## CASE STUDIES AND PATIENT TEACHING

*(Use a separate piece of paper for your responses.)*

### Case Study 1

*A 75-year-old man with known benign prostatic hypertrophy (BPH) has had numerous episodes of cystitis.*

1. If the patient develops flank pain, chills, fever, or other signs of infection higher in the urinary tract suggesting pyelonephritis, what actions should be taken?

2. The patient has been successfully treated with TMP-SMZ and has been prescribed nitrofurantoin (Macrodantin) to prevent recurrence of UTIs until he can be evaluated for surgery for his enlarged prostate. The nurse should teach the patient to be alert for what possible adverse effects from Macrodantin?

3. What nursing assessments and teaching can the nurse employ to prevent complications from nitrofurantoin (Macrodantin) therapy?

4. The patient calls to tell the office nurse that his urine has changed to a brown color. What should the nurse tell him?

5. Why is it important to monitor creatinine levels in this patient?

### Case Study 2

*A female student is seen at the college health center. She constantly feels that she needs to urinate, but does not want to because it hurts, and the urge to urinate persist after she voids. She denies fever, flank pain, and has not looked at her urine.*

1. What additional questions should the nurse ask the patient to assist the practitioner with diagnosing?

2. Why is it important to determine how frequently the patient has had urinary tract infections in the past?

3. The college health nurse knows that most urinary tract infections treated with sulfonamides are due to *Escherichia coli* infection. What instruction should the nurse provide the student to prevent future infections?

# 89 Antimycobacterial Agents: Drugs for Tuberculosis, Leprosy, and *Mycobacterium Avium* Complex Infection

## OBJECTIVES

See page 26 for the Objectives.

## CRITICAL THINKING AND STUDY QUESTIONS

1. Tuberculosis (TB)
   a. Infected but symptom free individuals cannot infect other people
   b. Infected individuals have a risk of developing active TB without additional exposure to the bacteria even if the infection has been dormant for many years
   c. Infected individuals in the USA usually do not develop symptoms of the disease
   d. Is an infection limited to the lungs
   e. Is caused by a fast-growing microbe
   f. Is more prevalent in jail and homeless populations than the general population
   g. Kills almost as many people as HIV
   h. Microbes can undergo a mutation resulting in resistance to multiple drugs
   i. Resistance to drugs is increasing
   j. Treatment of active infection should always include at least two drugs

▸ 2. What are nursing actions that can decrease the emergence of resistance of mycobacterium tuberculosis to drug therapy? (Select all that apply.)
   a. Advocating for better living conditions (sanitation, crowding) and access to healthcare for the poor, homeless, and penal populations to prevent the spread of resistant microbes.
   b. Identifying methods to maintain contact with suspected cases from time of obtaining culture specimen and getting results.
   c. Teaching the importance of taking the correct dose, for the correct time, of all of the prescribed medications.
   d. Insuring proper follow-up.
   e. Identifying obstacles for the individual to compliance with drug therapy and follow-up.

3. A patient who has been diagnosed with active tuberculosis (TB) has been prescribed isoniazid, rifampin, ethambutol, and pyrazinamide. The patient asks the nurse why he has to take so many drugs. The basis of the nurse's response should include that this multiple drug therapy: (Select all that apply.)
   a. confers immunity to the tuberculosis mycobacterium.
   b. decreases adverse effects.
   c. decreases the risk of relapse.
   d. does not increase the risk of suprainfection.
   e. eliminates actively dividing and resting tuberculosis mycobacteria.
   f. prevents the mycobacteria from developing resistance to a drug.

4. A patient asks the nurse why he has to continue to take medication after completion of the initial induction phase if he is his sputum is "clean"? The nurse explains that:
   a. dormant bacteria are still present inside cells and can become active at a later time.
   b. sputum cultures are not sensitive enough to ensure that the active bacteria are eliminated.
   c. sputum cultures are not specific for mycobacterium.
   d. the therapy is in case the person comes into contact with the person who originally infected him.

5. An HIV-infected patient who is receiving drug therapy including delavirdine (Rescriptor) and saquinavir (Fortovase) is diagnosed with an active tuberculosis infection. Because of the drug interaction that decreases the effect of these drugs for HIV infection, this patient should not be prescribed:
   a. ethambutol.
   b. isoniazid.
   c. pyrazinamide.
   d. rifampin.

6. A college student with no medical problems, no symptoms of disease, and no risk factors for contracting tuberculosis is being screened for TB before taking a course that requires contact with the public. She has a 20 mm area of erythema surrounding an 11 mm area of induration 48 hours after receiving a PPD tuberculin test. Chest x-ray and sputum culture are negative. The nurse would expect prophylactic treatment to involve:
   a. multiple drug therapy.
   b. watchful waiting.
   c. isoniazid.
   d. rifampin.

▶ 7. The nurse is receiving isoniazid therapy for latent tuberculosis. It would be most important to contact the prescriber if the nurse experiences:
   a. headache.
   b. dry mouth.
   c. right upper quadrant pain.
   d. heartburn.

▶ 8. The public health nurse would withhold administration of tuberculosis drug therapy with rifampin and pyrazinamide and contact the prescriber if the patient's laboratory testing results include:
   a. AST 75 International Units/L
   b. bilirubin, total 3.0 mg/dL
   c. BUN 22 mg/dL
   d. creatinine 1.0 mg/dL

9. The nurse should be particularly vigilant with monitoring intake and output and creatinine levels when a patient is receiving which of the following anti-tubercular drugs?
   a. Amikacin
   b. Cycloserine
   c. Ethambutol
   d. Ethionimide
   e. Gatifloxacin
   f. Kanamycin
   g. Isoniazid
   h. Pyrazinamide
   i. Rifampin
   j. Streptomycin

10. A patient with a history of peripheral vascular disease, type 2 diabetes mellitus, and latent TB is prescribed isoniazid and pyridoxine. The purpose of the pyridoxine is to:
   a. improve arterial blood flow.
   b. prevent hypoglycemia.
   c. prevent peripheral neuropathy.
   d. treat resting mycobacteria within cells.

11. The interaction of isoniazid and phenytoin is especially important because:
   a. isoniazid levels can become subtherapeutic.
   b. phenytoin has a narrow therapeutic range.
   c. phenytoin levels can become subtherapeutic.
   d. the risk of hepatotoxicity increases.

▶ 12. A paranoid schizophrenic patient who has been involuntarily committed to a psychiatric institution has been diagnosed with latent tuberculosis and is refusing drug therapy with isoniazid. An appropriate nursing response would be to:
   a. consult the prescriber and psychiatrist regarding possible intramuscular administration of isoniazid.
   b. explain the importance of drug therapy.
   c. withhold the drug and isolate the patient until he agrees to take the drug.
   d. withhold the drug, the patient cannot infect others.

13. The nurse knows that rifampin may not reach therapeutic levels if it is administered orally:
   a. on an empty stomach.
   b. with food.
   c. with other drugs that are metabolized by the hepatic cytochrome P450 enzymes.
   d. with protease inhibitors and NNRTIs for HIV infection.

▶ 14. A patient takes prophylactic warfarin because of a history of atrial fibrillation, which can cause the release of clots that become emboli. The patient has recently been diagnosed with tuberculosis and prescribed antimicrobial drugs including rifampin. Because of the interaction between warfarin and rifampin, it is important for the nurse to assess the patient for:
   a. abdominal pain.
   b. bleeding.
   c. change in level of consciousness.
   d. oliguria.

15. A patient has received instructions regarding TB therapy with rifampin. Which of these statements made by the client would indicate the patient needs further teaching?
    a. "I should contact my physician if I experience significantly decreased urine output."
    b. "I should contact my physician if I experience reddish colored urine."
    c. "I should contact my physician if I experience right upper quadrant pain."
    d. "I should contact my physician if I experience yellowish color to my skin or eyes."

▶ 16. The nurse is preparing to administer rifampin 420 mg intravenously. The solution was prepared by dissolving 600 mg of powdered rifampin in 10 mL of sterile water. Six mL of the prepared solution was added to a 500 mL intravenous bag of 5% dextrose. The infusion is to run over 3 hours. What is the hourly rate of infusion that the nurse should program into the intravenous infusion pump?

17. Matching (May use options more than once.)

| | |
|---|---|
| ___ a. rifabutin (Mycobutin) | 1. Administer on an empty stomach |
| ___ b. rifampin (Rifadin) | 2. Administer with food |
| ___ c. rifapentine (Priftin) | 3. Administer with or without food |
| | 4. Used to prevent disseminated MAC in HIV infected patients |
| | 5. Used to treat Hansen's disease (leprosy) |
| | 6. Used to treat tuberculosis |

18. Several second line agents for TB have the potential to damage the eighth cranial nerve. The nurse would assess for this damage by noting changes in: (Select all that apply.)
    a. balance.
    b. extraocular movements.
    c. facial movements.
    d. hearing.
    e. sense of smell.
    f. swallowing.
    g. vision.

19. Benefits of the new antitubercular drug R207910 include: (Select all that apply.)
    a. concentrates in lung tissue.
    b. does not interact with drugs for HIV.
    c. no known incidence of resistance.
    d. once a month dosing.
    e. safe for long term use.

20. Multidrug therapy for Hansen's disease (leprosy) is considered:
    a. curative.
    b. prophylactic.
    c. unnecessary.

21. Current recommendation for administration of rifampin for Hansen's disease (leprosy) is once a:
    a. day.
    b. week.
    c. month.
    d. year.

22. The nurse teaches a patient receiving dapsone for leprosy the importance of having blood specimens for complete blood count drawn if the patient has a history of:
    a. alcoholism.
    b. diabetes.
    c. G-6-PD deficiency.
    d. hypertension.

▶ 23. Which of these assessment findings, if identified in a patient who is receiving clofazimine, should the nurse report to the prescriber immediately?
    a. Absent bowel sounds in LLQ, hyperactive bowel sounds in RUQ
    b. Diarrhea
    c. Nausea
    d. Vomiting

## CASE STUDIES AND PATIENT TEACHING

*(Use a separate piece of paper for your responses.)*

### Case Study 1

*A 36-year-old, single mother, social worker is prescribed rifampin, isoniazid, ethambutol, and pyrazinamide after being diagnosed with active tuberculosis.*

1. Why is therapy for active infection always initiated with at least two drugs?
2. What information should the nurse provide to ensure that these medications are taken exactly as prescribed?
3. What obstacles might this patient face regarding compliance with drug therapy?
4. What will be necessary to determine the effectiveness of drug therapy?
5. The public health nurse is consulted regarding the need to identify all of the people who share facilities with the patient to screen them for TB and prophylactically treat the individual without active infection with isoniazid. Why is it essential to treat TB contacts prophylactically for TB?
6. When evaluating the contacts associated with an active TB patient, what considerations are made to determine whether they are candidates for isoniazid prophylactic therapy?
7. What is the drug of choice as the primary agent for treatment and prophylaxis of tuberculosis, and why is this true?
8. Two months into therapy, the nurse is reviewing laboratory results for this patient, which includes ALT 65 international units/L, AST 80 units/L, total bilirubin 0.3 mg/dL, creatinine 0.8 mg/dL, and uric acid 12 mg/dL. What questions should the nurse ask this patient?

### Case Study 2

*A homeless 45-year-old male comes to the emergency department with weight loss, lethargy, a low-grade fever, and a productive cough streaked with blood. His chest x-ray indicates a suspicious area in the middle right lobe. He is hospitalized, and sputum cultures are ordered. The sputum cultures reveal mycobacterium tuberculosis. His active TB is to be treated with a combination of drugs based on the sputum culture drug sensitivity. The patient is started on isoniazid, ethambutol, and pyrazinamide in the initial phase of therapy.*

1. What organ function is the nurse most concerned about when a patient is taking this combination of drugs? What symptoms would suggest this adverse effect?
2. What are the benefits of directly observed therapy (DOT) for this patient?
3. What interventions could the public nurse implement to improve compliance with drug therapy with this patient?
4. If this patient was found to be HIV positive, what drug-drug interactions may occur between the tuberculosis drug regime and his HIV drug therapy?
5. The nurse is evaluating the patient when he comes in for directly observed treatment. The patient reports vision changes where he feels like he is looking through a tunnel. What could possibly be causing this visual change? What should the nurse do?
6. The nurse is writing a letter to her legislator because of proposed cuts to funding for healthcare that would affect patients with tuberculosis. What could the nurse include in the letter to justify the expense of the government providing assistance for people who cannot afford to pay for therapy for TB?

# 90 Miscellaneous Antibacterial Drugs: Fluoroquinolones, Metronidazole, Daptomycin, Rifampin, Bacitracin, and Polymyxins

## OBJECTIVES

See page 26 for the Objectives.

## CRITICAL THINKING AND STUDY QUESTIONS

1. Ciprofloxacin is highly active against the microbe that commonly causes: (Select all that apply.)
   a. anthrax when used as postexposure prophylaxis.
   b. gastroenteritis from eating raw eggs.
   c. gas gangrene.
   d. methicillin resistant *Staphylococcus aureus.*
   e. pseudomembranous enterocolitis.
   f. tetanus.
   g. uncomplicated UTI.

2. The nurse assesses a 6-year-old child who is receiving ciprofloxacin (Cipro) for a complicated UTI. Which symptom is a common adverse effect of the drug?
   a. Diarrhea
   b. Pain and inflammation of the back of the heel
   c. Seizures
   d. Tooth discoloration

3. A consulting urologist orders ciprofloxacin 250 mg twice a day for a 72-year-old woman with a UTI. The patient is also receiving ferrous sulfate 300 mg for anemia and calcium carbonate 400 mg 4 times a day for osteopenia. The nurse should:
   a. administer the ciprofloxacin 1 hour before the other medications.
   b. administer the ciprofloxacin 2 hours after the other medications.
   c. consult with the prescriber regarding drug interactions.
   d. hold the ferrous sulfate and calcium during ciprofloxacin therapy.

4. The nurse is administering ciprofloxacin (Cipro) to a patient who receives theophylline for asthma. Because of potential drug interactions the nurse should monitor theophylline levels and assess for:
   a. constipation
   b. drowsiness
   c. tachycardia
   d. weakness

▶ 5. Because of common adverse effects of ciprofloxin in the elderly, a nursing priority is:
   a. altered sensory perceptions.
   b. fluid volume deficit.
   c. impaired urinary elimination.
   d. ineffective gas exchange.

6. The nurse teaches a patient who has been prescribed ciprofloxacin because of possible exposure to anthrax spores to take the medication as prescribed for a period of:
   a. 10 to 14 days.
   b. 30 days.
   c. 60 days.
   d. 6 months.

7. It is less of a priority than for other fluoroquinolones for the nurse to teach measures to prevent sunburn to a patient who is prescribed:
   a. ciprofloxacin (Cipro).
   b. lomefloxacin (Maxaquin).
   c. ofloxacin (Floxin).
   d. sparfloxacin (Zagam).

8. A common symptom of suprainfection that can occur with extended ciprofloxacin therapy is:
   a. circumoral cyanosis.
   b. high fever.
   c. pin-point maculopapular rash.
   d. white patches in the mouth.

9. Sparfloxacin (Zagam) is used for community acquired pneumonia because:
   a. absorption is not affected by dairy products, antacids, or iron.
   b. does not cause ECG changes.
   c. is effective against all common respiratory tract pathogens.
   d. is safe for children.

▶ 10. Trovafloxacin (Trovan) is reserved for life-threatening infections that cannot be treated with other antibiotics because of serious adverse effects. If the nurse is administering this drug, it is important to monitor and report the results of the:
   a. cardiogram for prolonged QT interval.
   b. liver function studies for elevations.
   c. BUN and creatinine for kidney function.
   d. CBC for agranulocytopenia.

▶ 11. When a patient is prescribed a fluoroquinolone that is known to cause prolongation of the QT interval on ECG, the nurse should monitor the electrolytes for which of the following results that are most likely to increase the risk of this adverse effect?
   a. Chloride less than 98 mEq/L
   b. Magnesium less than 1.3 mEq/L
   c. Potassium less than 3.5 mEq/L
   d. Sodium less than 135 mEq/L

12. Gemifloxacin (Factive) is generally not a preferred agent because unlike older fluoroquinolones it has a higher incidence of:
   a. interaction with dairy products.
   b. photosensitivity.
   c. prolonged QT interval.
   d. rash.

13. Metronidazole Flagyl, as an antibacterial agent:
   a. is effective against aerobic and anaerobic bacteria.
   b. is limited by rapidly developing resistance by microbes.
   c. is used as prophylaxis for gastrointestinal surgery.
   d. penetrates the CNS.
   e. should not be used if a patient ingests alcohol.

▶ 14. The nurse is preparing to administer daptomycin (Cubicin). The nurse should withhold the medication and contact the prescriber if:
   a. the patient is diagnosed with community acquired pneumonia.
   b. the patient's INR is 3.8.
   c. C&S identifies the infecting microbe as MRSA.
   d. peak and trough plasma levels have not been ordered.

▶ 15. A nursing measure to prevent the most common adverse effect of daptomycin (Cubicin) is to:
   a. dim the lights in the room.
   b. elevate the intravenous site.
   c. limit noise in the halls during the night.
   d. provide adequate fluid and fiber in the diet.

▶ 16. Which of the following laboratory tests should be monitored weekly to assess for the most common serious adverse effect if patient is prescribed daptomycin (Cubicin)?
   a. ALT
   b. CBC
   c. CPK
   d. Creatinine

▶ 17. The nurse is preparing to administer daptomycin (Cubicin). The patient has an intravenous infusion of 5% dextrose in 0.45% sodium chloride infusing at a rate of 125 mL/hr. What action should the nurse take?

18. The physician has asked the nurse to provide teaching for a 34-year-old female patient who has requested a prescription for rifaximin (Xifaxan) before a mission trip to Central America. Teaching should include not administering the drug if the patient experiences:
   a. amenorrhea
   b. bloody stool
   c. defecation urgency
   d. fever
   e. flatulence
   f. nausea

## CASE STUDIES AND PATIENT TEACHING

*(Use a separate piece of paper for your responses.)*

### Case Study 1

*A 68-year-old patient with a history of HF, diabetes, and chronic bronchitis presents to the emergency department with dyspnea, productive cough, and fever. Examination reveals pulse oximetry 89%, decreased breath sounds, thick, purulent sputum, tachycardia, and extensive use of accessory muscles of respirations. Home medications include glyburide, digoxin, and furosemide. The patient is diagnosed with acute bacterial exacerbation of chronic bronchitis. Intravenous gatifloxacin (Tequin) 400 mg once a day and methylprednisolone are prescribed.*

1. Intravenous gatifloxacin (Tequin) is supplied as 400 mg/200 mL. There are no specific directions for the amount of time for infusing the medication. What would be the minimum time for infusing this dose of gatifloxacin?

2. What are early symptoms of possible drug interactions that could occur?

3. Why is it particularly important for the nurse to assess renal functioning of this patient?

4. The patient's creatinine clearance is 35 mL/min. What action should the nurse take?

5. The patient stabilizes after 48 hours and is switched to oral gatifloxacin. Plans are made for discharge. What teaching should the nurse providing regarding the administration of this medication?

6. What symptoms of significant adverse effects of gatifloxcin should the nurse teach the patient to report to the prescriber?

### Case Study 2

*A 68-year-old female, returns to her physician after taking 10 days of ampicillin for her upper respiratory infection. She continues with a low-grade fever and does not seem to have improved. She has a productive cough and thick secretions. Her x-ray does not indicate pneumonia. The patient has a past history of atrial fibrillation, for which she takes an anticoagulant. She is given ciprofloxacin 250 mg, orally, 2 times a day for 7 more days. The nurse in the physician's office wants to be sure she understands this medication.*

1. What in the patient's history may contribute to potential drug-drug interactions?

2. What foods should the patient avoid when taking oral ciprofloxacin?

3. The patient calls the physician's office in two days to report that she is much better. She asks whether she can stop taking the medication since it is so expensive and she is improving so much. How should the nurse respond?

4. What new problem might the patient develop while taking this antibiotic?

# 91 Antifungal Agents

## OBJECTIVES

See page 26 for the Objectives.

## CRITICAL THINKING AND STUDY QUESTIONS

1. Amphotericin B: (Select all that apply.)
   a. causes some damage to the kidneys.
   b. doses must be decreased if creatinine clearance is less than 40 mL/min.
   c. fungal resistance is rare.
   d. has broad spectrum bacteriocidal activity.
   e. is toxic to human cells.
   f. readily penetrates the CNS.
   g. remains in human tissue more than a year after treatment is discontinued.

2. At what point is the patient most likely to experience fever, chills, rigors, nausea, and headache when receiving amphotericin B?
   a. Immediately after the infusion begins
   b. 20 to 30 minutes after the infusion begins
   c. 1 to 3 hours after the infusion begins
   d. 3 to 6 hours after the infusion begins

3. A patient receiving amphotericin B experiences sudden episodes of shaking chills after receiving a dose of amphotericin B. Which of the following drugs, which are ordered as needed for this patient, should the nurse administer at this time?
   a. acetaminophen
   b. dantrolene (Dantrium)
   c. diphenhydramine (Benadryl)
   d. lorazepam (Ativan)

4. The nurse is reviewing laboratory tests before preparing to administer a dose of amphotericin B. The patient's creatinine level is 3 mg/dL. The nurse should:
   a. administer the medication.
   b. administer the medication and assess intake and output.
   c. withhold the medication and assess skin color.
   d. withhold the medication and page the prescriber STAT.

5. Because amphotericin causes fungal death by increasing leakage of intracellular cations, it is important for the nurse to assess the patient for:
   a. abdominal cramps and peaked T waves on ECG.
   b. positive Chvostek's and Trousseau's signs.
   c. thirst and flushed skin.
   d. weakness and abdominal distention.

6. Which of the following laboratory results of an adult male patient suggest bone marrow suppression caused by amphotericin B?
   a. Hemoglobin 10 g/dL; hematocrit 30%; MCV 110 $\mu m^3$; MCH 28 pg/cell
   b. Hemoglobin 10 g/dL; hematocrit 30%; MCV 67 $\mu m^3$; MCH 30 pg/cell
   c. Hemoglobin 10 g/dL; hematocrit 30%; MCV 89 $\mu m^3$; MCH 28 pg/cell
   d. Hemoglobin 10 g/dL; hematocrit 30%; MCV 105 $\mu m^3$; MCH 20 pg/cell

7. A patient with a systemic fungal infection is prescribed amphotericin B and flucytosine. The nurse expects the drug interaction of:
   a. decreased risk of amphotericin toxicity.
   b. increased risk of renal damage.
   c. increased risk of rigors.
   d. potentiation of amphotericin effect.

8. Itraconazole is:
   a. always administered intravenously.
   b. capable of inhibiting hepatic metabolizing enzymes.
   c. effective against more fungi than amphotericin.
   d. nephrotoxic.

9. To achieve maximum absorption of itraconazole (Sporanox) capsules, the nurse administers the drug with:
   a. bread.
   b. milk.
   c. Pepsi-cola.
   d. water.

▶ 10. The nurse is reviewing test results for a patient who is prescribed itraconazole (Sporanox). Which of the following results would warrant immediate consultation with the prescriber?
   a. AST 35 International Units/L
   b. BNP 145 pg/mL
   c. Echocardiogram—ejection fraction 75%
   d. Potassium 3.8 mEq/L

▶ 11. The nurse is administering itraconazole (Sporanox) to a patient who has a history of hypertension treated with hydrochlorothiazide and diabetes treated with metformin and glyburide. Because of drug interactions the nurse should monitor the patient for symptoms of:
   a. hypoglycemia.
   b. hypotension.
   c. hyperglycemia.
   d. hypertension.

12. Which of the following drugs may prevent absorption of itraconazole (Sporanox) no matter when they are administered?
   a. cyclosporin (Sandimmune)
   b. digoxin (Lanoxin)
   c. esomeprazole (Nexium)
   d. ranitidine (Zantac)

▶ 13. Which of these patient findings would suggest a significant adverse effect when the nurse is administering fluconazole (Diflucan)?
   a. Abdominal pain
   b. Diarrhea
   c. Oral and ocular rash
   d. Nausea

▶ 14. The nurse is most concerned about alterations in metabolism of several of the antifungal drugs that are metabolized by the P-450 cytochrome system if a patient's diet includes:
   a. dairy products.
   b. grapefruit.
   c. green leafy vegetables.
   d. red meat.

▶ 15. The nurse reviews the laboratory results of a patient who is prescribed voriconazole (Vfend) 200 mg by mouth and notes that the creatinine clearance is 35 mL/min. The nurse should:
   a. administer the medication.
   b. consult the prescriber.
   c. withhold the medication.

▶ 16. A patient who has been receiving ketoconazole (Nizoral) for 5 days experiences nausea and vomiting. The initial response of the nurse should be to:
   a. administer the medication with food.
   b. assess the skin, abdomen, urine, and stool.
   c. consult the prescriber.
   d. withhold the medication.

▶ 17. When administering drugs that are potentially nephrotoxic, the nurse avoids administration of which over-the-counter drugs?
   a. Antacids
   b. Acetaminophen
   c. NSAIDs
   d. Laxatives

18. What can the nurse teach a patient who is prescribed flucytosine (Ancobon) to prevent nausea and vomiting?
   a. Take the medication over a 15-minute interval
   b. Take the medication with a cola beverage
   c. Take the medication with food
   d. Take the medication with milk

▶ 19. The nurse reviews the CBC of a patient who is prescribed flucytosine (Ancobon) and notes neutropenia. This patient is especially at risk for:
   a. fatigue.
   b. fluid volume deficit.
   c. impaired skin integrity.
   d. infection.

▶ 20. The nurse would be concerned that a patient who is receiving caspofungin is experiencing a histamine reaction if the patient reports:
a. coughing.
b. feeling flushed.
c. headache.
d. nausea.

21. Which of the following antifungal agents could cause adverse effects that are developmentally unacceptable to a 22-year-old male?
a. fluconazole (Diflucan)
b. itraconazole (Sporanox)
c. ketoconazole (Nizoral)
d. voriconazole (Vfend)

22. Matching: Site of fungal infection

| | |
|---|---|
| ___ a. Tinea capitis | 1. Body |
| ___ b. Tinea corporis | 2. Foot |
| ___ c. Tinea cruris | 3. Groin |
| ___ d. Tinea pedis | 4. Scalp |

23. A common cause of recurrence of tinea corporis is:

24. The medication administration record lists a clotrimazole troche to be administered at 0900. The nurse administers this medication by:
a. applying it to the skin.
b. dissolving it in 8 ounces of water.
c. instructing the patient to chew it.
d. instructing the patient to let it dissolve in the mouth.

▶ 25. A postoperative knee replacement surgery patient is prescribed Lovenox (low-molecular-weight heparin) to prevent clot formation related to immobility. The patient develops candidiasis under the breasts and in the groin. The physician prescribes miconazole cream. The nurse should:
a. administer both the Lovenox and miconazole.
b. administer the Lovenox, but consult the prescriber regarding the miconazole.
c. administer the miconazole but consult the prescriber regarding the Lovenox.
d. withhold both the Lovenox and miconazole and consult the prescriber.

26. What is a potential problem with using over-the-counter miconazole for vaginal discharge?
a. Local irritation
b. Systemic toxicity
c. The cause may not be a yeast infection
d. The treatment is usually not effective

## CASE STUDIES AND PATIENT TEACHING

*(Use a separate piece of paper for your responses.)*

### Case Study 1

*A 25-year-old female was recently diagnosed with acute myelogenous leukemia (AML). She is admitted for the induction phase of chemotherapy. Her platelet count is low, and she has vaginal candidiasis. Topical treatments for vaginal candidiasis are available over-the-counter.*

1. What problems might this produce?

2. The treatment of choice for this patient's fungal infection is clotrimazole. It is essential that extreme care be taken in providing nursing care to this patient because she is at high risk for additional infections that could now be lethal. There are many areas that the nurse must consider when treatment includes combining the treatment for fungus with the numerous other physical problems faced by a patient with AML. The nurse must teach this patient to report what possible adverse effects of intravaginal clotrimazole tablets used for vaginal infection?

3. The patient asks why she must use the vaginal tablets when she already has an IV for chemotherapy administration. What should the nurse tell her?

4. The patient's fungal infection has advanced because of her severely immunocompromised state. She now has systemic mycoses requiring amphotericin B for treatment. All of her medications must be carefully evaluated to determine whether they are toxic. What system is almost always damaged in some way by amphotericin B and can increase the risk of toxicity of other drugs?

5. What intervention can the nurse employ to reduce the risk of kidney damage by amphotericin B?

6. Why is it important for the prescriber to first order a 1-mg test dose of amphotericin B (Fungizone) before starting full therapy?

7. The drug book recommends after a successful test dose that the first dose of amphotericin B should be 0.25 mg/kg of drug. The patient weighs 110 lbs. The physician has prescribed 12 mg. Is this a safe dose?

8. The amphotericin B vial is dispensed as a powder. This 50 mg of powder must be reconstituted using 10 mL of sterile water that does not contain a bacteriostatic agent to a concentration of 5 mg/mL. This solution is further diluted in sterile water to provide a concentration of 0.1 mg/mL for infusion. Why must the drug be mixed this way?

9. How much solution will the nurse administer if the drug is diluted to 0.1 mg/mL, and the prescribed dose is 12 mg?

10. What nursing measures should the nurse take when infusing amphotericin to prevent infusion related adverse effects?

## Case Study 2

1. What can the nurse teach to decrease the incidence and complications of opportunistic infections in:
   a. the general population?
   b. debilitated patients?
   c. immunocompromised patients?

## Case Study 3

*A 42-year-old truck driver has been prescribed voriconazole (Vfend) for esophageal candidiasis secondary to immune deficiency caused by HIV.*

1. What teaching does the nurse need to provide this patient regarding drug therapy?

2. Why is this patient more at risk for hepatotoxicity and drug interactions than the average person?

# 92 Antiviral Agents I: Drugs for Non-HIV Viral Infections

## OBJECTIVES

See page 26 for the Objectives.

## CRITICAL THINKING AND STUDY QUESTIONS

1. A significant challenge to scientists who are trying to develop antiviral drugs is developing a drug that:
   a. can be administered orally.
   b. does not harm human tissue.
   c. is broad spectrum.
   d. is not metabolized by the liver.

2. When researching antiviral drugs and vaccines, epidemiologically, it is a priority for the researchers to identify if the drug decreases:
   a. active viral shedding.
   b. duration of illness.
   c. frequency of symptomatic episodes.
   d. symptoms.

3. A college student who has been diagnosed with her first genital herpes infection is discussing the disorder and prescribed topical acyclovir treatment with the college health center nurse. Which of the following statements, if made by the patient, would suggest that the patient needs teaching about this disorder and drug therapy?
   a. "I can get a different infection in the sores if I am not careful about cleaning after having a bowel movement."
   b. "I should use gloves when applying the ointment, immediately dispose of them, then wash my hands because I can spread the infection to other parts of my body."
   c. "If I apply the ointment as prescribed, it will decrease the chance that I spread the infection but the sores won't heal faster."
   d. "Using the ointment as soon as I feel the first signs of a new outbreak may decrease the severity of the outbreak."

▶ 4. What should the nurse teach a patient who is currently in a long-term committed monogamous relationship and who has been prescribed continuous oral acyclovir therapy for recurrent genital herpes regarding condom use?
   a. Condoms prevent the spread of infection, even during active outbreaks.
   b. Use a condom if any symptoms of outbreak are present.
   c. Use a condom with every sexual contact except if outbreak-free, and conception is desired.
   d. Your partner is already infected so condom use does not matter.

▶ 5. Which of the following actions by the nurse is most effective in preventing the most common complications of intravenous acyclovir (Zovirax) therapy?
   a. Assessing the intravenous site before infusing the drug
   b. Ensuring a fluid intake of 2500 to 3000 mL/24 hr
   c. Reporting vomiting to the prescriber
   d. Teaching perineal hygiene

▶ 6. The nurse is caring for a patient who is receiving intravenous acyclovir therapy. Which of the following assessment findings would be of most concern?
   a. Creatinine 0.9 mg/dL
   b. Dry, sticky mucous membranes
   c. Eight-hour urine output 750 mL
   d. Temperature 102° F

▶ 7. Which of the following laboratory results would be most significant to the nurse if a patient is receiving valacyclovir (Valtrex)?
   a. CD4 100/mm$^3$
   b. Hgb (Hb) 11 g/dL
   c. Platelets 220,000/mm$^3$
   d. WBC 12,800/mm$^3$

▶ 8. Because of possible organ damage, which of these factors identified in the history of an immunocompromised patient receiving ganciclovir for a CMV infection, would be of most concern to the nurse?
   a. Chronic obstructive pulmonary disease
   b. Diabetes mellitus
   c. Duodenal ulcer
   d. Hepatitis C

▶ 9. The nurse would withhold ganciclovir and notify the prescriber if patient laboratory test results include:
   a. BUN 20 mg/dL.
   b. HCG positive.
   c. neutrophils 2000/mm$^3$.
   d. platelets 75,000/m$^3$.

▶ 10. The nurse is discussing planned care with the certified nursing assistant who is assigned to a patient who is receiving oral ganciclovir for CMV retinitis. Which of the following precautions would the nurse include in instructions regarding care?
   a. Do not provide any food 1 hour before or 2 hours after drug administration.
   b. Elevate all 4 side rails.
   c. Turn and reposition the patient every 2 hours.
   d. Use an electric razor to shave the patient.

▶ 11. Which of the following steps is most important for the nurse to follow when administering valganciclovir?
   a. Administer with the patient in an upright position.
   b. Assess vital signs before administering the drug.
   c. Dissolve the drug completely in 8 ounces of water or juice.
   d. Wear gloves when handling the tablet.

▶ 12. When administering adefovir (Hepsera), which of the following assessments would suggest that therapy could be toxic?
   a. Decreased sperm count
   b. Nausea
   c. Oliguria
   d. Yellow-colored sclera

▶ 13. Laboratory results for a patient who is prescribed foscarnet (Foscavir) include FBS 90 mg/dL, AST 87 Units/L, potassium 3.6 mEq/L, calcium 8.4 mg/dL, and magnesium 2 mEq/L. The nurse should assess for:
   a. cool, clammy skin.
   b. headache.
   c. muscle spasms.
   d. thirst.

▶ 14. A patient is being seen for his weekly infusion of cidofovir for CMV retinitis. Which of the following assessment findings would warrant not administering the medication and consulting the prescriber?
   a. Dyspnea and distended neck veins
   b. Headache and tense muscles
   c. Photophobia and blurred vision
   d. Rhinorrhea and cough

15. When explaining prescribed pegylated interferon (peginterferon), the nurse should include that, compared with conventional interferon, this drug:
   a. can be administered orally.
   b. prevents relapse when discontinued.
   c. produces less adverse effects.
   d. produces more consistent therapeutic blood levels.

16. It is important for the nurse to assess for suicidal ideation if a patient is prescribed:
   a. interferon alfa.
   b. lamivudine.
   c. ribavirin.
   d. valacyclovir.

17. When administering ribavirin and interferon alfa for hepatitis C, loss of detectable serum HCV RNA for at least what period of time after cessation of treatment would indicate that therapy has achieved the desired effect?
   a. 6 weeks
   b. 6 months
   c. 1 year
   d. 5 years

18. When teaching a patient self-administration of subcutaneous interferon alfa, the nurse should stress the importance of:
   a. applying pressure to the site after injection to prevent hematoma formation.
   b. aspirating to check for blood before injecting.
   c. changing the needle after drawing the solution into the syringe.
   d. sterile technique.

19. The nurse teaches sexually active patients who are prescribed ribavirin of the need to use two reliable forms of contraception during treatment and for at least what period of time after treatment ends?
   a. 1 month
   b. 3 months
   c. 6 months
   d. 12 months

▶ 20. Which of these assessment findings, if identified in a patient who is receiving lamivudine (Epivir HBV), adefovir (Hepsera), or entecavir (Baraclude) for hepatitis B, should the nurse report to the prescriber immediately?
   a. Deep rapid breathing
   b. Fever
   c. Poor appetite
   d. Nausea

▶ 21. A patient is prescribed adefovir (Hepsera) 10 mg by mouth once a day. Results of her most recent laboratory tests include CrCl 62 mL/min. The nurse should:
   a. administer the medication as prescribed.
   b. consult the prescriber regarding the need for dose reduction.
   c. withhold the medication and contact the prescriber immediately.

▶ 22. The nurse would withhold administration of intranasal LAIV (FluMist) and consult the prescriber regarding which of the following patients?
   a. 7-year-old male with a seizure disorder
   b. 12-year-old female receiving aspirin for its cardioprotective effects
   c. 28-year-old male with type 1 diabetes
   d. 38-year-old female with multiple sclerosis

23. When preparing to administer a dose of LAIV (FluMist) for a 5-year-old child, who has never received a flu vaccine in the past, the office nurse notes a dose sitting on the counter. The seal is intact, and the expiration date is okay. On questioning, no other nurse remembers getting the dose out, and no other nurse needs the drug. The nurse should:
    a. administer 1 spray in each nostril.
    b. administer 1 spray in each nostril and remind the parents that a second dose will be needed in about 7 to 10 weeks.
    c. discard the dose and thaw a new dose, administering 1 spray in each nostril.
    d. discard the dose and thaw a new dose, administering 1 spray in each nostril and remind the parents that a second dose will be needed in about 7 to 10 weeks.

▶ 24. A priority of nursing teaching to a patient prescribed amantadine (Symmetrel) for influenza prophylaxis is:
    a. elimination.
    b. fluid volume.
    c. nutrition.
    d. safety.

25. The nurse is aware that the most significant factor in determining the effectiveness of oseltamivir (Tamiflu) in treating influenza is:
    a. administration with food.
    b. influenza A is the causative organism.
    c. starting therapy as soon as symptoms occur.
    d. vaccination for influenza has already been administered.

▶ 26. Which of the following new assessment findings would be most significant if noted in an infant who is receiving inhaled ribavirin for RSV?
    a. Coarse rhonchi (gurgles) in upper airways
    b. Pulse 120 beats/min
    c. Respirations 30 per minute
    d. Wheezing throughout lung fields

▶ 27. A child is scheduled for an appointment at 1000 at the pediatrician's office to receive a second dose of palivizumab (Synagis). When should the nurse prepare the drug for administration?
    a. 0940
    b. 1000
    c. When directed by the pediatrician
    d. When the parent and child arrives

## CASE STUDIES AND PATIENT TEACHING

*(Use a separate piece of paper for your responses.)*

### Case Study 1

*A 25-year-old married female graduate student comes to the college health center clinic complaining of painful sores in her genital region. She has a round ulcerated area on the labia minora and also on the cervix. She informs the nurse that she plans to get pregnant in the near future. She states she had these "sores" 3 months ago, but thought they were caused by the irritation of swimming every day. The CRNP diagnoses herpes simplex genitalis and prescribes oral acyclovir. The patient states that she hates to take pills and has heard that this drug is available in a cream.*

1. What information can the nurse provide as to why oral acyclovir was ordered instead of the topical acyclovir?
2. The patient asks whether this medication will cure the herpes. How should the nurse respond?
3. What information should the nurse provide regarding transmission of genital herpes?
4. How should the nurse respond to the woman's concerns about how this infection will affect her becoming pregnant?

### Case Study 2

*An elderly patient who has a history of smoking, DM, hypertension, and COPD has come to the flu shot clinic at the public health department to receive a flu vaccine.*

1. What questions should the nurse ask the patient before administering the vaccine?
2. If the patient complains of coughing and runny nose, should the vaccination be withheld?

3. The patient is complaining to the nurse about needing to get a flu shot every year. She hates the shot and has heard that people can still get the flu after receiving the shot. She asks why they cannot just come up with a pill that is effective to treat the infection. What could the nurse include in her explanation?

4. The patient asks why she cannot get the nasal spray that her grandson received yesterday. What is a possible explanation for why this drug is limited to people aged 5 to 49 years?

5. What teaching should the nurse provide regarding close contact with her grandson?

## Case Study 3

*The public health nurse receives a call from a school nurse questioning whether a child who received intranasal LAIV (FluMist) should be in school. The nurse is concerned because the child's teacher is pregnant.*

1. How should the nurse respond?

2. What intervention would be most important for the school nurse to emphasize when discussing with the teacher prevention of becoming infected with influenza from active cases or live vaccine?

# 93 Antiviral Agents II: Drugs for HIV Infection and Related Opportunistic Infections

## OBJECTIVES

See page 26 for the Objectives.

## CRITICAL THINKING AND STUDY QUESTIONS

1. Match drug and mechanism of action.

| | | |
|---|---|---|
| ___ a. Fusion inhibitor | 1. | Hampers the enzyme that promotes copying of RNA to DNA |
| ___ b. Protease inhibitors | 2. | Prevent HIV from maturing into infectious form |
| ___ c. Reverse transcriptase | 3. | Prevents joining of host and HIV cell membranes |

▶ 2. Which of the following assessment findings would best indicate that highly active antiretroviral therapy (HAART) is currently effective?
   a. CD4 T count 1100 cells/mm$^3$
   b. Neutrophils 2750/mm$^3$
   c. Plasma HIV RNA 100,000 virions/mL
   d. WBC 5000/mm$^3$

3. The nurse is teaching a patient about the need for multiple-drug therapy for HIV. Which of the following statements, if made by the patient, would indicate a need for further teaching?
   a. "If I don't take all of the drugs as prescribed, the virus is more likely to become resistant to drugs."
   b. "The higher the number of viruses in my body, the greater the chance one will become resistant."
   c. "The virus recognizes the antibiotic and is able to change to prevent being destroyed."
   d. "When the HIV is changing RNA into DNA within the host cell, genetic changes can occur spontaneously."

▸ 4. The nurse is caring for an AIDS patient admitted with *P. carinii* pneumonia. The patient's HAART includes zidovudine (Retrovir). Which of the following assessment findings would be of most concern to the nurse?
   a. Deep rapid breathing
   b. Rales (crackles) in lower lobes
   c. Temperature 101.6° F
   d. Warm, moist skin

▸ 5. Which nursing intervention can decrease the risk of lactic acidosis in a patient who is prescribed zidovudine (Retrovir)?
   a. Encouraging coughing and deep breathing
   b. Maintaining adequate hydration
   c. Monitor blood glucose
   d. Preventing skin breakdown

6. The prescriber has informed a patient who has been prescribed an NRTI of the risk of hepatic steatosis. The patient asks the nurse "What is hepatic steatosis?" The nurse should explain that this is a possible severe adverse effect involving:
   a. fatty degeneration of the liver.
   b. increased secretions of glands.
   c. infection of the liver.
   d. stools that are foamy and float.

7. The nurse is preparing to administer 60 mg of intravenous zidovudine to a patient who weighs 135 lbs. Before administering this dose, the nurse would ensure that it was diluted in at least:
   a. 2 mL of bacteriostatic water.
   b. 5 mL of sterile water.
   c. 15 mL of 5% dextrose for injection.
   d. 50 mL of normal saline.

▸ 8. An HIV-positive patient is prescribed trimethoprim-sulfamethoxazole for a urinary tract infection (UTI). Which of the following laboratory tests are extremely important for the nurse to monitor? (Select all that apply.)
   a. AST and ALT
   b. BUN and creatinine
   c. CBC and differential
   d. Electrolytes
   e. Lipids
   f. PT and INR

9. A patient has received instructions regarding administration of didanosine (Videx EC). Which of these statements made by the patient would indicate the patient understood the directions?
   a. "I can open this capsule and sprinkle the contents on applesauce."
   b. "I need to notify the prescriber if I cannot swallow this capsule whole."
   c. "I should keep the medicine in my bathroom medicine cabinet so I remember to take it every morning."
   d. "I should take this drug with meals."

▸ 10. Which of these nursing assessment findings would be most significant if a patient was receiving didanosine?
   a. Diarrhea
   b. Mental slowness
   c. Tremors
   d. Vomiting

▸ 11. A patient receiving HAART develops a sore throat and cough. Which of the following drugs, if part of the HAART, should the nurse immediately withhold and notify the prescriber?
   a. abacavir (Ziagen)
   b. didanosine (Videx)
   c. stavudine (Zerit)
   d. zidovudine (Retrovir)

12. Nursing interventions and teaching relating to the most common adverse effects of efavirenz (Sustiva) should focus on:
   a. circulation.
   b. nutrition.
   c. safety.
   d. skin integrity.

▸ 13. When a patient who is receiving nevirapine (Viramune) or delavirdine (Rescriptor) complains of muscle and joint pain, it would be important for the nurse to assess if the patient is also experiencing:
   a. dizziness.
   b. nausea.
   c. paresthesias.
   d. rash.

14. It would be a priority for the nurse to inform the prescriber that an HIV-positive patient has admitted to engaging in unprotected sex if the patient's HAART includes:
    a. efavirenz (Sustiva).
    b. emtricitabine (Emtriva).
    c. indinavir (Crixivan).
    d. zidovudine (Retrovir).

▶ 15. An HIV-positive patient who has recently been prescribed a HAART, including the NNRTI efavirenz, calls the prescriber's office and reports experiencing drowsiness and dizziness. An appropriate recommendation by the telephone triage nurse is for the patient to:
    a. discontinue all drugs and make an appointment to be seen as soon as possible.
    b. discontinue taking the drug, but continue the other drugs in the regimen.
    c. take the drug at bedtime.
    d. take the drug with food.

16. Weight-bearing exercise and adequate calcium intake are most important if HAART includes a:
    a. fusion inhibitor.
    b. nucleotide reverse transcriptase inhibitor (NRTI).
    c. nonnucleotide reverse transcriptase inhibitor (NNRTI).
    d. protease inhibitor (PI).

17. The nurse would be most concerned that the patient may not adhere to HAART therapy with which of the following classes of antiviral drugs if the patient verbalized that body image is an important priority?
    a. Fusion inhibitor
    b. Nucleotide reverse transcriptase inhibitor (NRTI)
    c. Nonnucleotide reverse transcriptase inhibitor (NNRTI)
    d. Protease inhibitor (PI)

18. The nurse is aware that the HIV-seropositive community often shares the belief that garlic supplementation decreases HIV reproduction and boosts the immune system. This belief can be particularly dangerous if the patient is prescribed:
    a. indinavir.
    b. lopinavir.
    c. nelfinavir.
    d. saquinavir.

19. Patients who are prescribed protease inhibitors (PI) should be instructed to not self-prescribe the herbal product St. John's wort because this product can increase the:
    a. MAO inhibitor effects of the St. John's wort.
    b. likelihood of suicidal ideation.
    c. likelihood of toxicity from the PI.
    d. rate of metabolism and decrease the blood levels of the PI.

▶ 20. Which of these assessment findings would be most significant if a patient was receiving the PI amprenavir (Agenerase)?
    a. Macular rash and perineal itching
    b. Nausea and vomiting
    c. Tachycardia and hyperventilation
    d. Tingling around the mouth and unusual taste to food

21. When taking a history from a 27-year-old woman who has just been prescribed amprenavir oral solution, which of the following methods of birth control used by the patient would be of most concern to the nurse?
    a. Diaphragm
    b. Latex condom
    c. Mirena IUD
    d. Yasmin 28 oral contraceptive

▶ 22. Which of the following, if identified in the history of a patient who has been taking atazanavir (Reyataz), would be most important for the nurse to report to the prescriber immediately?
    a. Diabetes treated with a sulfonylurea
    b. Erectile dysfunction treated with sildenafil
    c. GERD treated with a proton pump inhibitor
    d. Hyperlipidemia treated with a statin

23. The nurse has just provided instructions regarding administration of enfuvirtide (Fuzeon). Which of these statements made by the patient would indicate the need for further teaching?
    a. "I need to refrigerate the dissolved powder for up to 24 hours if I do not use it immediately after mixing."
    b. "I should discontinue using the drug if it causes a rash or itching at the injection site."
    c. "I should inject the drug into the fat beneath the skin of my belly or thigh."
    d. "I should inspect the solution for discoloration, bubbles, and undissolved particles before drawing it up into the syringe."

24. Which of these assessment findings, if identified in a patient who is receiving enfuvirtide (Fuzeon), should the nurse report to the prescriber immediately? (Select all that apply.)
    a. Chills
    b. Dizziness
    c. Headache
    d. Pain at injection site
    e. Positive pregnancy test
    f. Sudden muscle weakness in the legs

25. The recommended dose of enfuvirtide (Fuzeon) for an 8-year-old child who weighs 44 lbs is:
    a. 20 mg.
    b. 40 mg.
    c. 45 mg.
    d. 90 mg.

26. What is the most important role of the nurse when treatment failure occurs?
    a. Identifying individual factors that may have contributed to treatment failure
    b. Identifying the patient's immune status
    c. Supporting the patient emotionally
    d. Teaching the new drug regimen

27. Principles of treating HIV-seropositive pregnant women include: (Select all that apply.)
    a. administering the drugs to the neonate.
    b. benefits of treatment normally outweigh risks.
    c. considering C-section for delivery.
    d. HAART should not be used during pregnancy.
    e. the drugs are not teratogenic.
    f. the drug regimen should only include one drug at a time.

28. When emptying a urinal from an HIV-seropositive patient, the nurse splashes urine on intact skin. The nurse should:
    a. go to the emergency room at the end of the shift for blood work.
    b. immediately go to the emergency department for initiation of postexposure prophylaxis (PEP).
    c. make an appointment with his/her primary care provider on the next off day to discuss if postexposure prophylaxis (PEP) is appropriate
    d. report the incident immediately to a supervisor

## CASE STUDIES AND PATIENT TEACHING

*(Use a separate piece of paper for your responses.)*

### Case Study 1

*A 30-year-old female has been HIV seropositive for 4 years. She had been prescribed the highly active antiretroviral therapy (HAART), including zidovudine (Retrovir), indinavir (Crixivan), and lamivudine (Epivir), but until now she has never taken any antiviral agent.*

1. What are reasons for an HIV-seropositive patient, who does not feel ill, being prescribed drug therapy?

2. The patient asks if there are any reasons for not taking HAART when she still feels well. How should the nurse respond?

3. The patient asks the nurse why she feels better now than she did when she was first diagnosed. How can the nurse explain the presence of symptoms during the initial phase and lack of symptoms during the middle phase?

4. The patient asks why she needs so many drugs. She would rather take a large dose of one drug than multiple doses of different drugs. How should the nurse respond?

5. When consulting with the prescriber, what might the nurse discuss that might increase the chance that this patient will adhere to drug therapy?

6. The patient agrees to start taking the prescribed drugs. The original HAART included zidovudine (Retrovir), indinavir (Crixivan), and lamivudine (Epivir). The prescriber changes the HAART to zidovudine, saquinavir (Invirase), and lamivudine to improve the likelihood of adherence. The patient asks the nurse why the physician wants her to take saquinavir instead of indinavir. How can the nurse explain this change?

7. What symptoms of adverse effects of these NRTIs should the nurse teach the patient to report to the prescriber?
   a. zidovudine (Retrovir)
   b. lamivudine (Epivir)

8. What interventions can the nurse teach to prevent adverse effects from the protease inhibitor saquinavir (Invirase)?

9. The patient is sexually active. What teaching should the nurse provide to this patient regarding the possibility of pregnancy?

## Case Study 2

*A 38-year-old male who has been HIV seropositive for 12 years comes to the emergency department complaining of anorexia, nausea, chest and abdominal pain. He is currently prescribed a HAART of lopinavir, lamivudine, and stavudine.*

1. What factors relating to this drug therapy would support a triage nurse's decision to have this patient evaluated immediately?

2. During assessment the emergency department nurse notes a pale and anxious patient who weighs 147 lbs and is 5 feet 10 inches tall. Temperature is 103.2° F, BP 90/65 mm/Hg, pulse 118 beats/min, respirations 27 and labored. Crackles are noted throughout the lung fields with bronchial breath sounds in the upper lobes. The nurse notes a cough productive of purulent sputum and multiple enlarged lymph nodes. Chest x-ray, laboratory, and sputum specimens are obtained. Laboratory results include troponin I 0.01 ng/mL; troponin T 0.1 ng/mL; CPK 68 Units/mL; CK MB 0.2%; WBC 750/mm$^3$, neutrophil count 500/mL; CD4 T 180 cells/mL; hemoglobin 7.5 gm/dL; hematocrit 22.7%; AST 65 Units/L; BUN 27 mg/dL; and creatinine 1.4 mg/dL. What nursing concerns must the unit nurse address after receiving this report when planning for transfer of this patient to the nursing unit?

3. The patient is diagnosed with *P. carinii* pneumonia and dehydration and is prescribed for antibiotic therapy with pentamidine (Pentam) and intravenous fluids. What precautions must the nurse take when administering this antibiotic?

4. The patient develops rapport with the nurse and expresses his fears. He has heard from friends that there is a new injected drug that "works wonders." The nurse facilitates the patient in verbalizing his concerns and thoughts with his physician. What reason might the prescriber have for not prescribing enfuvirtide (Fuzeon) at this time for this patient?

## Case Study 3

*A 35-year-old male has been HIV seropositive for 12 years. His HAART includes zidovudine. When being interviewed by the nurse during a routine clinic appointment, he complains of declining vision, headaches, and daily temperature elevations. Physical examination findings include multiple enlarged lymph nodes and several white retinal patches.*

1. What complications of HIV are likely to be occurring?

2. The patient is diagnosed with CMV retinitis. The treatment of choice for CMV retinitis caused by cytomegalovirus (CMV) is ganciclovir. What concern does the nurse have about the addition of ganciclovir to a drug regimen including zidovudine?

3. The physician wants to begin with intravenous therapy. What strategies can the nurse employ when administering intravenous ganciclovir to reduce the risk of and identify possible damage to the patient's renal system?

4. The patient tells the nurse that he has no job or insurance at present. What would the nurse be concerned about?

## Case Study 4

1. What are important contributions that the nurse can make toward improving outcomes for patients infected with the human immunodeficiency virus (HIV)?

# 94 Drug Therapy of Sexually Transmitted Diseases

## OBJECTIVES

See page 26 for the Objectives.

## CRITICAL THINKING AND STUDY QUESTIONS

1. The nurse obtains the most accurate information about drug therapy for sexually transmitted diseases from the:
   a. Centers for Disease Control and Prevention.
   b. drug manufacturers.
   c. Food and Drug Administration.
   d. textbooks.

2. Annual screening for *Chlamydia trachomatis* is recommended for all sexually active women under the age of:
   a. 20 years.
   b. 25 years.
   c. 30 years.
   d. 35 years.

3. Doxycycline would not be prescribed for a female patient for whom pregnancy status is unknown because it:
   a. can damage fetal bones.
   b. causes nausea.
   c. is hepatotoxic.
   d. is not effective 25% of the time.

4. A patient asks why she has been prescribed doxycycline 100 mg twice a day for a chlamydia infection when a friend was prescribed a single dose of azithromycin. What factors must be considered when a prescriber is selecting an antibiotic for a patient?
   a. Sensitivity of the microbe to the antibiotic
   b. Patient allergies
   c. Possible adverse effects
   d. Other drugs the patient needs to take
   e. Pregnancy and breast-feeding status
   f. Patient conditions, such as renal or liver impairment, that might affect metabolism and/or excretion of a drug
   g. Developmental, lifestyle, and individual factors that affect the likelihood that a patient can adhere to the frequency and length of treatment
   h. Cost and whether the patient has insurance or other means of paying for the drug

▸ 5. The recommended safe dose of erythromycin succinate for a neonate who weighs 7 lbs is 50 mg/kg/day divided into 4 doses. The nurse calculates that the safe single dose for this neonate is approximately:
   a. 20 mg.
   b. 40 mg.
   c. 160 mg.
   d. 350 mg.

▸ 6. Which of these assessment findings would be most significant if a patient was receiving intramuscular ceftriaxone 1 gram every 12 hours for disseminated gonococcal infection?
   a. Fever
   b. Joint pain
   c. Petechial rash
   d. Stiff neck

▸ 7. The throat culture of a 6-year-old boy is positive for *Neisseria gonorrhoeae*. A nursing priority in this situation is:
   a. assessing for eye exudate.
   b. correctly calculating the dose of ceftriaxone to be administered.
   c. ensuring the safety of the child.
   d. removing the child from his home.

8. A patient is admitted to the hospital with a diagnosis of pelvic inflammatory disease (PID). She asks the nurse why her physician has recommended hospitalization and intravenous antibiotics instead of oral antibiotic therapy at home. The basis of the nurse's response is:
   a. inadequately treated PID is more likely to cause scarring of the uterine (fallopian) tubes.
   b. PID is very contagious, and she needs to be in isolation.
   c. the recommended antibiotic for PID is only available by intravenous route.
   d. women who have PID have a higher incidence of cervical cancer.

9. A 32-year-old woman develops septic arthritis. When obtaining a history, it is important to evaluate for previous infection with:
   a. *chlamydia trachomatis.*
   b. *Neisseria gonorrhoeae.*
   c. *treponema pallidum.*
   d. *trichomonas vaginalis.*

▶ 10. The nursery nurse is caring for a neonate whose mother has an active infection with *Chlamydia trachomatis*. A priority nursing outcome for the neonate would be that the neonate will:
   a. be free of conjunctival discharge.
   b. blink in response to direct light shined in the eyes.
   c. breast-feed for 10 to 15 minutes at least every 3 hours without becoming dyspneic.
   d. gain 2 ounces a week for the first 4 weeks after birth.

▶ 11. The current treatment recommendation for a pregnant patient who is allergic to penicillin and diagnosed with syphilis is:
   a. azithromycin.
   b. ceftriaxone.
   c. doxycycline.
   d. penicillin-allergy desensitization and penicillin.

12. The recommended treatment for acute epididymitis is different depending on the age of the patient because usually:
   a. older men have developed a resistance to the antibiotic used for younger men.
   b. the method and organism of infection is different.
   c. younger men have better kidney functioning.
   d. younger men are less likely to be adherent to multidose therapy.

▶ 13. The nurse teaches that the primary cause of recurrent sexually transmitted infections caused by the same organism is failure to:
   a. prescribe the correct antibiotic.
   b. seek treatment early in the disease.
   c. take the medication as prescribed.
   d. treat the sexual partner.

14. A 35-year-old woman comes to her gynecologist's office with the complaint of a yellow-green vaginal discharge. She is diagnosed with trichomoniasis and prescribed metronidazole (Flagyl). It is important for the nurse to teach the patient the importance of not consuming:
   a. alcohol.
   b. antacids.
   c. grapefruit juice.
   d. milk.

15. Clindamycin cream (Clindesse) requires only one dose of vaginal cream to treat bacterial vaginosis because:
   a. bacterial vaginosis is not a serious infection.
   b. clindamycin has a half-life of several days.
   c. the cream adheres to the vaginal mucosa for several days.
   d. the medication immediately kills the infecting microbes.

16. A major goal of therapy with famciclovir (Famvir) for genital herpes is:
   a. analgesia.
   b. to decrease length of active episodes.
   c. eradication of the virus.
   d. prevention of spread of the infection.

17. A patient has received instructions regarding administration of podofilox (Condylox). Which of these statements made by the client would indicate the patient needs further teaching?
   a. "After I complete this course of therapy and the skin completely heals over, I will no longer be contagious."
   b. "I must apply this twice a day for 3 days in a row."
   c. "It will take a long while before this medication has removed the wart."
   d. "This therapy may be painful."

## CASE STUDIES AND PATIENT TEACHING

*(Use a separate piece of paper for your responses.)*

### Case Study 1

*A sexually active, single, 19-year-old woman presents to the emergency department with a 2-week history of dull bilateral abdominal pain, low back pain, and mucopurulent vaginal discharge with increased pain today. She denies fever, nausea, vomiting, diarrhea, and urinary symptoms. She reports irregular periods since age 13. Her last menstrual period was 2 months ago. She does not use any measure of birth control. She was treated at the health department 3 months ago for a "female infection" and states she took the medication when she remembered and did not return for a follow-up examination. She has had two sexual partners in the past 6 months, one of whom was also treated for an infection 3 months ago at the health department. She is unsure whether he was adherent to his treatment plan or whether he is symptomatic at this time. She has no known medication allergies and takes no medication on a regular basis.*

*Her vital signs are as follows: BP 110/72 mm Hg, pulse 88 beats/min, respirations 20 breaths/minute, and temperature 99.4°F. The physician orders a CBC, sedimentation rate, RPR, serum pregnancy, and a catheterized urinalysis. He performs abdominal and pelvic examinations and obtains cervical cultures for gonorrhea and chlamydia and specimens for saline and KOH wet preps.*

*The physical exam reveals a soft abdomen, right and left lower quadrant tenderness without rebound, and normal bowel sounds. The pelvic exam reveals mucopurulent vaginal discharge and mild right and left adnexal tenderness with bimanual exam. The laboratory results reveal Hgb 11.1, WBC 7.0, negative results for urinalysis and pregnancy tests.*

*After review of the medical and social history, physical exam, and laboratory results (excluding the cultures), the physician makes a diagnosis of pelvic inflammatory disease (PID). Orders include administer ceftriaxone 250 mg IM now and prescriptions for doxycycline 100 mg twice a day for 10 days and Tylenol #3 1 tablet every 3 to 4 hours as needed for pain. The patient is told that she will be notified regarding the results of the cultures.*

1. Why is it important to determine whether the patient is pregnant before administering doxycycline or tetracycline?

2. The patient is to be observed for 30 minutes following administration of the cephalosporin injection and then discharged home. She is given instructions for bed rest for 2 days with a reexamination in 24 to 48 hours if the signs and/or symptoms increase or persist. What teaching regarding the prescribed medication and follow-up care should the nurse provide to this patient?

3. Why is it important for the patient to avoid all forms of alcohol?

4. The patient is instructed to inform her sexual partners of the need for examination. The patient's phone number and address are verified for notification purposes. She is also advised that the culture results will be reported to the health department if they are positive, and the health department will then follow-up with her. The patient states that she does not understand why she has to inform her sexual partners of her infection and why she has to take all of the medication if she is feeling better in a couple of days. What information and instructions can the nurse provide to the patient to help her understand the importance of adherence to her treatment plan?

5. After completing the teaching, the patient's verbalizations reflect that she still does not recognize the significance of her infection or importance of adhering to therapy. How might this alter the plan of care for this patient?

# 95 Antiseptics and Disinfectants

## OBJECTIVES

See page 26 for the Objectives.

## CRITICAL THINKING AND STUDY QUESTIONS

1. Antiseptics are:
   a. commonly used to treat superficial infections.
   b. effective when used properly to cleanse a new wound.
   c. more potent than disinfectants.
   d. only applied to nonliving tissue.

2. Why is it important for nurses to understand the time course of action of an antiseptic?

3. Which of the following is least significant in preventing a surgical incision-site infection?
   a. Preoperative scrubbing of surgical site with an antiseptic
   b. Preoperative scrubbing of scrub nurses' hands
   c. Rigorous disinfection of operating room and fixtures before surgery
   d. Sterilization of surgical instruments

4. To ensure effectiveness of ethyl alcohol (ethanol) as an antiseptic, the nurse should:
   a. apply the alcohol directly to open wounds after medicating the patient for pain.
   b. not use alcohol in combination with chlorhexidine.
   c. use an alcohol with a concentration greater than 75%.
   d. use foam that prolongs evaporation of the alcohol.

5. An adverse effect of wiping a subcutaneous heparin injection site with isopropyl alcohol immediately after injecting the medication is:
   a. bruising.
   b. lack of effect.
   c. poor absorption of the drug.
   d. significant pain.

6. When the nurse is preparing to cleanse a wound, which preparation would be most appropriate and effective?
   a. glutaraldehyde (Cidex)
   b. iodine solution
   c. iodine tincture
   d. povidone-iodine (Betadine)

7. The nurse knows that, when being used as a wound irrigant, sodium hypochlorate (household bleach) needs to be diluted with water in a ratio of 1 part bleach to:
   a. 1 part water.
   b. 5 parts water.
   c. 10 parts water.
   d. 20 parts water.

8. Hexachlorophene (PHisoHex):
   a. encourages the growth of gram-negative organisms.
   b. is bactericidal.
   c. is the antiseptic of choice for burns.
   d. is widely used as a preoperative scrub.

9. The benefit of applying hydrogen peroxide to a wound is: (Select all that apply.)
   a. killing of gram-positive bacteria.
   b. killing of gram-negative bacteria.
   c. killing of spores.
   d. killing of viruses.
   e. loosening of debris from the wound.

10. The surgical scrub that remains active on the skin after rinsing is:
    a. benzalkonium chloride (BAC).
    b. chlorhexidine (Hibiclens).
    c. hexachlorophene (PHisoHex).
    d. povidone-iodine (Betadine).

11. The operating room nurse is preparing to apply benzalkonium chloride (BAC) as a surgical scrub. Before applying the solution, it is important for the nurse to:
    a. rinse the skin with alcohol and water.
    b. shave the area.
    c. wash the skin with soap.
    d. warm the solution.

12. It is acceptable to use an alcohol-based handrub to cleanse the hands instead of soap and water: (Select all that apply.)
    a. after eating.
    b. after removing gloves.
    c. after taking linens into a patient's room.
    d. before patient contact.
    e. taking a pulse.
    f. using the restroom.
    g. when the hands have been exposed to wound drainage.

13. The nurse should scrub the hands and forearms with an antimicrobial soap for surgical scrub asepsis for:
    a. 1 to 2 minutes.
    b. 4 to 6 minutes.
    c. 8 to 10 minutes.
    d. 10 to 15 minutes.

14. The nurse professor is orienting student nurses to the intensive care unit. Hygiene instructions should include:
    a. alcohol handrub should be used when the hands are visibly dirty.
    b. all forms of jewelry are forbidden.
    c. do not wear artificial nails.
    d. trim natural nails to less than ½ inch beyond the fingertip.

## CASE STUDIES AND PATIENT TEACHING

*(Use a separate piece of paper for your responses.)*

### Case Study 1

*The delivery room nurse needs to prepare used instruments for disinfection with glutaraldehyde (Cidex) before being sent for sterilization.*

1. What steps should the nurse take before soaking the instruments?

2. How long do the instruments need to soak?

3. What precautions does the nurse need to take when disinfecting with glutaraldehyde (Cidex)?

4. Describe the hand-washing technique the nurse would use after completing this disinfection process.

# 96 Antihelmintics

## OBJECTIVES

See page 26 for the Objectives.

## CRITICAL THINKING AND STUDY QUESTIONS

1. Helminthiasis: (Select all that apply.)
   a. affects more people than any other infectious disorder.
   b. always produces symptoms.
   c. can go away without any treatment.
   d. can involve the liver and blood vessels.
   e. in some situations, teaching principles espoused by Florence Nightingale can be the most important nursing intervention.
   f. treatment with drugs is most important in situations where the patient is at high risk for reinfection.

2. A patient has just started treatment with mebendazole (Vermox) for hookworm infestation. The nurse assesses for the most common complication of hookworm infestation, which may be:
   a. feculent vomiting.
   b. pale conjunctiva.
   c. perianal itching.
   d. rectal prolapse.

3. A patient who has been treated with mebendazole (Vermox) for trichinosis is now prescribed prednisone. The purpose of this medication is to:
   a. kill larvae that have migrated.
   b. prevent calcification of dead larvae in skeletal muscle.
   c. prevent migration of larvae.
   d. reduce inflammation during larval migration.

4. Nursing examination of an elderly debilitated patient reveals severe scrotal and peripheral edema. What other assessment finding related to diagnosis, if present, is most important for the nurse to provide to the practitioner who is treating this patient?
   a. Limited range of motion of joints
   b. Multiple bruises
   c. Swollen lymph nodes
   d. Weak hand grasps

5. A patient, who works for the World Health Organization (WHO) and whose job duties include worldwide travel, complains of recent noticeable decreased visual acuity. Because of the possibility of contracting onchocerciasis from fly bites, the nurse should assess for recent travel to which of the following areas in the patient's history? (Select all that apply.)
   a. Argentina
   b. Australia
   c. Canada
   d. China
   e. Columbia
   f. Congo
   g. Guatemala
   h. Kenya
   i. Madagascar
   j. Mexico
   k. Mozambique
   l. Japan
   m. Peru
   n. Rwanda
   o. Venezuela

6. To prevent complications from therapy with praziquantel (Biltricide) prescribed for tapeworms, the nurse teaches the patient to:
   a. avoid hazardous activity.
   b. chew the tablet completely before swallowing.
   c. monitor daily urine output.
   d. take the medication on an empty stomach.

▶ 7. The nurse is administering albendazole (Albenza) to an elderly patient who has been diagnosed with the larval form of the pork tapeworm. Which of the following laboratory results would warrant consultation with the prescriber regarding administration of the medication?
   a. AST 95 units/L
   b. BUN 25 mg/dL
   c. Creatinine 1.4 mg/dL
   d. Potassium 3.4 mg/dL

▶ 8. A resident has just prescribed diethylcarbamazine (Hetrazan) for an infection with *Wuchereria bancrofti*. Which of the following symptoms, occurring after the start of administration of the drug, would be of most concern to the nurse?
   a. Dizziness
   b. Headache
   c. Nausea
   d. Personality change

## CASE STUDIES AND PATIENT TEACHING

*(Use a separate piece of paper for your responses.)*

### Case Study 1

*The mother of a 2½-year-old, who attends day care, notices that her child has been restless, is not sleeping well, has been scratching her perineal area, and wetting the bed. The mother calls her pediatric office and is told by the nurse to put a loop of transparent tape in the child's anal area in the early morning before the child awakens. The nurse further instructs the mother to remove the tape later in the morning, put it in a plastic bag, and bring it to the office. On examination of the tape sample, the pediatric nurse practitioner (PNP) diagnoses enterobiasis pinworms.*

1. What is the probable mode of transmission of the parasite in this case?

2. The PNP prescribes mebendazole (Vermox) for the entire family. What did the prescriber need to determine before prescribing the drug for the entire family?

3. How could the pinworm infestation have been transmitted from the child to other family members?

4. What teaching can the nurse provide these family members to prevent future infestation and spread of pinworms?

5. The entire family is adherent to the prescribed therapy. Why is there little problem with adherence with this therapy?

6. The mother is embarrassed and does not want to notify the day care of her child's infection. How should the nurse respond?

### Case Study 2

*A nurse is caring for victims exposed to contaminated floodwaters who have been brought into a makeshift clinic in a temporary shelter.*

1. The nurse knows that which segments of the population would be more at risk for helminthiasis?

2. Several children are experiencing vomiting and massive diarrhea. The nurse should be assessing for what symptoms of these possible fluid and electrolyte imbalances?
   a. Water
   b. Potassium
   c. Magnesium
   d. Sodium

3. Some patients are diagnosed with threadworm infestation. The only medication available for these patients is thiabendazole donated by a drug company. What actions should the nurse take to prevent complications of possible adverse effects of this drug?

4. What can the nurse do in this situation to prevent spread of these infections?

# 97 Antiprotozoal Drugs I: Antimalarial Agents

## OBJECTIVES

See page 26 for the Objectives.

## CRITICAL THINKING AND STUDY QUESTIONS

1. Malaria:
   a. deaths are most likely in children under the age of 5 years.
   b. does not occur in the United States or Canada.
   c. eradication has not been successful because the transmitting insect and the parasite have become resistant to the drugs.
   d. is most prevalent in the Sahara desert areas of Africa.
   e. is transmitted by the Anopheles fly.
   f. kills more people than any other infection except tuberculosis.
   g. vaccination has been effective for many years, but many African people are afraid of vaccinations.

▸ 2. The most important action by the nurse to prevent transmission of malaria is:
   a. administering drugs at the correct time.
   b. placing the patient in strict isolation.
   c. universal precautions.
   d. using a mask with all patient contact.

3. The repeating episodes of fever, chills, and profuse sweating that are characteristic of malaria are due to:
   a. infection at the site of the mosquito bite.
   b. ingestion of blood by the mosquito.
   c. red blood cell (RBC) rupture.
   d. toxicity of the suppressant drugs.

▸ 4. The most significant priority in the nursing care of a patient who has malaria caused by *Plasmodium. falciparum* to prevent a serious complication is:
   a. assessing for early changes in neurologic status.
   b. elevating the head of the bed.
   c. monitoring for elevations in liver function studies.
   d. providing adequate nutrition.

5. Primaquine is not used for relapse prevention of infection with malaria caused by *P. falciparum* because:
   a. it is a drug that is only used prophylactically to prevent infection of erythrocytes.
   b. *P. falciparum* is resistant to primaquine.
   c. the infection is mild, and relapses will decrease and disappear over time without treatment.
   d. there are no dormant forms of the organism in the liver to be eradicated.

6. A patient asks why prophylactic chloroquine (Aralen) is taken only once a week. The basis of the nurse's response is:
   a. absorption is very slow after oral administration.
   b. deposition in tissue is slowly released into the blood.
   c. it is administered IM as a depot preparation.
   d. it remains fat soluble and cannot be excreted by the kidneys.

▸ 7. Which of the following laboratory results of an adult female, if occurring during treatment with primaquine, should the nurse report immediately to the prescriber?
   a. G6PD 1.4 units/mL/RBC
   b. Hemoglobin 12 g/dL
   c. Hematocrit 36%
   d. RBC $4.2 \times 10^6/\mu L$

▶ 8. A patient with diabetes treated with metformin is prescribed quinine for malaria. It is most important for the nurse to assess for:
   a. excessive urination.
   b. hot, dry skin.
   c. palpitations.
   d. visual disturbances.

9. Quinine is categorized as category X. This means that the nurse should:
   a. administer the drug to a pregnant woman if prescribed because there are no known risks to the human fetus.
   b. administer the drug to a pregnant woman if the risk of not treating with the drug is greater than any risk to the fetus.
   c. administer the drug to a pregnant woman and carefully assess for any adverse effects.
   d. not administer the drug if the pregnancy status of the woman has not been determined.

▶ 10. Which of the following changes, if noted in a patient receiving mefloquine, is a reason for the nurse to withhold the drug and contact the prescriber?
   a. Headache
   b. Heartburn
   c. Lack of interest in things normally found to be pleasurable
   d. Nausea

▶ 11. Because of adverse effects, the nurse knows that developmentally which of the following American patients would be least likely to adhere to proguanil therapy?
   a. A 15-year-old girl
   b. A 35-year-old male
   c. A 55-year-old male
   e. A 75-year-old female

## CASE STUDIES AND PATIENT TEACHING

*(Use a separate piece of paper for your responses.)*

### Case Study 1

*A 45-year-old male has just returned from Africa after 4 years of service with the World Health Organization (WHO). During that time, he had been taking quinine prophylactically to prevent malaria in case he was bitten by an infected Anopheles mosquito.*

1. What does this treatment actually accomplish?

2. What other measures should he have been taught to decrease the risk of malarial infection?

3. Before his African service was completed, the man quit taking the quinine because he was experiencing ringing in his ears. Within a few months he started experiencing episodes of high fever followed by chills, then diaphoresis occurring every 2 days. He was seen by a physician and diagnosed with vivax malaria. He was advised that he should return home for treatment. Why was this patient not treated in Africa where he could continue his work?

4. The patient is prescribed a 3-day treatment of chloroquine for his acute attack of malaria. What are the adverse effects the nurse should teach the patient to be aware of during the acute attack treatment?

5. When the patient completes his acute treatment, he asks why he cannot continue taking the chloroquine to prevent recurrence of the malaria symptoms. What is the basis of the nurse's response to this question?

6. The patient informs the nurse that his physician prescribed primaquine for him to take after the acute attack. He wants to know why this particular medication was prescribed. How would the nurse respond?

# 98 Antiprotozoal Drugs II: Miscellaneous Agents

## OBJECTIVES

See page 26 for the Objectives.

## CRITICAL THINKING AND STUDY QUESTIONS

▶ 1. A nursing priority for a patient who is receiving high-dose prednisone for exacerbated COPD and who is diagnosed with cryptosporidiosis is at risk for:
   a. activity intolerance.
   b. fatigue.
   c. fluid imbalance.
   d. imbalanced nutrition.

▶ 2. An allergy to which of the following diabetic medications would be a reason for the nurse to contact the prescriber if a patient is prescribed trimethoprim plus sulfamethoxazole for *Pneumocystis carinii* pneumonia?
   a. glimepiride (Amaryl)
   b. rosiglitazone (Avandia)
   c. metformin (Glucophage)
   d. acarbose (Precose)

▶ 3. Which of the following symptoms, if present in a patient who is receiving iodoquinol (Yodoxin) for amebiasis, would be of most concern to the nurse?
   a. Anal itching
   b. Blurred vision
   c. Facial pustules
   d. Palpable thyroid

4. A patient asks why he has to take a second drug, iodoquinol (Yodoxin), after he finishes a course of metronidazole (Flagyl) for amebiasis. The best explanation for administration of the iodoquinol is:
   a. metronidazole does not adequately kill the amebae in the large intestine.
   b. iodoquinol is absorbed better than metronidazole.
   c. liver abscesses caused by the amebae are not affected by metronidazole.
   d. metronidazole is metabolized by the CYP3A4 hepatic enzyme.

▶ 5. The nurse teaches a patient who is prescribed metronidazole (Flagyl) that it is very important to report which possible adverse effect of the drug to the prescriber?
   a. Darkening of the urine
   b. Metallic taste
   c. Mouth ulcers
   d. Paresthesias

6. An emergency room nurse is providing discharge teaching to a breast-feeding mother who is prescribed metronidazole (Flagyl) for giardiasis after a camping trip where she drank water from a stream. It is important for the nurse to teach this patient to feed her baby formula and pump her breasts and discard the breast milk throughout the time the medication is being taken plus an additional:
   a. 1 day.
   b. 3 days.
   c. 1 week.
   d. 2 weeks.

7. A patient who has been prescribed metronidazole (Flagyl) asks why he should not drink any product that contains alcohol. The nurse's response is based on alcohol combined with metronidazole can cause:
   a. bradycardia.
   b. dangerous CNS depression.
   c. hypertension.
   d. psychotic symptoms.

8. Tinidazole (Tindamax) differs from metronidazole (Flagyl) in that tinidazole:
   a. does not interact with alcohol.
   b. has a longer half-life.
   c. is contraindicated in the last trimester of pregnancy.
   d. is less expensive.

9. The nurse notes yellowish discoloration of the sclera of a 7-year-old girl who is receiving nitazoxanide (Alinia) for giardiasis. The nurse should:
   a. administer the medication and continue nursing care.
   b. review the most recent BUN and creatinine.
   c. withhold the medication and review laboratory tests.
   d. withhold the medication and contact the prescriber.

10. For best absorption, the nurse teaches a patient who is prescribed atovaquone (Mepron) to administer the drug:
    a. crushed.
    b. on an empty stomach.
    c. with a full glass of water.
    d. with fatty food.

11. Which of the following laboratory results should be reviewed by the nurse before administering trimetrexate (Neutrexin)? (Select all that apply.)
    a. Alanine aminotransferase (ALT)
    b. Alkaline phosphatase (ALP)
    c. Arterial blood gases (ABG)
    d. Aspartate aminotransferase (AST)
    e. Creatine phosphokinase MB (CK-MB)
    f. Creatinine
    g. Complete blood count and differential (CBC/diff)
    h. Electrolytes
    i. Hemoglobin $A_{1C}$
    j. International normalized ratio (INR)

12. A female patient who is HIV positive is diagnosed with PCP. She has received instructions regarding drug therapy with trimetrexate (Neutrexin) and leucovorin (folinic acid) that is to be administered by a home health nurse. Which of these statements made by the patient would indicate the patient needs further teaching?
    a. "I must receive the leucovorin (folinic acid) for several days before I start therapy with trimetrexate (Neutrexin)."
    b. "I should contact the nurse or physician if I experience abdominal pain, nausea, dark urine, or clay-colored stool."
    c. "I should not get pregnant while on this drug."
    d. "I should store the trimetrexate (Neutrexin) powder in a dark cupboard."

13. The recommended adult dose of trimetrexate (Neutrexin) is 45 mg/m$^2$. What is the recommended dose for an adult who is 180 cm tall and weighs 60 kg?

## CASE STUDIES AND PATIENT TEACHING

*(Use a separate piece of paper for your responses.)*

### Case Study 1

*A 26-year-old patient with hemophilia is 5 feet 7 inches tall and weighs 140 lbs. Because of his hemophilia, he has received numerous transfusions since diagnosis at age 2 years. Three years ago, he was diagnosed as HIV positive and has been on azidothymidine (AZT) since then. He was hospitalized 3 days ago when he complained of a cough, dyspnea, and chest discomfort. The nurse notes that he is very pale and shows some cyanosis around his nail beds. He has been diagnosed with Pneumocystis carinii pneumonia (PCP). Drug orders include intravenous pentamidine isethionate (Pentam 300) 220 mg once a day for 14 days. The recommended dose is 4mg/kg/day.*

1. Is the prescribed dose safe and therapeutic?

2. The pentamidine must be dissolved in sterile water just before use. The vial is diluted to 100 mg/mL. How much pentamidine should be withdrawn from the vial to equal a dose of 220 mg?

3. The intravenous pentamidine is diluted to a total of 250 mL of 5% dextrose in water. What rate should be programmed into the infusion pump if the solution is to be administered over 60 minutes?

4. What nursing measures should be implemented to prevent complications of adverse effects of intravenous pentamidine?

5. The patient has received pentamidine before as an aerosol inhalation. He wants to know why he must have his medication through an IV instead of the inhaler. He says he is afraid that he will bleed if something happens to the IV. How should the nurse respond?

## Case Study 2

*A patient who has a history of diabetes, seizure disorder, atrial fibrillation, and bipolar disorder is prescribed metronidazole (Flagyl). The patient's home medication regimen lists metformin (Glucophage) 500 mg twice a day, phenytoin (Dilantin) 100 mg 3 times a day, warfarin (Coumadin) 2.5 mg once a day on Monday and Thursday and 2 mg once a day on the rest of the days, and lithium carbonate (Eskalith) 300 mg 3 times a day.*

1. What are the possible effects on drug levels of the interaction of each of these drugs with metronidazole (Flagyl)?

2. The nurse should assess for which symptoms of these drug reactions?

3. What are interventions the nurse should employ if symptoms occur?

## Case Study 3

*A school nurse who works in a rural farming area has noted an extremely high incidence of absences caused by severe diarrhea in children who live within a 1-mile radius of each other.*

1. What could possibly be causing these illnesses, and what can the nurse do to prevent these illnesses?

# 99 Ectoparasiticides

## OBJECTIVES

See page 26 for the Objectives.

## CRITICAL THINKING AND STUDY QUESTIONS

1. Matching (May use options more than once.)

___ a. Pediculosis
___ b. Scabies

1. Animals never infested
2. Common site of adult infestation is webs of fingers
3. Intense itching
4. Lice infestation
5. Mite infestation
6. Transmission possible via contact with objects
7. Treatment and how contracted differs by site
8. Visible lines where burrows

2. The nurse has taught a mother how to apply permethrin (Elimite) 5% cream to treat her 7-year-old son who has visible scabies burrows on his buttocks. Which of these statements made by the mother would indicate she understood the directions?
   a. "I should not apply the cream to his face or scalp."
   b. "The cream should be applied to the skin from head to the soles of the feet being careful to avoid eyes and mucous membranes."
   c. "The cream should be washed off after 10 minutes with warm water."
   d. "The cream should not be washed off."

3. Which of the following could be associated with a severe reaction when malathion (Ovide) has been prescribed for head lice?
   a. Absorption of the lotion through scratches on the scalp
   b. Administration concurrently with drugs that inhibit the P-450 hepatic cytochrome system
   c. Failure to use the fine-toothed comb to remove nits after application
   d. Smoking while applying the lotion

4. Which of the following treatments for scabies normally involves repeated applications?
   a. crotamiton (Eurax)
   b. ivermectin (Stromectol)
   c. lindane (Kwell)
   d. permethrin (Nix)

## CASE STUDIES AND PATIENT TEACHING

*(Use a separate piece of paper for your responses.)*

### Case Study 1

*A teacher consults the school nurse about a second-grade girl in her class. The child is one of three siblings attending the elementary school. The child has very long blond hair, and over the past week, the child has been constantly scratching her head. She has scratched her head so much that her hair is tangled and almost impossible to brush, and her scalp is bleeding. The school nurse notes small white spots on her hair shaft close to the scalp. Examination under the microscope reveals nits. The nurse contacts the girl's mother to report these nits (eggs), telling her it is probably Pediculus humanus capitis (head lice).*

1. How should the school nurse handle the possibility that other children in the school may be infested?

2. The girl's mother is quite upset about the lice. She wants to know how her child could have gotten "these bugs" and how to tell whether others in the family have them. How should the nurse respond?

3. The mother was told by a friend to cut all of Joan's hair to get rid of the lice. What are reasons why the nurse would not want the mother to do this to the child?

4. The mother contacts the pediatrician who orders permethrin (Nix) shampoo. What should the office nurse include in the explanation for using this product?

5. What is the purpose of the fine-toothed comb in head lice treatment?

6. The child's mother tells the nurse that when she had head lice as a child, her physician had her mother apply lindane (Kwell) shampoo. She wants to know why that is not used anymore. What would the nurse tell her?

# 100 Basic Principles of Cancer Chemotherapy

## OBJECTIVES

See page 26 for the Objectives.

## CRITICAL THINKING AND STUDY QUESTIONS

1. The best description of cancer cell reproduction is:
   a. abnormal.
   b. rapid.
   c. slow.
   d. unregulated.

2. A patient is admitted for surgical removal of a cancerous tumor of the colon. He is concerned about the prospect of living with a colostomy and asks the nurse why the physician cannot just give him some drugs to kill the cancer. The basis of the nurse's response is that solid tumors: (Select all that apply.)
   a. are disseminated.
   b. have fewer cells that are actively dividing.
   c. have fewer cells in the $G_0$ phase.
   d. have poor blood supply at the core.
   e. have normal DNA.

3. A spouse of a cancer patient asks why some tumors become resistant to chemotherapy. Which of the following would not be included in the explanation?
   a. A transport molecule may be stimulated to pump drugs out of the cancer cell.
   b. Cancer cells in the $G_0$ phase have time to repair drug-induced damage before it does serious harm.
   c. Chemotherapy drugs alter the cancer cell DNA making the cell resistant.
   d. Drug-resistant mutant cells have more nourishment because of the death of drug-sensitive cells.

4. The mother of a child with leukemia is concerned about her son's fear and discomfort during chemotherapy. She asks the nurse why he cannot receive one large dose of a single powerful drug instead of multiple doses of different drugs. After teaching, which statement if made by the mother, suggests that that this mother needs further explanation?
   a. "Different drugs kill cancer cells in different ways."
   b. "It is especially important for my son to receive multiple doses because one of the drugs that my son is getting only kills cancer cells at a particular point of cell reproduction."
   c. "If multiple drugs are used, the cancer is less likely to develop resistance to all of them."
   d. "My son will not experience adverse effects if he receives multiple drugs administered at different times."

5. The nurse would expect that when more than one anticancer chemotherapeutic agent is used together, the drugs:
   a. adverse effects primarily affect different organs.
   b. are less effective than if used alone.
   c. can be mixed in the same intravenous solution.
   d. have the same mechanism of action.

6. A patient with brain cancer asks the nurse why they are putting the drug into her back instead of a vein. The basis of the nurse's response should be that this route:
   a. allows higher doses of chemotherapy to be used.
   b. allows the drug to get to the tumor cells.
   c. prevents many adverse effects.
   d. prevents drug-resistant mutation of the cancer cells.

▶ 7. The nurse is caring for a 62-year-old female who developed pancreatitis during chemotherapy after mastectomy. Most recent laboratory results include RBC 2.8 $10^6/\mu L$, WBC $4100/mm^3$, neutrophils $18{,}000/mm^3$, and platelets $147{,}000/mm^3$. An expected nursing diagnosis, based on these laboratory results, would be:
   a. activity intolerance.
   b. decreased cardiac output.
   c. impaired gas exchange.
   d. ineffective cerebral tissue perfusion.

▶ 8. The nurse is caring for a chemotherapy patient with neutropenic precautions. The nurse washes her hands and dons gown, mask, and gloves in the anteroom before entering the actual patient room. The patient refuses care by the nurse until the nurse washes her hands at the sink in the room and puts on new gloves. The nurse should:
   a. explain that she is more likely to transmit an infection if she takes off her current gloves while in the room.
   b. explain that she washed her hands just outside the door before entering the room.
   c. rewash her hands in the room and put on new gloves.
   d. rewash her hands, put on new gown, gloves, and mask inside the room.

9. When teaching a cancer patient who is receiving chemotherapy, which of the following foods would be least likely to cause an infection if the patient develops neutropenia?
   a. Commercially canned fruit
   b. Fresh vegetables from the patient's garden
   c. Rare meat
   d. Yogurt

10. The nurse is administering subcutaneous insulin to a chemotherapy patient who is experiencing bone marrow suppression. Which of the following techniques would be best for the nurse to use to prevent an adverse effect from the bone marrow suppression?
   a. Administer the insulin via an existing IV port.
   b. Apply pressure to the injection site for a few minutes after injection.
   c. Delay the administration of insulin until after the patient has eaten his meal.
   d. Wipe the injection site with Betadine after injection.

11. A patient receiving chemotherapy develops hyperuricemia. A nursing priority addresses the effect of the urate crystals on the:
   a. blood.
   b. joints.
   c. kidneys.
   d. liver.

▸ 12. When administering a known vesicant chemotherapeutic agent, it is most important for the nurse to know:
   a. If the patient has been premedicated with an antiemetic.
   b. If an antidote is available should extravasation occur.
   c. The mechanism of action of the drug.
   d. Whether gloves are needed during administration.

## CASE STUDIES AND PATIENT TEACHING

*(Use a separate piece of paper for your responses.)*

### Case Study 1

*A 28-year-old female is admitted to the oncology unit with a diagnosis of suspected Hodgkin's disease. The diagnosis is confirmed after a biopsy. The patient is started on treatment, which consists of external radiation treatments and chemotherapy. The patient asks the nurse, "How does cancer spread?"*

1. What information can the nurse provide about the characteristics of cancer cells that promote growth and metastasis?

2. The patient asks why a person is more likely to get cancer if they have a family history of cancer. How are genetics linked to cancer?

3. The nurse is discussing strategies to minimize the adverse effects of chemotherapy, including mouth ulcer (stomatitis). The patient asks why these drugs cause mouth ulcers if they are given intravenously. How should the nurse respond?

4. What interventions can the nurse suggest to minimize the effects of chemotherapy on the patient's GI tract?

### Case Study 2

*A nurse has just lost a sister to breast cancer. Before her sister's death, her sister challenged her to use her knowledge and energy to prevent cancer suffering and death. The nurse networks with fellow nurses to identify what they can do to work toward fulfilling her sister's wishes.*

1. What actions could the nurse take?

### Case Study 3

*The oncology nurse is participating in a cancer support meeting for patients who are receiving chemotherapy and their families.*

1. What teaching can she provide regard minimizing harm and discomfort from these effects of the chemotherapy?
   a. Bone marrow suppression
   b. Reproductive toxicity
   c. Hyperuricemia

### Case Study 4

*Discuss with classmates interventions that address these nursing problems that may be experienced by a patient receiving chemotherapy.*

a. Activity intolerance and/or fatigue
b. Disturbed body image
c. Fluid volume deficit
d. Imbalanced nutrition: less than body requirement
e. Risk for infection

# 101 Anticancer Drugs I: Cytotoxic Agents

## OBJECTIVES

See page 26 for the Objectives.

## CRITICAL THINKING AND STUDY QUESTIONS

▶ 1. An important teaching relating to a common adverse effect of cytotoxic drugs would be:
   a. change positions slowly to prevent dizziness or fainting.
   b. night driving may not be safe.
   c. the importance of weight-bearing exercise.
   d. use an electric razor to prevent cutting yourself.

2. A cancer patient asks the nurse why so many drugs that are used to treat cancer cause infections. Which of the following should not be included in the nurse's response?
   a. Blood cells that protect from infection rapidly reproduce so they are easily affected by these drugs.
   b. Most drugs that kill cancer cells actually prevent them from reproducing.
   c. There are drugs available to help boost the body's production of infection-preventing and infection-fighting white blood cells.
   d. When a person has cancer, their blood cells are always invaded by the cancer so the drugs are killing cancerous blood cells.

3. To ensure that phase-specific anticancer drugs are present when cancer cells will be harmed by the drug, these drugs are administered:
   a. by prolonged infusion or at short intervals.
   b. combined with other drugs.
   c. in large doses spaced at least 3 weeks apart.
   d. when cancer cells are not resting.

4. Cell-cycle phase nonspecific drugs may not kill cells in $G_0$ phase because the:
   a. cell has time to repair damage.
   b. cell is not cancerous if it is in $G_0$ phase.
   c. cell is not reproducing.
   d. cell's DNA is not harmed.

5. The nurse is teaching a patient who has been prescribed oral cyclophosphamide (Cytoxan). Which of the following statements, if made by the patient, suggest a need for further teaching?
   a. "I need to notify my doctor if I develop a fever greater than 100.4° F."
   b. "I need to take a drug to prevent nausea at least an hour before I take this drug."
   c. "I should drink at least 12 glasses of fluids every day, especially water."
   d. "It is important for me to take this drug on an empty stomach with a full glass of water."

▶ 6. The nurse should perform which of the following assessments on a patient scheduled to receive ifosfamide (Ifex)?
   a. Hematest stool
   b. SMBG for glucose greater than 200 mg/dL
   c. Urine dip for blood
   d. Urine specific gravity for dehydration

▶ 7. The nurse should withhold chemotherapy with cisplatin (Platinol-AQ) and consult with the oncologist if a patient reports which of the following symptoms since the last infusion?
   a. Nausea
   b. Paresthesias
   c. Sensitivity to cold
   d. Tinnitus

8. Because of the danger of fetal malformation when receiving methotrexate, the nurse teaches a 38-year-old female the importance of using two reliable forms of birth control during:
   a. therapy.
   b. therapy and through at least 1 month after therapy.
   c. therapy and through at least 3 months after therapy.
   d. therapy and through at least 6 months after therapy.

9. Based on the complications of peripheral sensory neuropathy, the nurse would be most concerned if a patient who is receiving oxaliplatin (Eloxatin) reports?
   a. Clumsiness
   b. Difficulty swallowing
   c. Difficulty writing
   d. Intolerance to cold

10. A patient asks the nurse how methotrexate, a drug that her friend uses for rheumatoid arthritis, can be used to treat her cancer. The basis of the nurse's response should be:
   a. both cancer and rheumatoid arthritis cells are autoimmune disorders.
   b. both cancer and rheumatoid arthritis cells spend time in the $G_0$ phase.
   c. both cancer cells and rheumatoid arthritis joint changes require activated folic acid.
   d. the drug has two totally different mechanisms of action.

11. The nurse is reviewing the laboratory tests of a female patient who is scheduled to receive methotrexate. Which of the following results, especially if a change from a previous result, would be most important to report to the attending oncologist?
   a. ALT 55 International Units /L
   b. Creatinine clearance 45 mL/min
   c. Hemoglobin 10.8 gm/dL
   d. Sodium 134 mEq/L

12. A patient with throat cancer is receiving massive doses of methotrexate. Which of the following actions by the nurse would be most critical?
   a. Administering the prescribed ondansetron (Zofran) 30 minutes before the start of the methotrexate infusion
   b. Administering the leucovorin (folinic acid, citrovorum factor) as prescribed
   c. Infusing the methotrexate over exactly the prescribed time interval
   d. Monitoring for electrolyte imbalances because of the high risk of diarrhea or vomiting

13. Which of the following statements, if made by a patient who has been receiving teaching regarding prevention of adverse effects of methotrexate therapy, suggests understanding of the teaching?
   a. "Drinking cranberry juice will help protect my kidneys from damage by methotrexate."
   b. "I should increase my fluid intake to 30 ounces each day."
   c. "If I get a cough, I should report it to my doctor."
   d. "It is important to avoid grapefruit juice when taking this drug."

14. Based on body surface area recommendations, the dose of pemetrexed (Alimta) should be 600 mg/m$^2$ every 3 weeks. Which of the following doses of this drug would be within the therapeutic recommendations for a patient who is 5 feet 5 inches tall and weighs 135 lbs?
   a. 1 gm
   b. 850 mg
   c. 915 mg
   d. 925 mg

15. The nurse teaches a patient that dexamethasone is prescribed when a patient is being treated with pemetrexed (Alimta) in an attempt to prevent:
   a. anemia.
   b. infection.
   c. nausea.
   d. rash.

16. The oncology nurse is administering pemetrexed (Alimta) in 100 mL of 0.9% sodium chloride (NSS). While administering the drug, the nurse notes swelling at the intravenous catheter insertion site. The area is cool and pale. The most important action by the nurse is to:
   a. administer an antidote to prevent tissue necrosis.
   b. apply heat.
   c. apply cold.
   d. stop infusing the drug.

▶ 17. Which of the following symptoms of adverse effects of cytarabine (ara-C) would be of most concern to the nurse?
a. Anorexia, nausea, and bruising
b. Headache, fever, and vomiting
c. Mouth ulcers, inflamed conjunctiva, and nausea
d. Nausea, vomiting, and fever

18. The nurse should consult with the prescriber before administering which of the following chemotherapeutic agents if the patient reports diarrhea or mouth ulcers?
a. cladribine (Leustatin)
b. fludarabine (Fludara)
c. fluorouracil (Adrucil)
d. gemcitabine (Gemzar)

19. The nurse knows that palm and sole tingling, burning, redness, swelling, and blistering are possible adverse effects of some:
a. alkylating agents.
b. antimetabolites.
c. miotic inhibitors.
d. platinum compounds.

20. The nurse assesses for which of the following symptoms of the most common effects of mercaptopurine (Purinethol) toxicity?
a. Bleeding
b. Constipation
c. Diarrhea
d. Hair loss

21. A patient is receiving doxorubicin. The nurse should emphasize the importance of reporting symptoms of the most critical adverse effects including:
a. alopecia.
b. hyperpigmentation of extremities.
c. mouth ulcers.
d. shortness of breath.

22. The nurse is preparing to administer doxorubicin to a 24-year-old male with Hodgkin's lymphoma. The nurse would be most concerned if the patient admitted to not being adherent to taking his prescribed:
a. bupropion (Wellbutrin).
b. enalapril (Vasotec).
c. ibuprofen (Motrin).
d. lorazepam (Ativan).

▶ 23. A patient who is receiving an infusion of liposomal daunorubicin (DaunoXome) reports back pain and chest tightness within minutes of the start of the infusion. The nurse stops the infusion. The symptoms abate, and the patient's vital signs are within normal limits, but the patient voids bright red urine. The nurse would usually:
a. administer an antidote.
b. consult with the prescriber STAT.
c. hold the drug until the next scheduled dose.
d. restart the infusion at a slower rate and monitor for return of symptoms.

▶ 24. Which of the following information, if revealed by a patient who is scheduled to start chemotherapy with epirubicin (Ellence) for breast cancer, would be most important for the nurse to report to the prescriber before administering the drug?
a. Axillary nodes positive for cancerous cells
b. Desire to have children after therapy is completed
c. History of asthma
d. Recent episodes of hypoglycemia

25. The nurse should warn patients that they may experience a blue-green discoloration of their urine and the whites of their eyes if they receive which of the following antitumor antibiotics?
a. epirubicin (Ellence)
b. idarubicin (Idamycin)
c. liposomal daunorubicin (DaunoXome)
d. mitoxantrone (Novantrone)

▶ 26. The nurse is preparing to administer bleomycin (Blenoxane) to a patient with testicular cancer. Which of these test results would warrant withholding the drug and consulting with the prescriber?
a. Erythrocyte sedimentation rate (ESR) 10 mm/hr
b. Hematocrit (Hct) 38%
c. Peak expiratory flow (PEF) 54% of best
d. Platelets 180,000/mm$^3$

27. When teaching a patient who is receiving mitomycin, the nurse explains that the greatest danger of contracting an infection caused by the effect of the drug on the immune system usually occurs:
a. 3 to 4 weeks after the infusion.
b. 6 to 8 days after the infusion.
c. 24 to 48 hours after the infusion.
d. during the infusion.

28. A patient is scheduled to receive gemtuzumab ozogamicin (Mylotarg). Before administering the drug, the nurse should consult with the prescriber regarding premedication with:
   a. aspirin.
   b. dexamethasone.
   c. diphenhydramine.
   d. leucovorin.

▶ 29. Which of the following assessments would warrant stopping the infusion of paclitaxel (Abraxane) and consulting the prescriber?
   a. Pulse 58 beats/min
   b. Pulse 98 beats/min
   c. Respirations 15 per minute
   d. Respirations 24 per minute

▶ 30. Which of these assessment findings would be most significant if a patient was receiving docetaxel (Taxotere)?
   a. Blood pressure 147/90 mm/Hg
   b. Eight-hour output of 850 mL of very dark amber urine
   c. Three soft formed stool in 8 hours
   d. Two plus pitting edema of the ankles

▶ 31. The wife of a patient who received a treatment of irinotecan (Camptosar) 3 days ago calls the oncology clinic nurse to report that his wife has been up all night with diarrhea. She is currently in bed and is too weak to stand up. He asks the nurse what he should do. The nurse should advise the husband to:
   a. administer 1 loperamide (Imodium AD) tablet to his wife after each unformed stool.
   b. allow his wife to rest.
   c. get his wife to take frequent sips of a sports drink with sugar and electrolytes.
   d. take his wife to the hospital for evaluation.

▶ 32. The oncology clinic nurse is administering chemotherapy to several patients. Which of the following would warrant closest monitoring?
   a. 37-year-old female receiving carboplatin (Paraplatin) for ovarian cancer
   b. 78-year-old male receiving cyclophosphamide for non-Hodgkin's lymphoma
   c. 64-year-old female receiving gemcitabine (Gemzar) for pancreatic adenoma
   d. 54-year-old male receiving pemetrexed (Alimta) for mesothelioma

## CASE STUDIES AND PATIENT TEACHING

*(Use a separate piece of paper for your responses.)*

### Case Study 1

*A 41-year-old female is admitted to the outpatient area for her first course of adjuvant chemotherapy for metastatic breast cancer. Four weeks ago, she underwent a left modified radical mastectomy and axillary lymph node dissection for infiltrating ductal carcinoma of the breast. Two of 20 nodes sampled were positive for cancer. The patient will be receiving standard dosage therapy of Adriamycin, Cytoxan, and 5-FU (mg/m$^2$) IV bolus. Premedications include Zofran 32 mg as IV push bolus (IVPB) and Decadron 20 mg IV. In addition, she will receive filgrastim 300 mcg SQ daily for 10 days beginning 24 hours after chemotherapy completion.*

1. What techniques should the nurse use when administering these cytotoxic chemotherapy agents to prevent personal harm?

2. What administrative techniques should the nurse use to prevent patient injury from a vesicant anticancer drug?

### Case Study 2

*Chemotherapy prescribed for a 53-year-old male for advanced non-Hodgkin's lymphoma includes vincristine. The nurse is preparing a plan of nursing care relating to probable adverse effects from this drug.*

1. What nursing diagnoses should the nurse consider?

### Case Study 3

*The nurse is preparing to administer paclitaxel (Taxol) to a 38-year-old patient with ovarian cancer.*

1. Developmentally, what effect of this drug would be a priority for the nurse to prepare this patient to experience?

2. What teaching should the nurse provide relating to the likelihood of the drug causing neutropenia?

3. Filgrastim (Neupogen) is prescribed 5 mcg/kg/day. The patient weighs 132 lbs. What dose should be administered?

4. Dexamethasone, diphenhydramine, and cimetidine are prescribed "before treatment." What information can the nurse research to determine how soon after administering these drugs should the chemotherapy infusion be initiated?

5. What actions should the nurse take when administering paclitaxel to prevent harm to the patient relating to this specific drug?

6. The patient experiences a tingling sensation around her lips 10 minutes after the paclitaxel infusion is started. What action should the nurse take at this time?

7. The patient returns 3 weeks later. She is very concerned when the nurse informs her that prescribed therapy still includes paclitaxel (Abraxane). What explanation by the oncologist can the nurse reinforce?

# 102 Anticancer Drugs II: Hormonal Agents, Biologic Response Modifiers, and Targeted Drugs

## OBJECTIVES

See page 26 for the Objectives.

## CRITICAL THINKING AND STUDY QUESTIONS

1. An important nursing concern for patients receiving drugs that deprive prostate tumors of testosterone involves the risk of:
   a. constipation.
   b. impaired skin integrity.
   c. ineffective breathing pattern.
   d. sexual dysfunction.

2. The nurse is reinforcing the prescriber's teaching about the expected effects of leuprolide (Lupron), which has been prescribed for a 62-year-old male with advanced prostate cancer. Which of the following statements, if made by the patient, suggests a need for further teaching?
   a. "I might have more trouble passing my water for a short time after I start this drug."
   b. "I need to be careful to avoid going out in crowds while taking this drug."
   c. "I should pick up throw rugs in my house so I don't trip and fall."
   d. "It is important for me to try to walk regularly."

▸ 3. A patient with advanced prostate cancer treated with the GnRH analog triptorelin has been depressed and has a poor appetite. The nurse is sitting with the patient to encourage him to eat his lunch. Based on adverse effects of this drug therapy, which of the following foods on the patient's lunch tray would be most important for the patient to eat?
   a. Ham sandwich
   b. Orange
   c. Tossed salad
   d. Yogurt

▸ 4. Which of these laboratory tests would be most important for the nurse to assess when a patient is receiving goserelin (Zoladex) and flutamide (Eulexin)?
   a. Alkaline phosphatase (ALP)
   b. Blood urea nitrogen (BUN)
   c. Platelets
   d. Neutrophils

5. An important teaching for a patient who has been prescribed nilutamide (Nilandron) is:
   a. change positions slowly to prevent dizziness or fainting.
   b. limit your fluid intake in the evening so you do not need to get up to go to the bathroom.
   c. night driving may not be safe.
   d. use an electric razor to prevent cutting yourself.

6. Which of the following teachings would not be necessary when the nurse is teaching a patient regarding adverse effects of abarelix (Plenaxis)?
   a. Avoid stimulation for several hours before bedtime to improve sleep.
   b. Blood pressure monitoring for hypertension is important.
   c. Eating whole grains, fruits, and vegetables can prevent constipation.
   d. You must stay in the office for at least 30 minutes after the injection because this drug has been known to cause allergic reactions.

▶ 7. Because diethylstilbestrol diphosphate (Stilphostrol) can cause hypercalcemia, the nurse assesses patients receiving this drug for:
   a. abdominal cramps and borborygmi.
   b. bleeding gums and bruising.
   c. muscle weakness and constipation.
   d. positive Chvostek's and Trousseau's signs.

▶ 8. The nurse would withhold administering estramustine (Emcyt) and consult the prescriber if a patient is experiencing unexplained:
   a. chest pain.
   b. nausea.
   c. sore throat.
   d. weight gain.

▶ 9. Which of the following nursing actions would be most likely to support patient adherence to taking antiestrogen drug therapy for breast cancer?
   a. Demonstrating administration techniques
   b. Emphasizing benefits of therapy
   c. Identifying patient concerns
   d. Teaching mechanism of action of the drugs

10. When taking a history from a 52-year-old woman with high risk for breast cancer for whom tamoxifen therapy is being considered, which of the following questions would be most important for the nurse to ask?
    a. "Has anyone in your family ever had breast cancer?"
    b. "Have you ever been told that your cholesterol is high?"
    c. "Have you had your bone density measured recently?"
    d. "Have you had a hysterectomy?"

11. Tamoxifen therapy is prescribed for a patient who takes carbamazepine (Tegretol) and phenytoin (Dilantin) for a seizure disorder. These drugs induce the CYP3A4 hepatic enzyme needed for metabolism of tamoxifen. The nurse is aware that dosage of tamoxifen for this patient will be:
    a. the same as usual, but may be less effective.
    b. the same as usual, but may be more likely to produce adverse effects.
    c. higher than usual.
    d. lower than usual.

12. A patient who is receiving tamoxifen read in the newspaper that a STAR study is being conducted on a similar drug (raloxifene) Evista. The patient asks the nurse why they are studying this drug if it is so similar to tamoxifen. The basis of the nurse's response is that research suggests that raloxifene:
    a. does not cause hot flashes.
    b. does not increase the risk of uterine cancer.
    c. does not promote clot formation.
    d. improves bone density better than tamoxifen.

13. The nurse is preparing to administer fulvestrant (Faslodex). Based on current recommendations for IM injections and the incidence of injection-site pain, the best site for this 5-mL intramuscular injection would be:
    a. one 5-mL injection in either dorsogluteal site.
    b. two 2.5-mL injections in bilateral dorsogluteal sites.
    c. one 5-mL injection in either ventrogluteal site.
    d. two 2.5-mL injections in bilateral ventrogluteal sites.

14. The teaching plan regarding expected adverse effects for a patient who is prescribed the aromatase inhibitor anastrozole (Arimidex) should include:
    a. change positions slowly to prevent dizziness.
    b. limit your intake of dairy products to prevent hypercalcemia.
    c. report chest pain.
    d. safety precautions to prevent falls in the home.

15. Nursing interventions for a patient receiving letrozole (Femara) for breast cancer should focus on:
    a. adequate nutrition.
    b. comfort.
    c. maintaining tissue perfusion.
    d. preventing the spread of cancer cells.

16. Trastuzumab (Herceptin) is prescribed for a patient with a breast cancer tumor that produces excessive HER2. The nurse would notify the prescriber immediately if patient laboratory results included:
    a. ALT 65 units/L.
    b. BNP 876 mcg/mL.
    c. creatinine 1.5 mg/dL.
    d. WBC 11,000/mm$^3$.

17. A patient asks the nurse how interferon alfa-2a (Roferon-A) is fighting his cancer. The basis of the nurse's response is that this drug: (Select all that apply.)
    a. alters DNA preventing cancer cell reproduction.
    b. blocks microtubule assembly.
    c. causes nonreproducing cancer cells to stay nonreproducing.
    d. deprives cancer cells of hormones needed for survival.
    e. disrupts cellular protein synthesis.
    f. improves the body's ability to fight cancer cells.
    g. promotes cancer cells' change into forms that do not reproduce.
    h. suppresses cancer genes.

18. To prevent some of the most common adverse effects of interferon alfa-2a (Roferon-A), the nurse teaches the patient about administering which of the following drugs?
    a. acetaminophen (Tylenol)
    b. dexamethasone (Decadron)
    c. diphenhydramine (Benadryl)
    d. ondansetron (Zofran)

19. The oncology nurse is infusing aldesleukin (Proleukin) when the patient suddenly becomes very short of breath. The first response by the nurse should be to:
    a. assess the patient's vital signs.
    b. elevate the head of the bed.
    c. notify the oncologist.
    d. stop the drug infusion.

20. Nursing preparation for administration of BCG vaccine includes:
    a. accessing a central venous line.
    b. assessing the intravenous site for patency.
    c. inserting a urethral catheter.
    d. identifying the appropriate landmarks for intramuscular infusion.

21. The nurse teaches a patient who is receiving BCG vaccine to use precautions to protect from contamination with excreted urine for 6 hours after the end of therapy, including cleaning the toilet with:
    a. alcohol.
    b. ammonia.
    c. bleach.
    d. peroxide.

22. The oncology clinic nurse is monitoring the chemotherapy infusions of the following patients. The patient receiving which of the following drugs would warrant close observation and access to epinephrine and cardiopulmonary resuscitation because of the known risk of an anaphylactic reaction? (Select all that apply.)
    a. bevacizumab (Avastin)
    b. bexxar (Tositumomab with I$^{131}$ Tositumomab)
    c. bortezomib (Velcade)
    d. cetuximab (Erbitux)
    e. denileukin diftitox (Ontak)
    f. erlotinib (Tarceva)
    g. gemtuzumab ozogamicin (Mylotarg)
    h. rituximab (Rituxan)

23. The teaching plan for patients receiving EGFR-tyrosine kinase inhibitors should include the importance of reporting sudden onset of which of the following symptoms to the oncologist?
    a. Fever
    b. Irritability
    c. Nausea
    d. Shortness of breath

▶ 24. Which of the following symptoms, if occurring 12 to 24 hours after the first infusion of rituximab (Rituxan), suggests possible drug induced renal failure?
a. Hypotension and cool, clammy skin
b. Muscle spasms and tingling around the mouth
c. Nausea and constipation
d. Weakness and thirst

▶ 25. A patient is receiving rituximab (Rituxan). The nurse should teach the patient to observe for critical adverse effects that warrant immediate medical attention, including:
a. fever and chills.
b. muscle aches and pains.
c. stomatitis and widespread rash.
d. vomiting and diarrhea.

26. Teaching should include prompt reporting of abdominal pain, chest pain, shortness of breath, change in mental status, and blood in sputum when a patient is receiving treatment with:
a. bevacizumab (Avastin).
b. bortezomib (Velcade).
c. gemtuzumab ozogamicin (Mylotarg).
d. rituximab (Rituxan).

27. The priority nursing consideration for the visiting nurse when caring for a patient who has started therapy with bevacizumab (Avastin) after a colon resection and who spends long periods of the day in bed is the risk for:
a. altered nutrition related to loss of appetite and nausea.
b. altered tissue perfusion, altered coagulation, and sluggish circulation.
c. constipation related to decreased mobility and loss of appetite.
d. fluid imbalance caused by decreased intake of fluids and possible diarrhea.

▶ 28. The nurse notes a 2-lb weight gain in 24 hours when assessing a hospitalized patient who has been receiving imatinib (Gleevec) for CML. It is a priority for the nurse to assess this patient's:
a. cardiopulmonary status.
b. gastrointestinal status.
c. musculoskeletal status.
d. neurologic status.

▶ 29. A patient who has been receiving arsenic trioxide (Trisenox) for promyelocytic leukemia is hospitalized with pleural and pericardial effusions. High-dose glucocorticoid therapy is initiated. When assessing the patient, the nurse notes that the patient is confused; his skin is hot and dry, and he is breathing rapidly. When reporting the patient's condition to the physician, it would be particularly important to also include results of:
a. BUN levels.
b. deep tendon reflexes.
c. metered blood glucose.
d. urine output.

## CASE STUDIES AND PATIENT TEACHING

*(Use a separate piece of paper for your responses.)*

### Case Study 1

*The nurse works in a busy gynecologic practice. She is responsible for assisting the patients with completing an initial patient history and highlighting abnormalities to alert the primary care provider.*

1. What information on the history would suggest an increased risk for breast cancer?

2. A 53-year-old patient has a sister who died at age 48 of metastatic breast cancer. The patient is 5 feet 4 inches and 187 lbs. She asks the nurse how losing weight can decrease her risk of breast cancer. How should the nurse respond?

3. The patient has been advised to consider tamoxifen (Nolvadex) therapy because of her high risk for breast cancer. She asks the nurse how this drug will help prevent breast cancer. What explanation can the nurse provide?

4. Why is it important for the nurse to assess the patient's smoking status and recommend smoking cessation if the patient smokes and is considering tamoxifen therapy?

5. The patient has not had a menstrual period for 2 years. Why would the nurse advise this patient to come in to be seen if she experiences any vaginal bleeding?

6. What other symptoms or serious adverse effects of tamoxifen would the nurse teach the patient to report immediately?

7. Adherence to tamoxifen therapy is affected by the patient's ability to cope with adverse effects. What information can the nurse provide to this patient to assist her in dealing with the following adverse effects?
   a. Hot flushes
   b. Fluid retention
   c. Nausea and vomiting

## Case Study 2

*A 76-year-old male with a history of non-Hodgkin's lymphoma, COPD, type 2 diabetes mellitus, atrial fibrillation, and hypothyroidism is admitted to the nursing unit with a diagnosis of community acquired pneumonia. He is prescribed intravenous tobramycin 120 mg 3 times a day, metformin 500 mg twice a day, diltiazem (Cardizem CD) 240 mg once a day, levothyroxine (Synthroid) 0.075 mg once a day, and tiotropium (Spiriva) inhalation once a day. Respiratory therapy is ordered every 4 hours and PRN. The patient's primary cancer site was in his lung 20 years ago, and he has experienced 7 relapses and/or metastases that have been treated with partial lung lobectomy, gastric and duodenal resection, and cytotoxic chemotherapy. His most recent site of metastasis is the esophagus at which time he had pleural and pericardial effusions, requiring thoracotomy and chest tube insertion. He is currently being treated with rituximab (Rituxan). The patient's wife is very attentive, and the nurse believes that she has been a major factor in the patient's survival. The patient's wife tells the nurse that the patient's most recent prostate-specific antigen (PSA) was 8 (ng/mL). She is concerned because the oncologist is not considering surgery and has not ordered any additional chemotherapy.*

1. How should the nurse respond?

2. The oncologist discusses concerns that additional chemotherapy would not be effective and that the patient's overall condition makes surgery a greater risk than the cancer. He discusses therapy with tamsulosin (Flomax) for symptom relief. Why is androgen deprivation therapy not being offered in this case?

3. What nursing diagnoses should the nurse consider for this patient and his wife?

# 103 Drugs for the Eye

## OBJECTIVES

See page 26 for the Objectives.

## CRITICAL THINKING AND STUDY QUESTIONS

1. The most important thing that a nurse can do to prevent blindness from primary open-angle glaucoma (POAG) is:
   a. administer eye medications as ordered.
   b. explain the importance of regular eye screening per guidelines.
   c. identify individuals at high risk for glaucoma.
   d. teach the common symptoms of glaucoma.

▸ 2. The nurse is providing telephone guidance as a service of an insurance company. Which of the following calls most warrants referral for immediate care?
   a. Blurring of peripheral vision
   b. Copious eye exudate with crusting
   c. Halos appearing around lights
   d. Severe eye pain that started 10 minutes ago

▸ 3. When performing an assessment on a patient who is receiving timolol optic drops (Timoptic) for POAG, which of the following findings would be a reason for the nurse to withhold the medication and contact the prescriber? (Select all that apply.)
   a. Audible wheezing
   b. Blood pressure 170/100 mm/Hg
   c. Clouding of lens of eye
   d. End inspiratory crackles
   e. Keyhole appearance to pupil
   f. Pulse 50 beats/min

▸ 4. If a brown discoloration of the eyelid is noted on a patient receiving latanoprost (Xalatan), the nurse should:
   a. administer the medication and document the finding.
   b. assess for symptoms of a migraine headache.
   c. teach the patient proper eye cleansing hygiene.
   d. withhold the medication and contact the prescriber.

▸ 5. Which of these symptoms, if identified in a patient who is receiving brimonidine (Alphagan), should the nurse report to the prescriber immediately?
   a. Red, congested conjunctiva
   b. Dizziness with position changes
   c. Foreign body sensation
   d. Headache

▸ 6. It is important for the nurse to assess for which of the following symptoms when administering dipivefrin (Propine) drops for POAG?
   a. Blurred vision
   b. Bradycardia
   c. Hypotension
   d. Sudden eye pain

▸ 7. A patient who has been prescribed oral acetazolamide (Diamox) for refractory POAG and experiences the adverse effects of severe vomiting and diarrhea should be monitored by the nurse for:
   a. calcium greater than 11 mg/dL.
   b. capillary blood glucose less than 70 mg/dL.
   c. potassium less than 3.5 mEq/L.
   d. sodium greater than 145 mEq/L.

8. A patient asks the nurse why his physician does not advise using the ocular decongestant tetrahydrozoline (Visine) for his allergic conjunctivitis. Which of the following would be included in the nurse's explanation?
   a. Benefits take several days to develop.
   b. Rebound congestion is likely.
   c. The drug can cause cataracts.
   d. The drug can elevate intraocular pressure.

9. The nurse can help decrease the progression of age-related macular degeneration (ARMD) by teaching patients at risk to:
   a. have preventative laser surgery.
   b. have adequate light when reading.
   c. take specific supplements of vitamins C and E, betacarotene, zinc, and copper.
   d. wear sunscreen and sunglasses in bright light.

10. Patients with ARMD should be taught to protect their skin from light for 5 days after therapy that includes the drug:
   a. brimonidine.
   b. pegaptanib.
   c. phenylephrine.
   d. verteporfin.

11. It is important for the nurse to teach a patient who has been prescribed pegaptanib (Macugen) to immediately report:
   a. blurred vision and halos.
   b. light sensitivity and pain.
   c. conjunctival redness and edema.
   d. floaters and decreased visual acuity.

## CASE STUDIES AND PATIENT TEACHING

*(Use a separate piece of paper for your responses.)*

### Case Study 1

*A 62-year-old female is seen by her ophthalmologist at the direction of her PCP. She has a history of chronic obstructive lung disease, psoriasis, and breast cancer. She is accompanied by her daughter and is reluctant to seek care because her eyes are "fine." A topical anesthetic is placed in the eye, and the ophthalmologist measures her intraocular pressure (IOP) to be 23 mm Hg. Tropicamide (Tropicacyl) drops are applied, and the patient is sent to wait until mydriatic and cytoplegic effects occur.*

1. What are mydriatic and cytoplegic effects, and what are their purposes in this situation?

2. After further examination, the patient is diagnosed with primary open-angle glaucoma (POAG). Her daughter asks how she could have this disease, glaucoma, and not be aware of it. How should the nurse respond?

3. The patient is prescribed latanoprost (Xalatan) 1 drop to each eye at bedtime. The prescription is denied by the patient's insurer. The prescriber changes the order to betaxolol (Betoptic) 1 drop in each eye twice a day. Why had the prescriber originally chosen latanoprost (Xalatan) instead of betaxolol (Betoptic) for this patient?

4. What teaching should the nurse provide the patient regarding the betaxolol (Betoptic) prescription and her glaucoma?

5. The patient returns to the ophthalmologist to have her IOP checked. Her IOP measures at 25 mm Hg. The prescriber adds brimonidine (Alphagan) 1 drop instilled in each eye 3 times a day and dorzolamide (Trusopt) 1 drop 3 times a day. The patient asks why the physician did not just increase the drops of latanoprost (Xalatan). How should the nurse respond?

6. What teaching should the nurse provide about therapy with brimonidine (Alphagan) and dorzolamide (Trusopt)?

# 104 Drugs for the Skin

## OBJECTIVES

See page 26 for the Objectives.

## CRITICAL THINKING AND STUDY QUESTIONS

1. The nurse is teaching the parents of a $2\frac{1}{2}$-year-old child about administration of topical glucocorticoid therapy prescribed for their son's eczema. Which of the following statements, if made by a parent, would suggest a need for further teaching?
   a. "I should apply a thick film when using the cream on his chin."
   b. "I should not cover the area of the skin where the cream was applied with a bandage or any type of plastic item unless the doctor tells me to."
   c. "It is important that I only apply the cream to areas with the rash."
   d. "The cream can help stop itching so he won't scratch and get it infected."

▶ 2. The nurse is teaching an adolescent about expected and adverse effects of applying prescribed salicylic acid. Which of the following changes after starting to use this drug would be most important for the nurse to teach the patient to report?
   a. Constant restlessness
   b. Flaking of skin
   c. Headache
   d. Itching in the area where the drug was applied

▶ 3. The nurse is teaching a 12-year-old who has been prescribed salicylic acid for acne. The nurse should tell the patient and his mother that it is best to not use this product if the patient experiences symptoms of which of the following types of illness?
   a. Cold
   b. Flu
   c. Hay fever
   d. Urinary tract infection

▶ 4. The nurse is responsible for answering telephone questions in a dermatology practice. A patient who has recently been prescribed benzoyl peroxide calls because she has been experiencing scaling and swelling at the site of application. An expected protocol for the nurse's response normally would include:
   a. continue to use the benzoyl peroxide and try an oil-based moisturizer to relieve the severe dryness.
   b. continue to use the benzoyl peroxide as prescribed because this is an expected therapeutic effect.
   c. continue to use the benzoyl peroxide, but use it less often.
   d. stop using the benzoyl peroxide.

▶ 5. A 24-year-old college student with acne asks the health center nurse if she can use her brother's unopened topical clindamycin because she does not have health insurance to pay for the clindamycin-benzoyl peroxide (BenzaClin) that has been prescribed. The basis of the nurse's response should be that the combination product:
   a. causes less drying and peeling of the skin.
   b. decreases the chance that antibiotic resistance will occur.
   c. prevents allergic reactions.
   d. prevents systemic absorption of the drug components.

6. A 56-year-old patient asks the nurse what she can tell her about using tretinoin (Retin-A) to prevent wrinkles. The nurse could share research that suggests that tretinoin:
   a. causes the skin to feel softer.
   b. eliminates deep wrinkles.
   c. prevents sunburn.
   d. repairs sun-damaged skin.

7. A patient has been prescribed adapalene (Differin) for acne. Which of the following would the nurse include in teaching? (Select all that apply.)
   a. An increase in acne lesions is common early in therapy.
   b. Apply a sunscreen, such as zinc oxide, before applying the cream.
   c. Apply the cream twice a day, morning and bedtime.
   d. Expect a decrease in blackheads, whiteheads, and inflamed lesions.
   e. Stop the drug if a burning sensation or peeling of the skin occurs.
   f. Use a sunscreen every morning, even if you are not going to be outside.

8. It would be particularly important for the nurse to teach patients with a dark complexion who have been prescribed azelaic acid (Azelex) to apply the cream:
   a. evenly over the face.
   b. only at bedtime.
   c. only to active lesions.
   d. to every area that is red.

▶ 9. Which of the following should the nurse teach a patient to report to the prescriber when prescribed isotretinoin for severe acne? (Select all that apply.)
   a. Back pain and muscle stiffness
   b. Burns easily when out in sun
   c. Frequent nosebleeds
   d. Missed menstrual period
   e. No longer interested in normally pleasurable activities
   f. Peeling of skin from palms and soles
   g. Severe headache followed by transient blurred vision

▶ 10. The oral contraceptive, Estrostep, is prescribed for a 17-year-old female with acne who desires contraception. Developmentally, which of the following effects of the estrogen component of this drug is most likely to be a concern to this patient?
   a. Anorexia
   b. Nausea
   c. Swollen breasts
   d. Weight gain

▶ 11. A patient has been prescribed Ortho Tri-Cyclen and spironolactone (Aldactone) for contraception and treatment of acne that has been resistant to topical treatments. It is important for the patient to be instructed to report which of the following symptoms of the most likely electrolyte disturbance related to this therapy?
   a. Persistent abdominal cramps and diarrhea
   b. Persistent bone pain and constipation
   c. Persistent fatigue and cool, clammy skin
   d. Persistent thirst and flushed skin

12. Recent research suggests that psoriasis is caused by:
   a. an inflammatory disorder.
   b. excessive production of sebum.
   c. excessive reproduction of keratinocytes.
   d. poor hygiene.

13. A patient asks the nurse why he should not use his high-potency glucocorticoid on his face. The basis of the nurse's response is that the face is especially prone to what effect of topical glucocorticoids?
   a. Acne-like eruptions
   b. Changes in pigmentation
   c. Sensitivity to sunlight
   d. Thinning of the skin

14. A patient is admitted with leukocytosis, high fever, nausea, vomiting, and constipation. The nurse notes red patches with silvery, flaking scales on a patient's knees, elbows, and scalp. It is important for the nurse to determine the dose and frequency of medication if this patient is being treated for psoriasis with:
   a. anthralin.
   b. calcipotriene (Dovonex).
   c. tars.
   d. tazarotene (Tazorac).

▸ 15. The nurse would be most concerned about adherence to psoriasis treatment with anthralin if a 28-year-old female patient is experiencing symptoms of:
a. fatigue.
b. impaired physical mobility.
c. sexual dysfunction.
d. urge urinary incontinence.

▸ 16. Which of the following laboratory results for a 57-year-old female patient who is receiving methotrexate for psoriasis would be of most concern to the nurse?
a. Alanine aminotransferase 35 International Units/L
b. Hemoglobin 12 gm/dL
c. Platelet count 8000/mm$^3$
d. White blood cell (WBC) count 10,000/mm$^3$

▸ 17. The nurse would be especially vigilant with thorough assessment of the cardiovascular system if an obese patient with severe psoriasis being treated with acitretin (Soriatane) has a history of:
a. COPD.
b. DM.
c. GERD.
d. OA (DJD).

18. Matching: Drugs for psoriasis and common adverse effects (Some items have more than one answer.)

| | |
|---|---|
| ____ a. acitretin (Soriatane) | 1. Alopecia |
| ____ b. alefacept (Amevive) | 2. Assess for bleeding |
| ____ c. efalizumab (Raptiva) | 3. Chills |
| ____ d. etanercept (Enbrel) | 4. Damage to liver |
| ____ e. methotrexate | 5. Decreased RBC count |
| | 6. Increased risk of cancer |
| | 7. Increased risk of infection |
| | 8. Teratogenic |

▸ 19. The most important intervention that a nurse can provide to prevent squamous cell carcinoma is teaching people to:
a. avoid chronic exposure of the skin to sunlight.
b. examine moles for irregular borders.
c. report rough scaly red-brown papules to PCP.
d. use sunscreen.

20. The nurse in a long-term care facility is administering topical fluorouracil (Carac) to an actinic keratosis lesion. Which of the following assessments suggests that therapy has achieved the desired effect and treatment can be stopped?
a. Burning and vesicle formation
b. Erosion, ulceration, and necrosis
c. Mild inflammation with redness
d. Severe inflammation and stinging

21. An important nursing teaching for patients using diclofenac gel (Solaraze) or imiquimod cream (Aldara) is to:
a. avoid sun exposure.
b. cover the treated area with an occlusive dressing.
c. discontinue treatment if redness or itching occur.
d. that the medications may stain clothing.

▸ 22. The nurse would consult with the pediatrician before administering which of the following immunizations if a child is prescribed topical tacrolimus (Protopic) for atopic dermatitis?
a. Prevnar (pneumococcal)
b. Recombivax HB (hepatitis B)
c. Tripedia (DTaP)
d. Varivax (varicella)

▸ 23. Which of the following laboratory results for a 27-year-old female patient who is receiving podophyllum (Podocon-25) for genital warts would be most important for the nurse to report to the gynecologist administering treatment?
a. Alanine aminotransferase 35 International Units/L
b. HCG positive
c. Hemoglobin 12 gm/dL
d. White blood cell (WBC) count 5000/mm$^3$

24. A patient is convinced that the aluminum in antiperspirants causes breast cancer and asks a nurse how deodorants work. The basis of the nurse's response is that deodorants:
a. cover odor with a pleasant fragrance.
b. decrease flow of apocrine but not eccrine sweat glands.
c. inhibit release of acetylcholine.
d. slow growth of skin bacteria.

25. The principle of treatment for seborrheic dermatitis is suppression of:
    a. cellular reproduction.
    b. growth of yeasts.
    c. histamine release.
    d. scalp oil production.

26. A patient asks the nurse why botulinum toxin (Botox) injections have to be repeated. The best answer to this question includes:
    a. discussion of the half-life of the drug.
    b. enzyme degradation of the toxin.
    c. neurons grow new terminals.
    d. reactivation of vesicles.

▶ 27. The nurse is providing information to a patient who regularly takes aspirin and is considering botulinum toxin (Botox) injections. It is recommended that a patient avoid aspirin for a week preceding treatment. It would be important for the nurse to inform the patient not to discontinue taking aspirin without consulting a physician if the aspirin is being taken for:
    a. analgesia.
    b. fever reduction.
    c. joint pain.
    d. platelet inhibition.

## CASE STUDIES AND PATIENT TEACHING

*(Use a separate piece of paper for your responses.)*

### Case Study 1

*The nurse identifies that body image is a priority concern when collecting data from a 46-year-old patient who is being seen in the dermatology practice. The patient has heard of friends using tretinoin (Renova) to prevent aging of the skin. She asks if this drug really works.*

1. What information can the nurse provide?

2. The patient is concerned about cost and asks if tretinoin is better than face creams that you can buy in the drugstore. What does research suggest on this topic?

3. The patient and physician agree that tretinoin (Renova) is appropriate for this patient. What information can the nurse provide when she asks how this differs from the tretinoin (Retin-A Micro) prescribed for her daughter's acne?

4. What teaching should the nurse provide about use of tretinoin products?

5. The patient reports that she has always used a sunscreen of at least SPF 30 and reapplies it regularly because she enjoys activities out in the sun. What teaching about skin protection should the nurse provide to this patient?

### Case Study 2

*An 18-year-old female high school senior is being seen at the dermatology office after treatment with antibiotics, benzoyl peroxide, tretinoin (Rein-A Micro), and adapalene (Differin) over the past 2 years have failed to provide acceptable results.*

1. What data needs to be collected when the prescriber is considering treatment with isotretinoin (Accutane?)

2. The dermatologist has decided to prescribe isotretinoin (Accutane) and has asked the office nurse to reinforce teaching regarding this drug. What are some nursing diagnoses that should be included when planning teaching relating to this patient, this diagnosis, and this treatment?

3. How should the nurse respond to the patient's question of how isotretinoin therapy differs from tretinoin?

4. Because patients do not always remember what is explained to them, what teaching methods besides oral explanation should the nurse provide to this patient?

5. What teaching must the nurse provide this patient regarding the iPLEDGE program?

# 105 Drugs for the Ear

## OBJECTIVES

See page 26 for the Objectives.

## CRITICAL THINKING AND STUDY QUESTIONS

1. Which of the following is true regarding otitis media?
   a. It can be caused by eustachian tube malfunction.
   b. Presence of otalgia suggests serious complications have occurred.
   c. It primarily occurs in children aged 5 to 12 years.
   d. Treatment of bacterial infection should include antibiotics.

2. The nurse is caring for a 2-year-old child. When bathing the child, the nurse notes sticky, crusting exudate filling the right external ear canal. The nurse would use which of the following terms when documenting this finding?
   a. Otalgia
   b. Otitis media
   c. Otorrhea
   d. Otosclerosis

▸ 3. The recommended dose of amoxicillin for a 6-month-old child who weighs 15 ½ lbs is 300 mg/day administered in 2 divided doses. The pharmacy supplies an oral suspension of 125 mg/mL. The nurse administers a dose of:
   a. 0.8 mL measured in a needleless 1-mL syringe.
   b. 1.2 mL measured in a needleless 3-mL syringe.
   c. 1.6 mL measured in a needleless 1-mL syringe.
   d. 2.4 mL measured in a needleless 3-mL syringe.

4. Which of the following assessment findings in a child receiving amoxicillin would be a reason for the parent to contact the prescriber?
   a. Allergy to clarithromycin
   b. Diarrhea
   c. Facial rash that is maculopapular and does not itch
   d. Multiple intensely itchy and swollen raised areas on the skin of the chest and back

5. The most significant reason why prophylactic antibiotic therapy for recurrent otitis media is not currently recommended is because it:
   a. increases the development of antibiotic resistance.
   b. involves the use of drugs that stain the teeth.
   c. frequently causes diarrhea.
   d. is too expensive.

6. Recommendations for acute otitis externa include instilling into the ear canal a 2% solution of:
   a. alcohol.
   b. ascorbic acid.
   c. peroxide.
   d. vinegar.

▸ 7. The nurse is doing telephone triage in a primary care office. A patient calls complaining of ear pain. Which of the following information would warrant the patient being seen immediately? (Select all that apply.)
   a. Child less than 12 years of age
   b. Elderly diabetic
   c. History of impacted cerumen
   d. Immunocompromised
   e. Pain when the outer ear is touched
   f. Purulent otic discharge
   g. Uses cotton swabs regularly to clean ear canal

8. Amoxicillin-clavulanate is used for antibiotic-resistant acute otitis media because the clavulanate:
   a. allows for a lower dose of amoxicillin.
   b. decreases incidence of adverse effects.
   c. increases antibacterial action against *Streptococcus pneumoniae*.
   d. prevents destruction of the antibiotic by bacterial enzymes.

## CASE STUDIES AND PATIENT TEACHING

*(Use a separate piece of paper for your responses.)*

### Case Study 1

*A pregnant mother has brought her 2 ½ year-old child to the pediatrician because he was fussy all last night. The pediatric nurse practitioner (PNP) diagnoses acute otitis media (AOM), but does not prescribe an antibiotic.*

1. What factors did the PNP consider when deciding whether or not to treat with an antibiotic?

2. The mother is upset and complains to the office nurse that she always received a prescription in the past when her son had an ear infection. What should the nurse include in the explanation of why antibiotics are not being prescribed?

3. What drug treatment should be provided for this child?

4. What symptoms should the nurse teach the mother to report regarding the need for the child to be brought back for reevaluation?

5. The nurse notes that this child has had multiple episodes of otitis media. What teaching can the nurse provide that may decrease the incidence of otitis media for this child and the new sibling when born?

### Case Study 2

*A patient has been prescribed Cipro HC drops for otitis externa.*

1. What information should the nurse include when teaching about administration of these drops?

2. What technique should the nurse use to evaluate the learning if the child's mother does not appear to understand oral instruction?

3. The patient asks if she can use old drops from a previous infection. What should the nurse include in her response?

4. The nurse notes that the patient has had repeated episodes of otitis externa. What teaching can the nurse provide that might decrease the number of episodes?

# 106 Miscellaneous Noteworthy Drugs

## OBJECTIVES

See page 26 for the Objectives.

## CRITICAL THINKING AND STUDY QUESTIONS

1. A priority nursing diagnosis for a patient receiving epoprostenol (Flolan) is:
   a. decreased cardiac output.
   b. fatigue.
   c. fluid volume excess.
   d. ineffective airway clearance.

2. When administering bosentan (Tracleer) to a patient admitted with pulmonary artery hypertension, which of the following nursing assessments would indicate that therapy is achieving the desired effect?
   a. Blood pressure 110/70 mm/Hg
   b. Jugular venous pulsation 2.5 cm above sternal angle
   c. Lower extremity peripheral edema decreased from 3+ to 2+ bilaterally
   d. Peak expiratory volume (PEV) 75% of best

3. A priority nursing teaching for a patient with pulmonary artery hypertension who is receiving iloprost (Ventavis) is:
   a. change positions slowly.
   b. cough and deep breathe.
   c. do not cross your legs.
   d. pursed-lip breathing.

4. Which of these laboratory test results, if identified for a patient who is receiving bosentan (Tracleer), should the nurse report to the prescriber immediately?
   a. BNP 87 pg/mL
   b. Creatinine 1.4 mg/dL
   c. HCG positive
   d. Urine leukocyte esterase positive

5. The most recent ALT result for a patient receiving bosentan (Tracleer) is 85 International Units/L. The nurse should:
   a. administer the drug as prescribed.
   b. withhold the drug and consult with the prescriber regarding a dose decrease or interruption.
   c. withhold the drug and consult with the prescriber regarding discontinuing the drug.

6. The nurse is performing an abdominal assessment on a septic patient who is receiving drug therapy with drotrecogin alfa activated (DrotAA, Xigris). Which of the following assessment findings suggests a critical complication of therapy with this drug warranting immediate consultation with the prescriber?
   a. Distended abdomen
   b. Hyperactive bowel sounds
   c. Hypoactive bowel sounds
   d. Rigid abdomen

7. The recommended dose of drotrecogin alfa activated (DrotAA, Xigris) is 24 mcg/kg/hr. What is the recommended hourly dose for a patient who weighs 137.5 lbs?

8. A patient is prescribed 1.5 mg of drotrecogin alfa activated (DrotAA, Xigris). The drug is reconstituted in normal saline solution (NSS) at a concentration of 100 mcg/mL. The infusion pump is calibrated in mL/hr. What rate of infusion should be programmed into the pump?

9. Which of the following laboratory results would warrant withholding drotrecogin alfa activated (DrotAA, Xigris) and consulting the prescriber?
   a. ALT 400 International Units/L
   b. INR 3
   c. Platelet count 40,000,000/mL
   d. RBC 4.5 $10^6$/µL

10. The nurse is administering intramuscular (IM) dexamethasone to a pregnant woman who is at risk for premature delivery of the fetus. The patient's skin is hot and dry, and the patient is voiding 200 to 250 mL every hour. Which diagnostic test results should the nurse check at this time?
    a. BUN
    b. Creatinine
    c. SMBG
    d. Urine specific gravity

11. A priority nursing diagnosis relating to administration of beractant (Survanta) to a premature neonate is related to the risk of:
    a. airway clearance impairment.
    b. deficient fluid volume.
    c. hypothermia.
    d. ineffective breast-feeding.

12. For maximal therapeutic results, dornase alfa (Pulmozyme) should be administered to patients with cystic fibrosis:
    a. after chest physiotherapy.
    b. after meals.
    c. before chest physiotherapy.
    d. before meals.

13. The nurse is caring for a 15-year-old girl who has been admitted in a sickle cell crisis. The patient complains of severe joint pain (10 of 10). The nurse notes that the child is sitting quietly in bed conversing with her parents. Intravenous morphine 0.5 mg and ibuprofen 200 mg are ordered every 3 hours as needed. The patient has not had any analgesic medication in the past 3 hours. The nurse should:
    a. administer the ibuprofen.
    b. administer the morphine.
    c. assess for other physiologic indicators of pain.
    d. provide nonpharmacologic pain relief measures.

14. A 19-year-old with sickle cell anemia has been prescribed hydroxyurea (Droxia). Developmentally, which nursing diagnosis would be of most concern relating to this drug therapy?
    a. Body image
    b. Adherence
    c. Infection
    d. Tissue perfusion

15. A toddler has come to the outpatient oncology clinic for an infusion of rasburicase (Elitek) to be administered daily for 5 days before the start of chemotherapy. The nursing plan of care should address prevention and relief of the most common adverse effect of this therapy, including the possible need for an:
    a. analgesic.
    b. antidiarrheal.
    c. antiemetic.
    d. antihistamine.

16. When a patient is receiving riluzole (Rilutek) for amyotrophic lateral sclerosis (ALS), it is most important for the nurse to assess for which of the following symptoms of the underlying condition?
    a. Dizziness
    b. Nausea and vomiting
    c. Respiratory distress
    d. Weakness

## CASE STUDIES AND PATIENT TEACHING

*(Use a separate piece of paper for your responses.)*

### Case Study 1

*A 14-year-old female with cystic fibrosis has come to the emergency room because of sudden onset of shaking chills, fever 102.5° F, and greenish-colored sputum. She tells the nurse that she is worse than she was 6 months ago. Her last airway studies show a decreased vital capacity and increased residual volume. She appears very depressed. The patient is 5 feet tall and weighs 80 lbs. She is being admitted to the adult unit since the adolescent unit has no beds. This upsets the patient because she is a frequent patient and knows the adolescent unit staff well. The nurse begins planning care.*

1. What are some possible nursing diagnoses for this patient?

2. The nurse is having difficulty reaching the patient's primary care provider to obtain orders for the patient's routine enzymes. Why is this so important?

3. The patient snaps at the nurse when she brings the enzymes one-half hour after lunch was served. How should the nurse respond?

### Case Study 2

*A 22-month-old African-American child is admitted to a pediatric hospital because of fever, irritability, jaundice, and unremitting malaise. Laboratory test results reveal anemia and presence of hemoglobin S, confirming the diagnosis of sickle cell disease. The boy's mother asks the nurse why his eyes are so yellow.*

1. What would be the logical explanation for jaundice in sickle cell disease?

2. The mother has heard of a new drug, hydroxyurea, and asks why it has not been prescribed for her child. The best explanation is that:
   a. The drug has adverse effects.
   b. The drug has only been approved for age 18 and older.
   c. The drug is an orphan drug.
   d. The drug is only used as a last resort.

3. The mother asks the nurse if there is anything that she can do to prevent her child from experiencing sickle cell crises. How should the nurse respond?

### Case Study 3

*A 38-year-old female patient who is prescribed thalidomide (Thalomid) for multiple myeloma complains to the nurse of the need to obtain a pregnancy test within 24 hours before the first dose, every 2 weeks for a month, then once a menstrual cycle. She states that she has had regular periods and has been using the same oral contraceptives without problems for many years.*

1. What information should the nurse provide to this patient?

# 107 Herbal Supplements

## OBJECTIVES

See page 26 for the Objectives.

## CRITICAL THINKING AND STUDY QUESTIONS

1. Matching: Herbal products and primary use

| | | |
|---|---|---|
| ___ | a. Aloe | 1. Benign prostatic hyperplasia |
| ___ | b. Black cohosh | 2. Constipation |
| ___ | c. Echinacea | 3. Decrease triglycerides |
| ___ | d. Feverfew | 4. Depression |
| ___ | e. Garlic | 5. Improve memory |
| ___ | f. Gingerroot | 6. Migraine headache prophylaxis |
| ___ | g. Ginkgo biloba | 7. Morning sickness of pregnancy |
| ___ | h. Goldenseal | 8. PMS and menopause symptoms |
| ___ | i. Kava | 9. Prevent colds |
| ___ | j. Ma Huang (ephedra) | 10. Promote sleep |
| ___ | k. St John's wort | 11. Skin therapy |
| ___ | l. Saw Palmetto | 12. Treat URI and UTI |
| ___ | m. Valerian | 13. Weight loss |

2. The nurse should be concerned about the patient's use of herbal products because before the regulation proposed in the USA in 2003: (Select all that apply.)
   a. products marketed as dietary supplements did not require rigorous evaluation before marketing.
   b. the FDA could not remove the product from the market even if there is evidence that it causes harm.
   c. the product may have contained harmful ingredients such as arsenic, mercury, and lead.
   d. the product may not have contained the stated ingredients in the amount listed on the label.
   e. their labels could claim to treat disease without adequate research supporting the claim.
   f. there was no evidence that any of these products are effective or safe.

3. Lack of oversight of the accuracy of a herbal product's label can be particularly dangerous for patients who are:
   a. allergic to inert ingredients often found in pills.
   b. in lower socio-economic groups.
   c. using a generic brand of a product.
   d. using the product to promote health.

4. Regulations proposed in the USA in 2003 (CGMPs) seek to correct the problem of: (Select all that apply.)
   a. eliminating contaminants in herbal products.
   b. ensuring accuracy of labels on herbal products.
   c. ensuring the herb produces the effect that it claims to produce.
   d. ensuring potency of the herbal product.
   e. ensuring the herbal product is safe.

5. The nurse should teach a patient who chooses to use a herbal product to:
   a. always buy the more expensive brand.
   b. take the herb with at least 8 ounces of water.
   c. use products that have the seal of approval from the USP or NSF.
   d. use the lowest dose possible.

▶ 6. The most important intervention when a nurse discovers that a patient self-prescribes herbal products is to:
   a. assess for the symptoms they are trying to relieve.
   b. be an advocate for the patient's right to make choices.
   c. convince the patient to stop taking the products.
   d. teach the patient the importance of informing all healthcare providers of all products being used.

7. A patient who is taking metronidazole is at risk for a drug interaction if also taking a herbal product in which of the following forms?
   a. Decoctions, teas, and infusions
   b. Fluid extracts and tinctures
   c. Glycerites
   d. Solid extracts

8. It is important for the nurse to assess for symptoms of which of the following adverse effects in a patient who reports self-prescribing with aloe latex?
   a. Electrolyte loss
   b. Excessive bruising
   c. Fluid retention
   d. Suprainfection of the skin

9. Based on German studies, it is important for the nurse to teach postmenopausal women who are taking black cohosh for hot flashes and insomnia to:
   a. avoid prolonged exposure to the sun.
   b. change positions slowly.
   c. drink adequate amounts of fluids.
   d. stop taking the herb if you experience a headache.

10. Pregnant nurses should wear gloves if they are administering which of the following herbal supplements?
   a. Aloe
   b. Feverfew
   c. Ginger
   d. Saw Palmetto

11. Echinacea: (Select all that apply.)
   a. can aggravate autoimmune disorders.
   b. can produce an allergic reaction the first time taken in patients allergic to ragweed.
   c. can stimulate the immune system.
   d. can suppress the immune system.
   e. decreases the severity of the common cold.
   f. prevents symptoms of the common cold.
   g. should be avoided by people with immune suppression.

▶ 12. The nurse is assessing a new admission. The patient lists echinacea, garlic, and kava among the products that she uses regularly. On first observation, the nurse notes that the patient's skin has a yellowish color. The most appropriate action for the nurse to take next is to:
   a. continue to assess the patient.
   b. document jaundice in the nursing note.
   c. notify the physician of the findings stat.
   d. tell the patient to stop taking the herbal products.

13. A patient who regularly takes feverfew to prevent migraine headaches stopped taking the herb before elective surgery. The nurse should assess the patient for possible adverse effects of discontinuation of this therapy including:
   a. bleeding
   b. flatulence
   c. insomnia
   d. nausea

14. The nurse is aware that a patient who takes ginkgo biloba and antihistamines increases their risk of experiencing the adverse effect of:
   a. bleeding.
   b. dizziness.
   c. headache.
   d. seizures.

15. The emergency room nurse admits a 2-year-old child who has ingested an unknown amount of goldenseal. A nursing priority is:
   a. gas exchange.
   b. nausea.
   c. pain.
   d. safety.

16. The nurse is aware that which of the following herbal supplements has a potential for abuse?
   a. Black cohosh
   b. Ginger
   c. Kava
   d. Valerian

17. The nurse is caring for a patient who regularly uses Ma Huang (ephedra) for weight loss. It is important for the nurse to:
    a. assess mental status.
    b. monitor vital signs.
    c. not administer any other sedatives.
    d. weigh the patient daily.

18. The nurse should monitor the patient for bleeding if the patient uses which of the following herbal products? (Select all that apply.)
    a. Aloe
    b. Black cohosh
    c. Echinacea
    d. Feverfew
    e. Garlic
    f. Ginger
    g. Ginkgo biloba
    h. Goldenseal
    i. Kava
    j. Ma Huang (ephedra)
    k. St John's wort
    l. Saw Palmetto
    m. Valerian

## CASE STUDIES AND PATIENT TEACHING

*(Use a separate piece of paper for your responses.)*

### Case Study 1

*A 52-year-old man is admitted with chest pain. Assessment findings include height 5 (feet) 8 (inches), weight 220 lbs, waist circumference 42 inches, BP 145/86 mm/Hg, and pulse 78 beats/min. Lab results include triglycerides 380 mg/dL, LDL 240 mg/dL, and HDL 34 mg/dL. He is diagnosed with GERD and metabolic syndrome. He informs his physician that he wants to try natural therapy and has heard that garlic can help many things. The physician asks the nurse to discuss therapy with garlic with this patient.*

1. What are possible positive effects of garlic supplementation for this patient?

2. The physician recommends enteric coated garlic supplement. What can the nurse teach the patient to ensure that the product that he purchases contains effective amounts of allicin?

3. The patient insists on using raw garlic. What information should the nurse provide about raw garlic therapy?

4. Why is it important for the patient to inform all healthcare providers and his pharmacist that he is using garlic therapy?

### Case Study 2

*An 85-year-old with atrial fibrillation is being treated with digoxin (Lanoxin) and warfarin (Coumadin). At times, she is fatigued and forgetful. Her friend suggests that she take ginkgo to give her more energy.*

1. What possible complications can occur with this combination of drugs and herbs?

2. What teaching should the nurse provide this patient regarding the use of herbal products?

3. The patient informs the nurse that she is not going to get her annual flu shot because she has purchased a bottle of echinacea. How would the nurse respond?

# 108 Management of Poisoning

## OBJECTIVES

See page 26 for the Objectives.

## CRITICAL THINKING AND STUDY QUESTIONS

▶ 1. The priority of nursing care of a patient with a suspected poisoning is:
   a. administering an antidote.
   b. identifying the poison.
   c. maintaining airway and circulation.
   d. preventing absorption of poison that has not been absorbed.
   e. removing residual poison that has not been absorbed.

▶ 2. A person with an unknown medical history has ingested an unidentified poison. The patient is comatose when arriving at the emergency room. After circulation and respiration are well established, the nurse should assess for:
   a. capillary refill and pedal pulses.
   b. diaphoresis and tachycardia.
   c. dizziness with position changes.
   d. dry mucous membranes and poor skin turgor.

3. The nurse knows that the most accurate and efficient method of identifying the poison and the dose is:
   a. analysis of body fluids by a laboratory.
   b. evaluation of patient symptoms.
   c. examining the container.
   d. interviewing the caregiver.

4. The purpose of an antidote to a poison is to:
   a. increase renal excretion of the poison.
   b. prevent absorption of the poison.
   c. remove residual poison from the GI tract.
   d. reverse the effects of the poison.

5. Over-the-counter sale of syrup of ipecac for noncaustic poisoning is no longer routinely recommended because it:
   a. causes electrolyte imbalances.
   b. does not work.
   c. involves complicated directions.
   d. may delay seeking time-sensitive professional care.

6. Charcoal is most effective in binding with poisons in the GI tract and preventing absorption if administered:
   a. after syrup of ipecac.
   b. after the patient has vomited.
   c. within 30 minutes of poison ingestion.
   d. with fat soluble poisons.

7. A patient has been treated for poisoning by hemoperfusion, which passes blood over an absorbent resin. The nurse should monitor the patient for:
   a. bleeding.
   b. dehydration.
   c. hyperglycemia.
   d. seizures.

8. Matching: Chelating agents and metal[s] they bind

| | |
|---|---|
| ___ a. deferoxamine (Desferal) | 1. Arsenic |
| ___ b. dimercaprol (BAL in oil) | 2. Copper |
| ___ c. edetate calcium disodium (Calcium EDTA) | 3. Ethylene glycol (antifreeze) |
| ___ d. fomepizole (Antizole) | 4. Gold |
| ___ e. penicillamine (Depen) | 5. Iron |
| ___ f. succimer (Chemet) | 6. Lead |
| | 7. Mercury |

9. A patient is being treated for acute ferric iron poisoning with deferoxamin (Desferal). The nurse knows that this drug works by:
   a. binding with iron in the blood, causing excretion in the urine.
   b. binding with iron in the GI tract, preventing absorption.
   c. flushing the GI tract.
   d. inducing vomiting.

▶ 10. A nurse assesses the vital signs of a patient who is being treated for ferric iron poisoning with intravenous deferoxamin (Desferal). Which of the following findings suggests that the administration rate of the drug might be too rapid?
   a. Blood pressure 150/85 mm/Hg
   b. Pulse 95 beats/min
   c. Respirations 15 per minute
   d. Temperature 100.4° F (38° C)

▶ 11. Which of the following would be an appropriate technique when the nurse is administering dimercaprol (BAL in oil)?
   a. Deep injection into the dorsogluteal muscle
   b. Subcutaneous injection into abdominal fat
   c. Subcutaneous injection above the vastus lateralis
   d. Z track injection into the ventrogluteal muscle

▶ 12. The nurse is caring for a 3-year-old who weighs 15 kg and is scheduled to receive an intramuscular dose of edetate calcium EDTA for lead poisoning. The child's urinary output has averaged 15 mL/hour for the last 4 hours. The nurse should:
   a. administer the drug and continue nursing care.
   b. consult the prescriber regarding the need for additional fluids.
   c. withhold the medication and consult the prescriber.
   d. withhold the medication and assess for renal failure.

▶ 13. To detect serious adverse effects, it is most important for the nurse to monitor the results of which laboratory test when caring for a patient with Wilson's disease who is receiving pencillamine (Depen)?
   a. Alanine aminotransferase
   b. Blood urea nitrogen
   c. Complete blood count and differential (CBC and diff)
   d. Creatinine

▶ 14. The nurse calculates, using BSA ($m^2$), the recommended dose of succimer (Chemet) for a child with acute lead poisoning who weighs 18 kg and is 100 cm tall. The prescribed dose is 200 mg. The nurse should:
   a. administer the drug.
   b. withhold the drug and consult the prescriber.

15. A child who was admitted after ingesting antifreeze is treated with fomepizole (Antizole). The prescriber orders a loading dose followed by doses every 12 hours. The child's kidneys are failing and hemodialysis is ordered. The nurse should consult the prescriber regarding:
   a. extending the time between doses.
   b. shortening the time between doses.
   c. lowering the dose of fomepizole (Antizole).
   d. raising the dose of fomepizole (Antizole).

16. The nurse teaches parents that dialing 1-800-222-1222 will connect them with:
   a. the national poison center.
   b. a pharmacist.
   c. a local certified poison center.
   d. a specially trained nurse.

## CASE STUDIES AND PATIENT TEACHING

*(Use a separate piece of paper for your responses.)*

### Case Study 1

*A 4-year-old, who has been playing outside in her yard, comes in the house and says she doesn't feel well. Her mother notices a purple stain on the child's face. Knowing that they do not have any grape juice in the house, the mother asks her daughter what she has eaten. The child tells her about some berries she found in the yard. The mother calls the poison control center and the child is rushed to the emergency department of the hospital.*

1. Why didn't the poison control center recommend syrup of ipecac?

2. When the nurse questions the mother, she describes "weeds" growing at the back of the yard with blueberry-size purple berries that her daughter may have ingested. What should be done to identify the ingested substance?

3. The stomach contents contain a noncaustic neurotoxin. What data can the nurse collect to assist the emergency physician with deciding if charcoal, gastric lavage, or whole bowel irrigation is the best approach for this poisoning?

4. The mother is sure that the ingestion of the poison occurred less than 30 minutes ago. Gastric lavage and aspiration is ordered. What is the nurse's role?

5. The child is stabilized and observed overnight. What instruction should the nurse provide this family before discharge?

## Case Study 2

*A patient has been admitted after being accidentally sprayed with a toxic liquid.*

1. What procedure should the nursing staff take to decontaminate the patient while protecting themselves?

# 109 Potential Weapons of Biologic, Radiologic, and Chemical Terrorism

## OBJECTIVES

See page 26 for the Objectives.

## CRITICAL THINKING AND STUDY QUESTIONS

1. The nurse would be concerned about a patient who exhibits which of the following symptoms because, if caused by a specific biologic weapon infection, it has no effective treatment?
   a. Headache, high fever, chills, and rigors
   b. Multiple red spots on the tongue and buccal mucosa
   c. Painless ulcers with a necrotic core that develop black eschar
   d. Tender, enlarged, inflamed lymph nodes

2. The basis of nursing actions to prevent transmission when *Bacillus anthracis* presence is suspected is based on:
   a. dividing bacteria produces spores when adequate nutrition is present
   b. mature bacteria can survive for long periods in a moist, dark environment
   c. spores can survive for long periods in many environmental conditions
   d. the bacteria is easily transmitted from person to person

3. Which of the following statements, if made by a patient receiving ciprofloxacin for cutaneous anthrax, would indicate understanding of drug therapy teaching?
   a. "I must take all of the prescription as directed because if I do not serious illness and death could occur."
   b. "I should take the antibiotic until the scabs fall off."
   c. "If I start the antibiotic immediately, there is a chance that I will not experience itchy vesicles."
   d. "My prescription needs to be changed if I get pregnant."

4. The community health nurse, who works in areas known to have the presence of *Bacillus anthracis*, promotes routine vaccination with anthrax vaccine (BioThrax) for:
   a. police.
   b. postal workers.
   c. receptionists.
   d. sheep shearers.

▶ 5. Intramuscular streptomycin 0.5 gm twice a day is prescribed for a 150-lb adult male who has been diagnosed with tularemia. The drug is provided in a solution of 100 mg/mL. Nursing assessments before administration of the drug include BP 140/72 mm/HG, pulse 88 beats/min, respirations 24, moist cough, and end inspiratory crackles in upper lobes. The nurse should:
   a. administer the drug and consult the prescriber regarding the dose.
   b. administer the drug as one injection in the dorsogluteal site.
   c. wear a high-efficiency particulate mask when administering the drug.
   d. withhold the drug and consult the prescriber.

▶ 6. A patient is admitted with a diagnosis of pneumonic plague. Which of the following precautions would be needed to prevent spread of this infection?
   a. Airborne precautions.
   b. Contact precautions.
   c. Droplet precautions.
   d. Prophylactic vaccination of staff.

7. The public health nurse is administering smallpox vaccine (Dryvax) to police officers. Which of the following statements, if made by a vaccination recipient, would indicate a need for further teaching?
   a. "I should keep the site covered to avoid spreading the live vaccine."
   b. "I should report any drainage that occurs from the vaccination site."
   c. "It is important that I not get pregnant for at least 4 weeks after receiving this vaccination."
   d. "This vaccination should be effective even if I was exposed to smallpox yesterday."

▶ 8. The nurse is preparing to vaccinate a person who has been exposed to the smallpox virus. The patient states that she is pregnant. The nurse should:
   a. administer the vaccine.
   b. administer cidofovir before administering the smallpox vaccine.
   c. assess if the patient has been informed of benefits and risks of vaccination.
   d. withhold the vaccine.

▶ 9. The most important nursing priority for a patient with botulism poisoning is:
   a. effective breathing.
   b. impaired mobility.
   c. swallowing ability.
   d. visual acuity.

▶ 10. The nurse is providing emergency care after a disaster at a nuclear power plant that caused the release of radioactive material. Which of the following doses of potassium iodide should be administered to a 17-year-old pregnant female?
   a. None
   b. 65 mg daily
   c. 130 mg daily
   d. 195 mg daily

▶ 11. To prevent magnesium deficiency when receiving zinc trisodium (Zn-DTPA), the nurse teaches a patient to include adequate amounts of which of the following foods?
   a. Eggs
   b. Liver
   c. Red meat
   d. Whole grains

12. Which of the following statements, if made by a patient who has been prescribed Ca-DPTA therapy for americium poisoning, would suggest understanding of teaching?
   a. "I cannot receive these drugs if my kidneys are not functioning properly."
   b. "I need to take a pill every day for at least 2 months."
   c. "I should drink 100 ounces of fluid, especially water, each day."
   d. "I will need to provide a urine specimen every day while on treatment."

13. The nurse knows that adverse effects of ferric hexacyanoferrate (Prussian blue) used to increase excretion of nonradiaoctive thallium can increase the risk of toxicity of which of the following medications?
    a. Acetaminophen
    b. Atenolol
    c. Digoxin
    d. Furosemide

## CASE STUDIES AND PATIENT TEACHING

*(Use a separate piece of paper for your responses.)*

### Case Study 1

*People died from inhalation of anthrax spores in the United States in October 2001. The nation was on alert for terrorist attacks.*

1. What are possible reasons for the infections not being promptly diagnosed and treated in time to prevent all deaths?

2. How can the nurse contribute to early recognition of infections caused by biologic agents?

3. People who were possibly exposed to the *Bacillus anthracis* were offered prophylactic drug therapy. What teaching should be provided by the community health nurses assisting with this mass prophylaxis?

### Case Study 2

*A patient has come to the emergency department because of exposure to an unknown powder.*

1. If this person was exposed to anthrax bacilli, how can the infection spread to other people?

2. What precautions should the nurse take to prevent the spread of anthrax infection?

### Case Study 3

*The military nurse is participating in a mock drill imitating exposure of soldiers to mustard gas.*

1. What would be the first action that the nurse should take?

2. How can the nurse prevent additional exposure to the agent for the soldiers and healthcare providers?

3. What questions about the episode would the nurse ask to determine which persons probably received the most exposure to the gas?

4. What symptoms would the nurse expect to occur first?

5. What should the nurse assess to determine if the most serious consequences could be occurring?